WITHDRAWN FROM
NORTHERN ARIZONA
UNIVERSITY LIBRARY

AF327340

DISEASES OF THE ORAL CAVITY AND SALIVARY GLANDS

A GUIDE TO THE CLINICAL AND RADIOGRAPHIC DIAGNOSIS WITH SUGGESTIONS FOR THERAPY

BY

PROFESSOR Dr. G. BOERING

Professor of Oral Surgery, University of Groningen, The Netherlands

FIRST ENGLISH EDITION

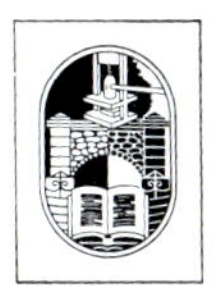

BRISTOL: JOHN WRIGHT & SONS LTD.

1971

Original Title (now in Second Edition)
"Aandoeningen van de Mond en de Speekselklieren"

© Stafleu's Wetenschappelijke Uitgeversmaatschappij
N.V. Leiden

Distribution by Sole Agents:
United States of America: The Williams & Wilkins Company, Baltimore
Canada: The Macmillan Company of Canada Ltd., Toronto

ISBN 0 7236 0291 3

PRINTED IN GREAT BRITAIN BY JOHN WRIGHT & SONS LTD.,
AT THE STONEBRIDGE PRESS, BRISTOL BS4 5NU

PREFACE

THE general medical practitioner is often consulted about diseases or deformities of the mouth, the dentition, the jaws, and the salivary glands. A good survey of the commonly occurring lesions of this part of the body is lacking in modern medical literature. It is the purpose of this monograph to rectify this deficiency. The identification of the different lesions which may occur in practice is covered. To make reading easier the text has been amply illustrated. Treatment of the greater part of the described lesions is briefly discussed. For more extensive information reference is made to the literature.

As tooth extractions and other purely dental treatment are no longer performed by medical practitioners, these subjects are not described.

Modern dentistry has now reached a high degree of development. Except for the occasional, lone dental practitioner there is a tendency to work together as a group, assisted by dental hygienists or dental nurses.

Specialization in orthodontics and oral surgery is possible in many dental training centres. Oral surgeons are incorporated in the staff of many hospitals. Close co-operation between general surgeons, plastic surgeons, tumour surgeons, E.N.T. surgeons, and many other specialists exists.

I wish to acknowledge the contribution to the text by Dr. A. Löwenberg (general medical practitioner) and the constructive criticism provided by Professor Dr. H. N. Hadders (pathologist), Professor Dr. A. J. C. Huffstadt (plastic surgeon), Professor Dr. O. Backer Dirks (cariologist), Dr. J. Boersma and Mr. C. Booy (orthodontists), Professor Dr. T. Huizinga (pharmacotherapist), and Professor Dr. J. Oldhoff (tumour surgeon).

I also wish to acknowledge the assistance of Mr. W. D. Lange; it was his photographic ability which made the high quality of the illustrations possible.

Last but not least I wish to thank the staff of the Groningen Oral Surgery Clinic for their help and stimulating words.

Groningen, June, 1971

G. BOERING

CONTENTS

I. *THE ORAL CAVITY*

II. *THE SALIVARY GLANDS*

I

THE ORAL CAVITY

CHAPTER 1

THE DENTITION

Dental Caries.—Dental caries is the most frequently occurring disease of the dentition and is mainly seen in countries in which there is a high consumption of refined sugar. In areas where 'natural' food is consumed, consisting of meat or uncooked food (which has a cleaning effect), dental caries is relatively rare. The average diet in western Europe is cariogenic to a high degree; it is estimated that about 98 per cent of the total population over 5 years of age is suffering from this disease. The use of sugars between meals (e.g., tough and sticky sweets) is especially conducive to dental caries. In bakers dental caries is practically an occupational disease.

Past investigations provide few reasons for presuming that there is an enhanced susceptibility to dental caries during pregnancy. It is very improbable that resorption of calcium from the dentition takes place endogenously during this period. All investigations to date (e.g., in cases of osteomalacia) reveal that calcium is not resorbed from the tooth. Presumably a lower standard of mouth hygiene during this period, the tendency to eat more sweets, the vomiting by some women, together with failure to obtain regular dental examination, are important aetiological factors.

Caries prophylaxis is aimed at a good oral hygiene (brushing teeth properly and rinsing well after each meal) and at a reduction of the consumption of sugar between meals, although nutritional customs are hard to change. Sugar is one of the most important factors in the aetiology of dental caries. It is converted by cariogenic streptococci into organic acids, mainly lactic acid. Moreover, the glucose polymer *dextran*, a syrupy substance, which is an essential part of the bacterial plaque, is predominantly made out of sugar. This bacterial plaque, a whitish deposit on the enamel surface, makes the pH value fall locally to such a degree that the enamel is decalcified. Frequent eating of sweets causes a continuously high sugar level in the saliva, a continuous production of acid, and deposition of plaque resulting in a high caries frequency.

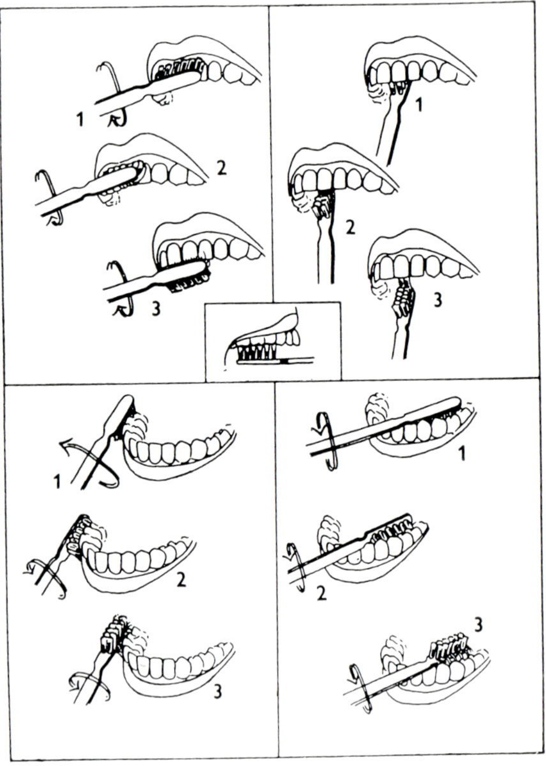

Fig. 1.—Brushing teeth according to the roll method (*het ivoren kruis*, 'the ivory cross') (*Netherlands Association for Mouth and Tooth Hygiene*).

It is important to treat existing defects as early as possible in order to prevent their extension.

When brushing the teeth the toothbrush should be put on the gums and brought towards the crown by means of a rolling movement (*Fig.* 1). The brush should not be too large and should be regularly replaced by a new one.

Besides the observance of good mouth hygiene, 6-monthly examination by the dentist is necessary. Regular treatment of the deciduous dentition is also desirable, but, unfortunately, this cannot yet be done on a large scale universally owing to a shortage of man-power.

Preservation of the deciduous dentition is amongst the factors of importance in the prevention of irregularities of the permanent dentition. Premature loss of deciduous teeth is followed by mesial drifting in the dental arch, especially of teeth sited furthest away from the midline. The result may be lack of space and impaction of permanent teeth or eruption of canines outside the dental arch. The deciduous teeth are space maintainers for their permanent successors. The preservation of the second deciduous molar is of particular importance in preventing drifting of the first permanent molar. Unfortunately, extraction of deciduous teeth cannot always be avoided. If these teeth are severely affected by dental caries and cause inflammation, it is undesirable to retain the remnants.

The object of the organized dental care of schoolchildren is:—

a. To educate children by providing a better understanding of the value of a sound dentition and to teach them how to apply independently and accurately all those measures which have an influence on keeping their dentition in good condition.

b. To propagate as widely as possible among children, parents, guardians, and teachers knowledge of the principles of oral hygiene and the measures which can be taken to further the health of the dentition.

c. By prophylaxis, to prevent affection of the dentition by caries, to recognize affection early, and to promote treatment as soon as possible.

d. To trace other defects in the dentitions of the children and to promote, if necessary, treatment by specialists.

School dentistry is mainly aimed at the preservation of the first permanent molars. The conservation of these teeth is of great importance for the rest of the dentition as well. Treatment of these molars only, often already grossly affected by caries soon after eruption, takes a relatively large part of the total available time and manpower.

Administration of calcium in any form in the case of an already formed dentition, for instance in the case of high caries frequency, is of no use, as the calcium cannot be absorbed by the tooth, nor are there indications that extra calcium *during* tooth formation promotes later caries resistance. The ideal calcium and phosphate sources are still milk and milk products.

One of the latest prophylactic measures with greater success is the fluoridation of drinking water. Investigations in America and also in the Netherlands (Tiel, Culemborg) have demonstrated that fluorides added to drinking water strongly reduce the caries susceptibility during the whole life. In Tiel as well as in America a caries reduction was found of 50–70 per cent. The concentration of fluorides in water, which is normally about 0·06–0·15 mg. per l., is increased to 1·0–1·2 mg. per l. Fluorides reduce the solubility of the enamel and presumably exercise a restraining influence on the fermentation of lactic acid on the tooth surface. It may be taken for granted that this measure, which is recommended by the W.H.O. (World Health Organization), is harmless to general health.

Local application of highly concentrated fluoride (stannous fluoride) on teeth, carefully cleaned and dried beforehand, has also a caries-preventing effect. This method is rather laborious and can therefore only be applied with difficulty on a large scale. Application of a mixture of organic fluorides (Elmex) is said to be less complicated.

Little is known with certainty about the effect of fluoride-containing toothpastes and the application of fluoride in tablet form. With regard to the latter the following scheme of administration is sometimes given:—

First year of life	0·25 mg. per day	
Second year of life	0·50 mg. per day	
Third to sixth years of life	0·75 mg. per day	calculated as fluoride
Seventh to tenth years of life	1·00 mg. per day	
Eleven years and older	1·25 mg. per day	

If deciduous teeth have erupted it is advisable to melt the tablets slowly in the mouth; there is also a direct local effect. The tablets, normally containing 0·25 mg. fluoride (sodium fluoride), have to be applied after brushing the teeth and must be taken throughout the day. Warn emphatically against overdose!

Administration of fluoride to pregnant women for the foetus's dentition is probably of little use; to date no effect of fluoride administered during pregnancy has been demonstrated. When the permanent dentition has erupted administration of fluoride is of lesser importance.

As a matter of fact administration of extra fluoride is undesirable in those areas where fluoride is added to the drinking water.

Malformations.—Malformations of teeth may be either congenital or the result of disturbed calcium metabolism during enamel formation (e.g., rickets, viral infection, intestinal disturbances). Enamel formed in this period may show many small pit-like defects running band-like around the tooth.

As a result of trauma a deciduous tooth may be wedged in the jaw and may cause either displacement or damage of the germ of the permanent tooth, and consequently an abnormal position or malformation of the crown.

The so-called 'Hutchinson's teeth' resulting from congenital syphilis (barrel-like crown with crescent-shaped notches in the incisal edge of the permanent teeth) are extremely rare.

Discolorations.—A black, green, or even orange film may occur on the tooth surface near the gingiva, especially in children. This is probably caused by pigment-forming micro-organisms. From a clinical point of view this abnormality is insignificant.

Differences in colour due to malformation of dentine or enamel (dentino- or amelogenesis imperfecta) are rare.

An overdose of fluoride may cause white or, in serious cases, brown spots in the enamel (mottled enamel). These discolorations occur, for instance, in areas where the natural drinking water contains more than 2 mg. of fluoride per l.

A property of the antibiotic *tetracycline* is that it rapidly accumulates in growing bone or tooth tissue, presumably by binding to calcium phosphate. Administered to pregnant women after the fourteenth week and to children before their eighth year of life, i.e., during the formation of the deciduous or permanent dentition, it may cause brown discolorations or malformations of the teeth (*Fig.* 2). They are, however, rare in the permanent dentition. It is believed that there is less chance of these abnormalities occurring if oxytetracycline (Terramycin) is used instead of tetracycline.

Disturbances in the Eruption of Teeth.—The deciduous dentition erupts from about 6 months (lower incisors) until 2 years after birth (upper second molar) and is lost between the seventh and twelfth years of life. The first permanent molars erupt when the child is

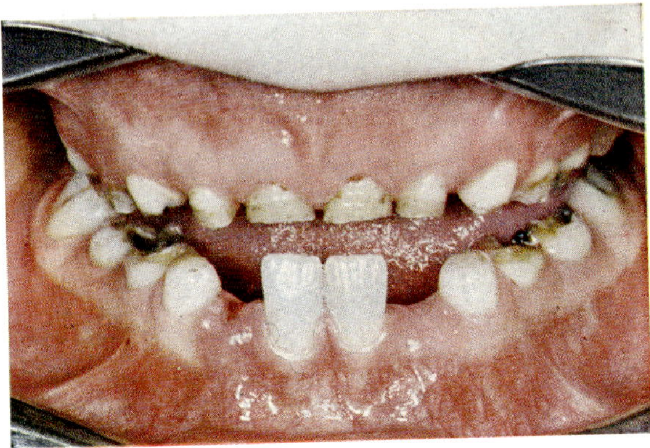

Fig. 2.—Discoloration and malformation of deciduous teeth in a $7\frac{1}{2}$-year-old boy, due to administration of tetracycline immediately after birth. The permanent lower central incisors are sound. (*P. H. G. Kremer.*)

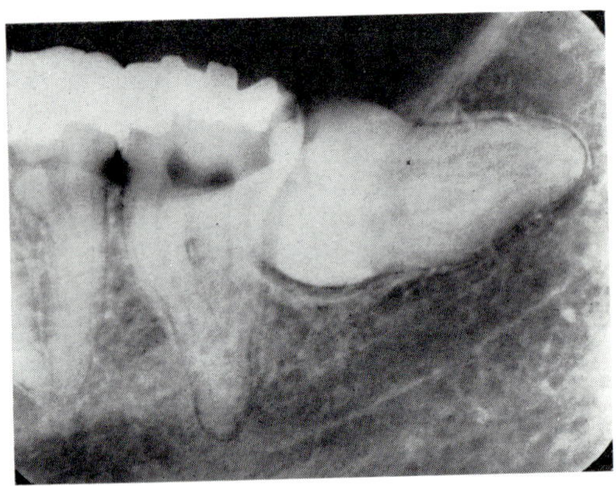

Fig. 3.—Third molar horizontally in the jaw. Surgical removal is indicated.

about 6, dorsally of the deciduous dentition. A few years later these molars are so grossly affected by caries in many children that they are often mistaken for carious deciduous molars. At an age of about 12 shedding is completed. Between 17 and 21 years of age, finally, wisdom teeth may erupt; sometimes, however, they are agenetic or have an abnormal position (*Fig.* 3).

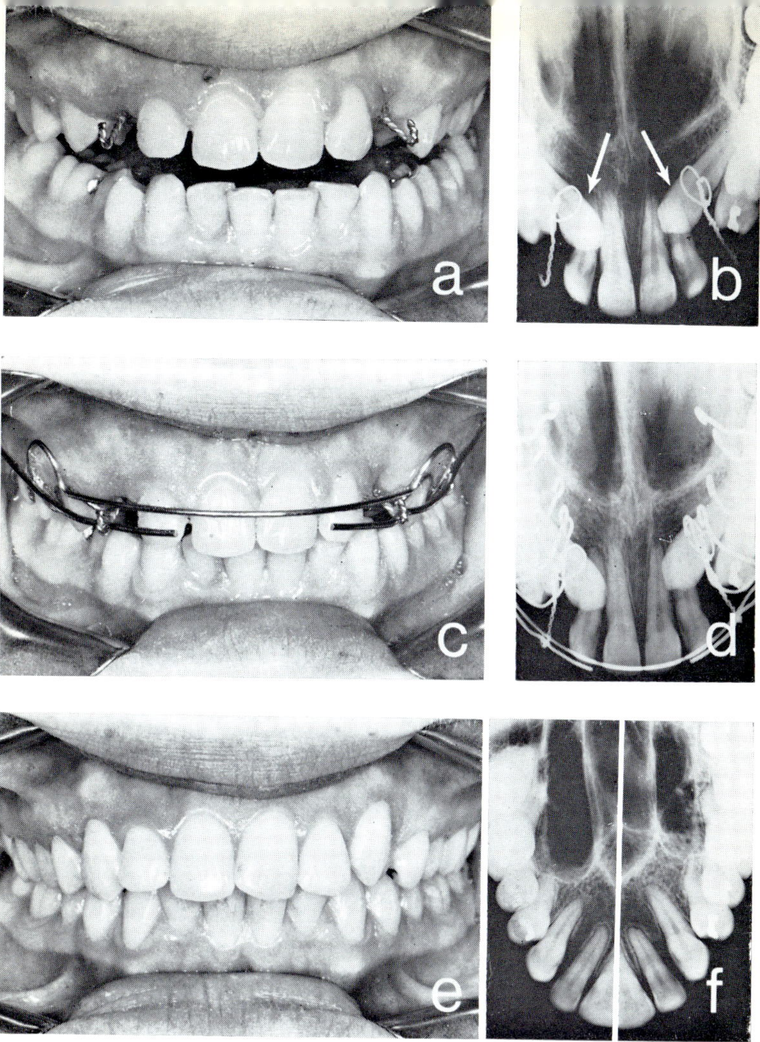

Fig. 4.—a, Both impacted upper canines are provided surgically with thin steel ligatures. The twisted ends, passing through the mucosa, are bent into a hook. b, The radiograph shows the position of the canines and the ligatures around the necks of the teeth. c, On either side a spring is attached to the hooks and fixed to an orthodontic appliance, thus continuously exerting a slight force in the incisal direction. d, A radiograph in which the connexion between labial springs and canines is clearly visible. The other wires and loops in the radiograph serve as a fixation of the orthodontic apparatus to the dentition. e, Result after a period of treatment and retention of 2 years in a 17-year-old patient (*Orthodontic Department, University of Groningen*). f, Canines in the right position, the bone is completely adapted.

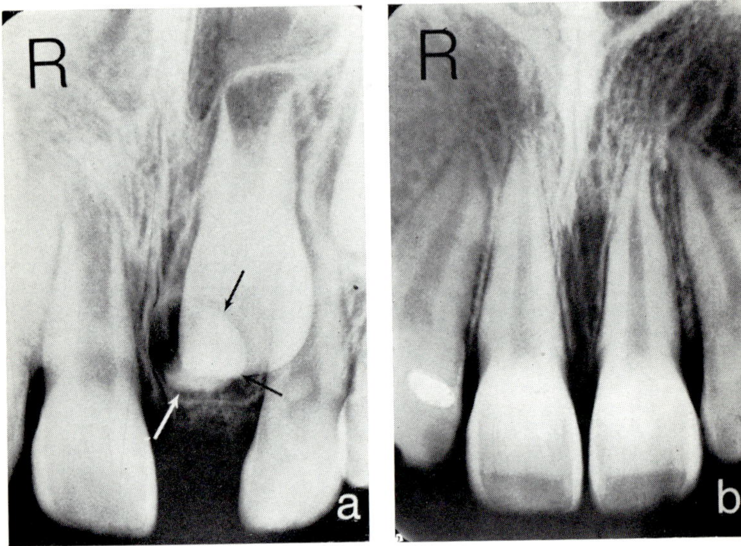

Fig. 5.—A supernumerary tooth (*see* arrows) in the path of eruption of the upper left central incisor. Four years after removal of this mesiodens the incisor has attained its correct position.

If the upper lateral incisor fails to erupt we must consider agenesis and, where an upper canine is concerned, lack of space or an abnormal position (often more or less horizontally in the palate). If non-eruption of the canine is caused by lack of space, the tooth can often be trained into the right position by means of orthodontic treatment (*Fig.* 4). To provide space it is often necessary to sacrifice a pre-molar. If the position of an impacted canine, and especially the root, is very abnormal, or if the root is strongly curved or connected ankylotically with the jaw, it is impossible to regulate the tooth orthodontically. Sometimes transplantation of the canine may be considered.

When an upper central incisor does not erupt at the proper time this is often caused by a supernumerary tooth (mesiodens) situated in the line of eruption (*Fig.* 5), while in rare cases a damaged germ or abnormal position caused by trauma to the deciduous dentition can also play a part.

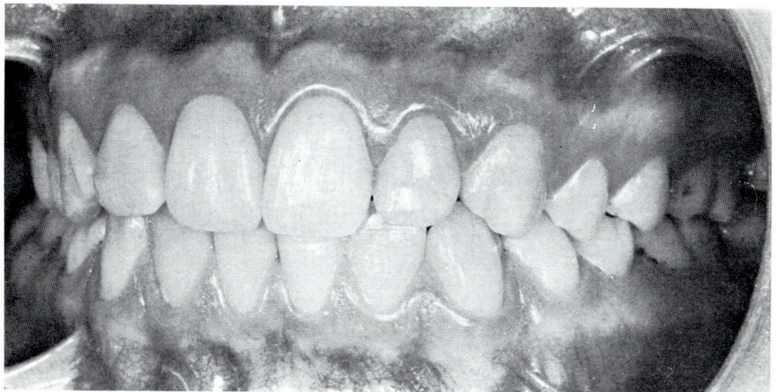

Fig. 6.—Normal (ideal) dentition as to position of teeth and occlusion of lower and upper dentition (*Orthodontic Department, University of Groningen*).

Agenesis may sometimes be explained from a phylogenic reduction of the dental arches; familial occurrence may be encountered, but in most cases there is no explanation at all. In cases of partial or total anodontia ectodermal dysplasia has to be considered (ectodermal structures, such as hairs, nails, sweat-glands, and sebaceous glands, are here underdeveloped or completely absent; the enamel of the dentition is also ectodermal). When several teeth do not erupt at all or when eruption is very much delayed, cleidocranial dysostosis (agenetic clavicles) (*see* p. 45 and *Fig.* 29) must be borne in mind.

Occlusal Disharmonies.—The contact between the dental arches of the lower and upper jaws is called 'occlusion'. In normal cases the lower incisors contact the upper incisors palatally, about 1–3 mm. from the incisal edges of the maxillary incisors; the lower premolars and molars are placed more ventrally so that they bite with their buccal cusps between the buccal and palatal cusps of the upper teeth. *Fig.* 6 shows an example of a normal dentition.

The most common occlusal disharmonies are:—

a. Angle's Class II, division 1, characterized by a narrow upper arch, often combined with strongly protruding upper incisors and a dorsal position of the mandible. It is of common occurrence in western Europe (*Fig.* 7).

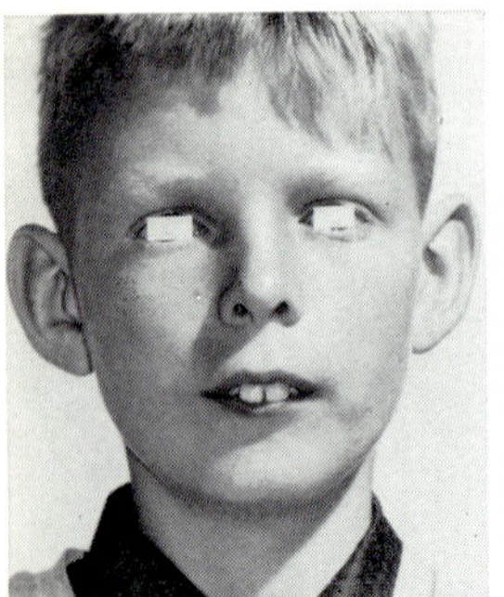 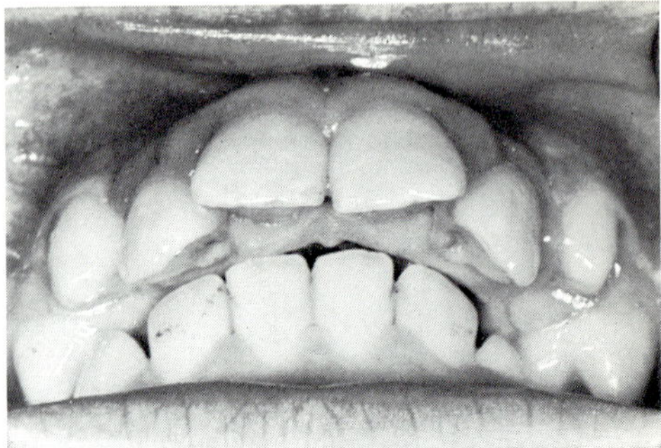

Fig. 7.—Angle's Class II, division 1. Narrow upper arch, protruding upper incisors (sagittal overbite), deep overbite (almost against the palate), lack of space for the teeth, and a too short and non-functioning upper lip.

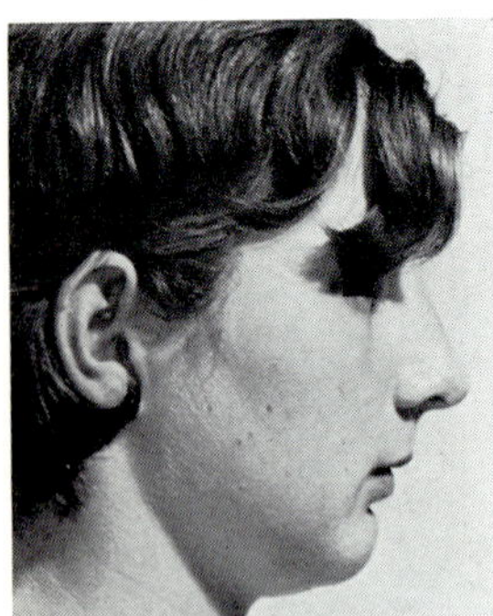 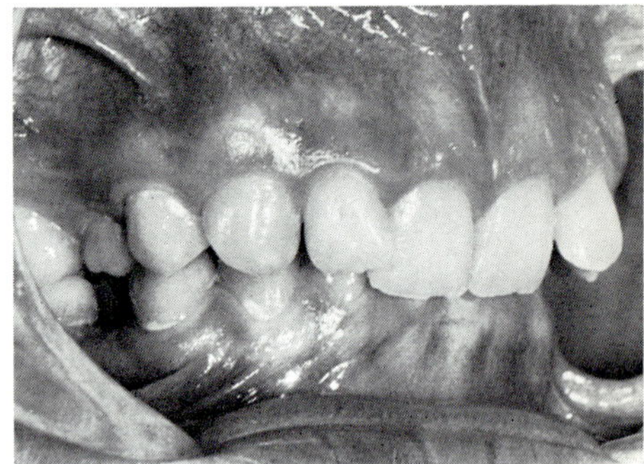

Fig. 8.—Angle's Class II, division 2. Linguoversion of the upper frontal teeth, deep vertical overbite, prominent nasal part of the face, and deep mentolabial sulcus (*Orthodontic Department, University of Groningen*).

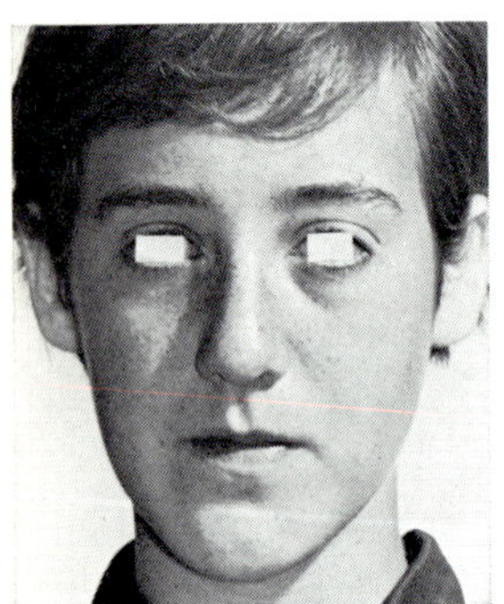 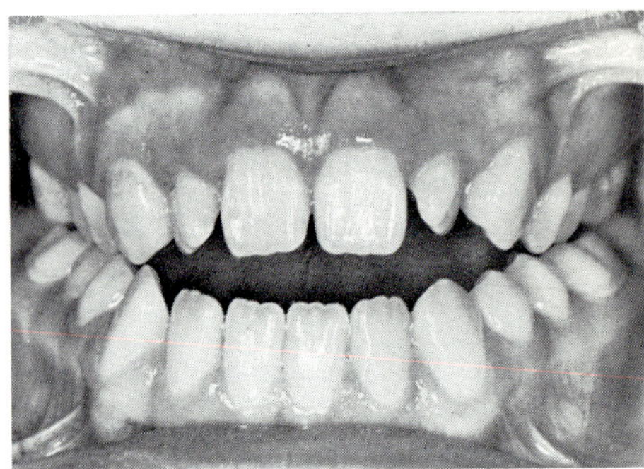

Fig. 9.—Open bite. In a vertical direction there is no contact between the incisal edges of lower and upper frontal teeth.

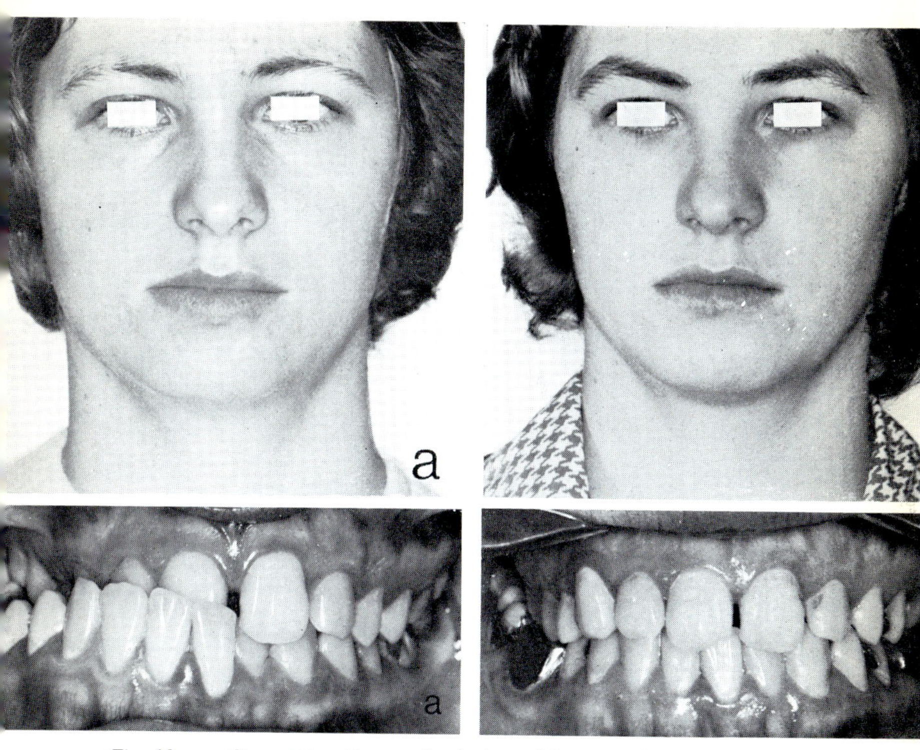

Fig. 10.—a, Cross-bite. Reversed relation of lower and upper arch in transverse direction from lower right second molar to lower left lateral incisor. The lower frontal teeth are overerupted. There is a deviation of the chin-point towards the right and an oblique lip fissure. b, After orthodontic treatment (*E. J. Ponten*). Improved occlusion. The obliqueness of the face is corrected.

b. Angle's Class II, division 2 (linguoversion of the upper frontal teeth, mostly the central incisors only, a square upper arch, wide palate, and a deep vertical overbite) (*Fig.* 8).

c. Open bite. The lower and upper frontal teeth do not contact (in vertical direction) (*Fig.* 9). The mandibular angle is often obtuse. The rachitic open bite, especially, may be very serious and difficult to treat, but is fortunately of rare occurrence.

d. Angle's Class III. An anterior relationship of the lower jaw to the upper jaw, which means reversed overbite; in characteristic cases there is a straight mandibular angle and a protruding chin. This type of malocclusion was hereditary in the Habsburg royal family (*Fig.* 13).

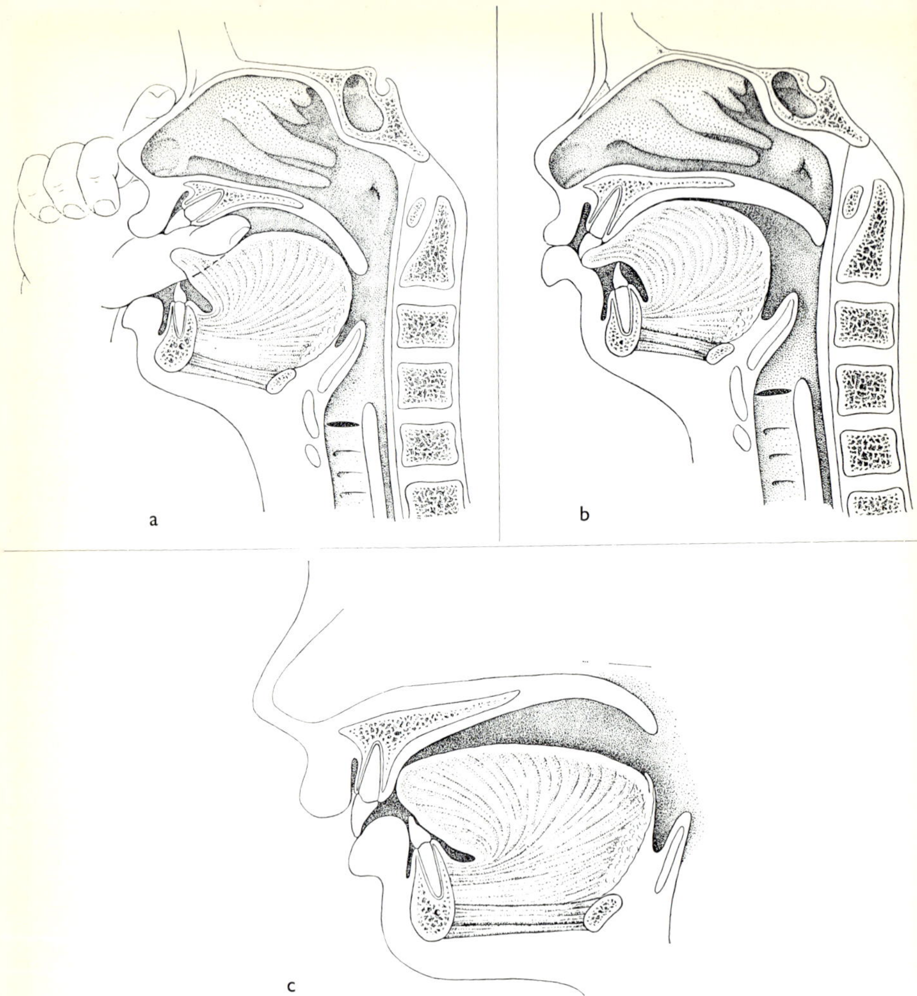

Fig. 11.—a, Thumb-sucking. The upper frontal teeth are protruded and the lower front flattened and tilted dorsally. An open bite in the vertical direction may be the result and the upper jaw may be compressed. Partly owing to the too narrow upper arch the lower jaw develops insufficiently in a ventral direction. b, Abnormal swallowing habit. By bringing the tongue between the teeth during swallowing movements an open bite can be effected or an existing open bite may be stimulated. c, Abnormal lip relation. This situation is found in patients with the orthodontic anomaly known as Angle's Class II, division 1, with sagittal overbite (*Fig.* 7). The (too) short upper lip, the absence of lip contact, the location of the tongue between the teeth, the frequently overdeveloped mental muscle (owing to swallowing without lip contact), and the abnormal tongue position are contributory to the maintenance or the aggravation of this anomaly.

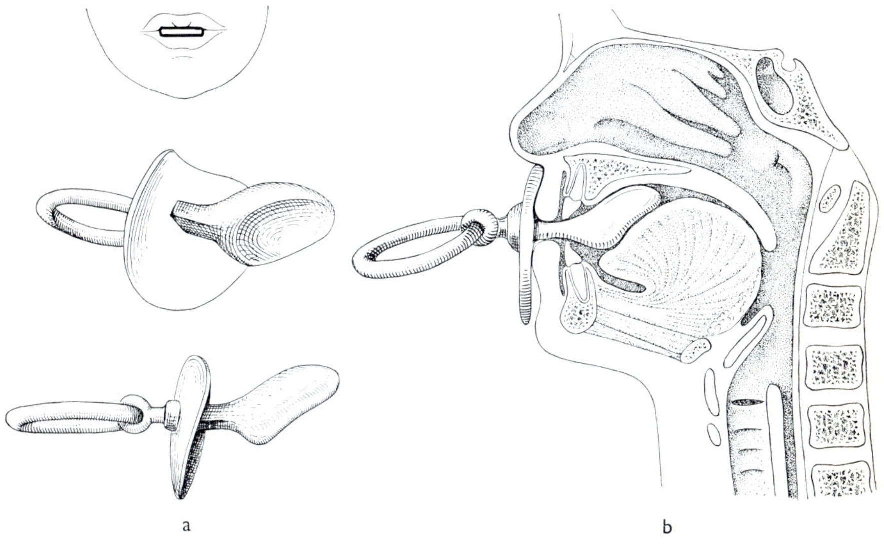

a   b

Fig. 12.—a, Well-shaped comforter. b, The deforming effect on the dentition is less serious than in the case of thumb- or finger-sucking.

e. Cross-bite. Characterized by a disturbed relation of the dental
arches in transverse direction. Deviation of the point of the chin
is often seen (*Fig*. 10).

Presumably hereditary factors play the most important part in
the origin of these malocclusions, but there are also a number of
exogenous influences, such as premature loss of deciduous teeth
(caries) and masticatory habits (thumb- or finger-sucking, abnormal
swallowing movements or tongue habits, and so on; in the orthodontic literature known as 'bad masticatory habits') (*Fig*. 11). It
may be very difficult to stop thumb- or finger-sucking. Strictly
speaking, the habit should be dropped when the child is 5 years of
age (beginning of eruption of the permanent dentition), because
later on abnormalities in the dentition may become irreversible.
There is little chance that stopping the habit will give rise to psychological difficulties. Presumably psychological difficulties are often
responsible for the persistence of these habits. The number of

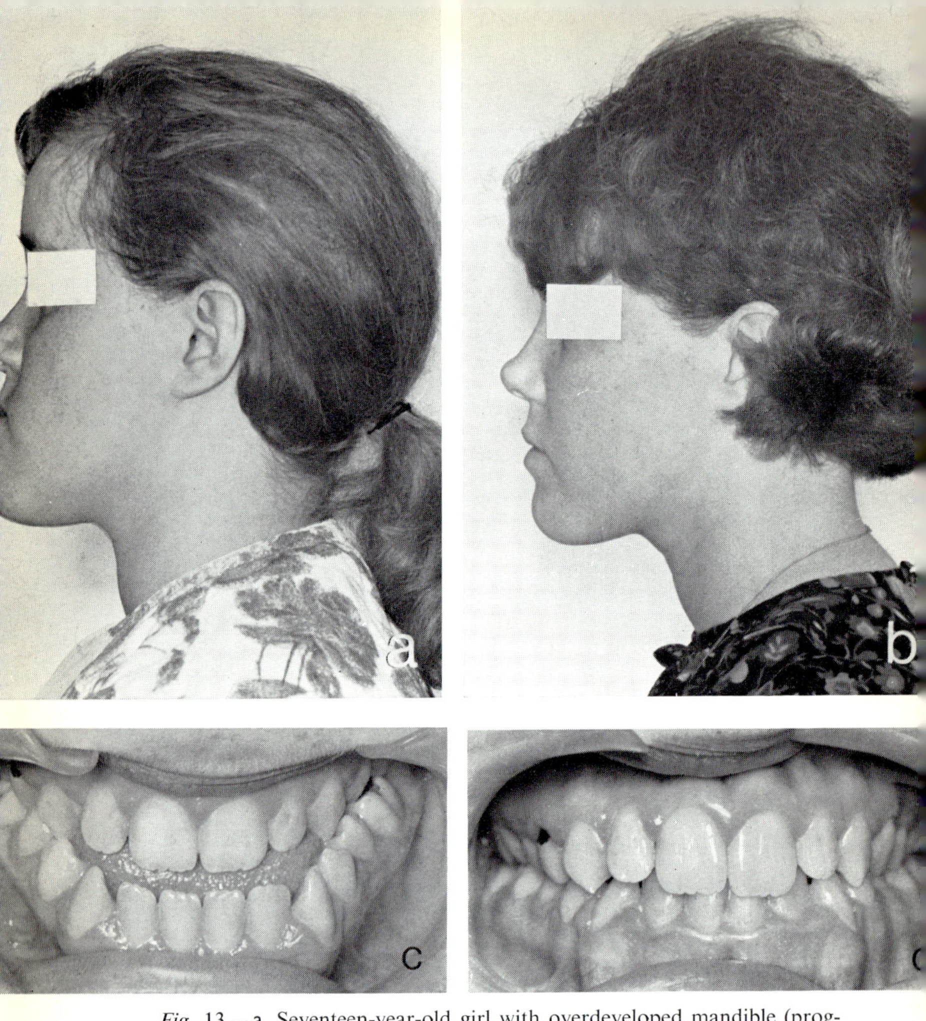

Fig. 13.—a, Seventeen-year-old girl with overdeveloped mandible (prognathic appearance). b, After bilateral osteotomy in the mandibular ascending ramus the profile is normal (*Professor C. A. Merkx*). c, Pre-operatively the lower teeth bite far anterior of the upper teeth. Biting off is impossible and chewing is defective. d, Postoperatively ideal occlusion of the dentition.

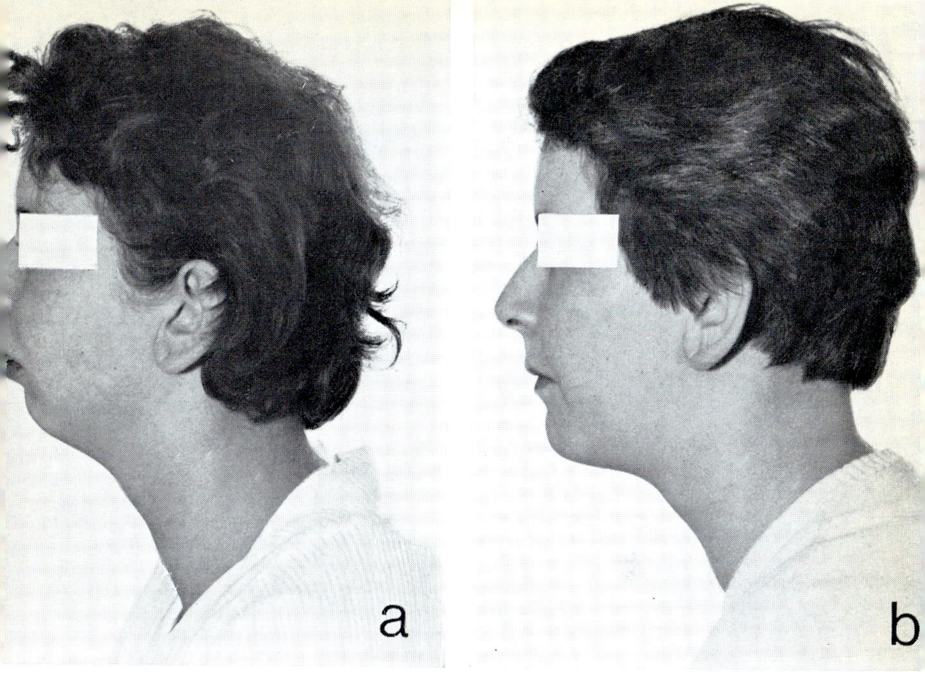

Fig. 14.—a, Bird face, 19-year-old woman. b, Accentuation of the chin prominence by a pedicled bone transplant from the lower mandibular border, combined with alveolotomy in the upper jaw and exercises for the too short upper lip resulting in a very good profile (*Professor C. A. Merkx*).

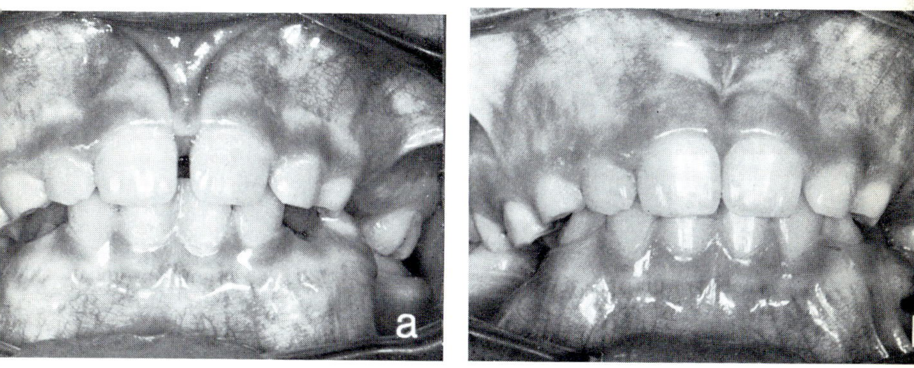

Fig. 15.—a, Hypertrophic fraenulum of the upper lip with a central diastema in a 9-year-old boy. b, Four months after removal of the fraenulum the diastema is closed.

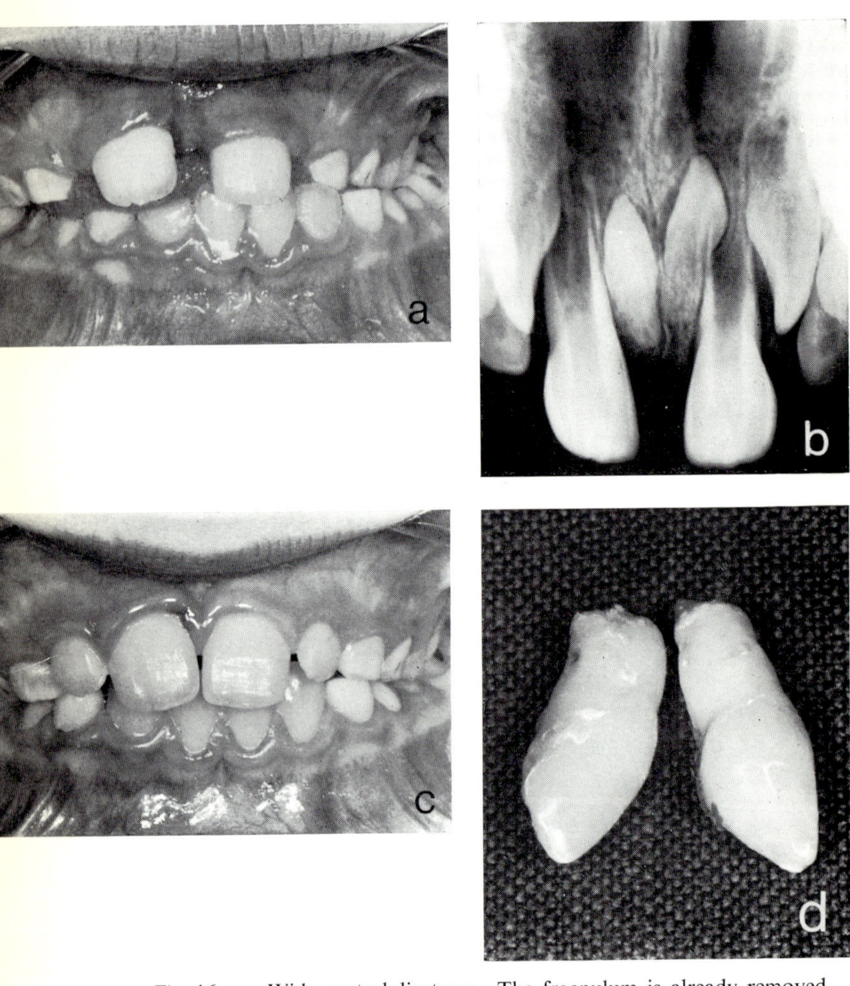

Fig. 16.—a, Wide central diastema. The fraenulum is already removed. b, On the dental radiograph two supernumerary teeth are visible, which are located in the jaw upside down. c, Over a year after removal of the mesiodentes the diastema is nearly closed. d, The two removed mesiodentes ($\times$ 3).

methods used to break the children of the sucking habit is manifold (e.g., woollen glove pinned to the pyjamas, evil-tasting substance on the 'sucking-thumb', cuffs around the arm which make it impossible to bend the elbows (in bed), and many others). If growing girls are concerned it may be of help to let them use nail varnish and make an appeal to their sense of honour by insisting that they should not damage the varnish. In case of persistent young 'suckers' it may be possible to change thumb-sucking into sucking on a well-shaped comforter (*Nuk-Beruhigungssauger* or *Nuk-Kieferformer*) (*Fig.* 12). The harmful influence on the dentition is then reduced to a minimum and, moreover, it is easier to break a child of the comforter-sucking habit. When the child is treated orthodontically the orthodontic apparatus fixed in the mouth usually makes sucking impossible and the patient is rapidly cured of the habit.

Treatment of these occlusal disharmonies is the responsibility of a dentist or orthodontist. In extreme cases (e.g., Angle's Class III) operative correction may be necessary (osteotomy). If osteotomy is considered, the operation should not be performed before the growth of the jaw has stopped (17–21 years of age) (*Figs.* 13 and 14).

A *central diastema* between the upper central incisors may be caused by, or persist owing to, a hypertrophic fraenulum of the upper lip (*Fig.* 15) or by a supernumerary tooth (*Fig.* 16). Fraenectomy may result in early closure of the diastema. In general, however, fraenectomy can be postponed until the upper lateral incisors have erupted. When the child is younger than 8 years of age there is a fair chance of spontaneous closure and surgical treatment is not necessary.

Traumatic Injuries.—Excessively protruding upper incisors in children are easily damaged by trauma. The *crown* may be fractured so that the pulpal chamber is opened. Endodontic treatment is necessary, after which a dowel crown can be made (and fixed with a pin in the root canal). If a permanent tooth is involved and its pulp has remained vital and corrective grinding does not provide a solution, a jacket crown can be made later (at the age of about 17).

In case of a *root fracture* (seen on dental radiograph) therapy depends on the location of the fracture; when the coronal part has insufficient support, the tooth can be splinted; when the pulp has become necrotic it is advisable to remove the (small) apical fragment and to fill the root canal. When the support of the coronal part

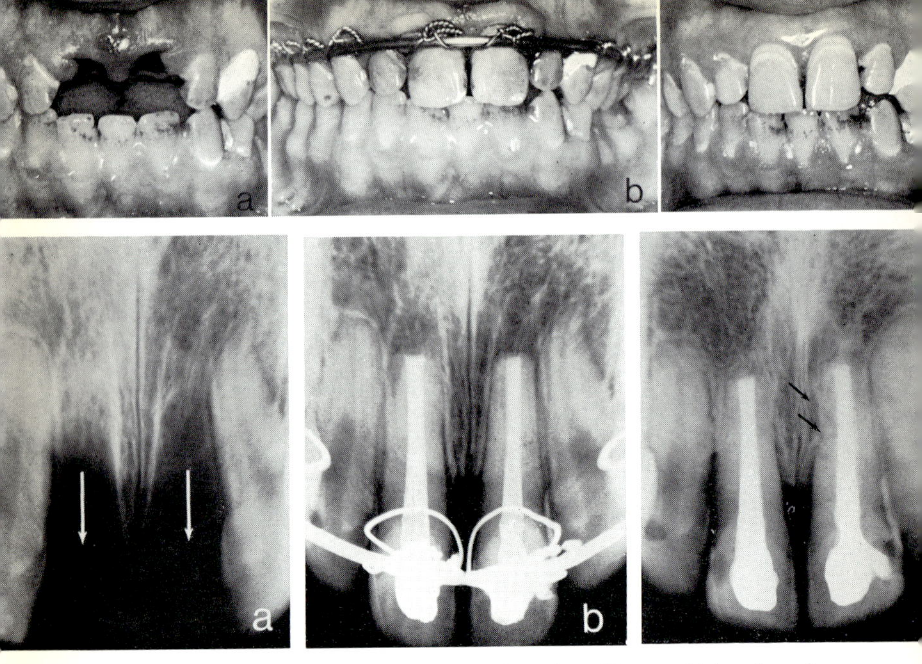

Fig. 17.—a, Both upper central incisors in a 15-year-old boy have been knocked out. b, Replantation 1 day after sterilization (by boiling water) and root-canal treatment. Fixation by means of a metal arch bar. c, Six months after replantation. The two teeth have resettled. Slight root resorption (*see* arrows).

is insufficient, extraction and removal, including the fractured root tip, is indicated.

In case of *luxation*, repositioning (manually) and fixation of the tooth must be done as soon as possible by a dentist or an oral surgeon. For this purpose a metal arch bar is used, being fixed to the rest of the dentition by means of stainless-steel ligatures. As a rule after 6–8 weeks the involved tooth is firm again. If there is marked dislocation the apical blood-vessels and nerve systems are often torn off. As a result the pulp becomes necrotic and the tooth may discolour in due course to blue or grey, especially in the case of haemorrhage in the pulpal chamber. Therefore, tooth luxation must be followed in almost all cases by good endodontic treatment. Only in very young persons when the luxated tooth has a wide apical foramen may the pulp remain vital.

The prognosis is usually good as far as the viability of the tooth is concerned.

Luxated *deciduous* teeth can be repositioned manually and splinted if the child is easy to treat. If the teeth are very loose their removal is indicated. Extraction is also indicated in cases in which root resorption has taken place to a large extent already. It is advisable not to reposition slightly intruded deciduous teeth (wedged into the jaw) which are still rather firm and show only slight dislocation, while damage to the germ of the permanent successor is unlikely (dental radiograph); it is better to let them reattach in their new position.

When the tooth is completely knocked *out of the mouth*, the best thing to do is to pick it up, put it into the mouth, and keep it under the tongue or behind the molars. This has to be done to keep the periodontium fragments on the root vital and to enable primary healing. The patient should see his dentist or oral surgeon to have the tooth replanted, if he wishes to retain the tooth. When the trauma has happened more than $1\frac{1}{2}$ or 2 hours before, or when the tooth is very soiled, it is cleaned and the periodontium fragments are removed, because they are no longer vital. The root tip with its many ramifications of the root canal is resected and the canal itself is cleaned. Before the tooth is replanted it is sterilized (in boiling water) and the root canal is filled. This completely non-vital tooth resettles by resorption of the root surface and bone apposition in the lacunae (ankylosis). Because this substitution of dentine by bone is gradually taking place, it takes about 5 years, on an average, to substitute the whole root and then the crown will fall out. Yet in children and adults, who value preservation of their dentition, replantation is almost always effective (*Fig.* 17). In the case of lack of space or a large sagittal overbite it has to be decided whether orthodontic closure of the diastema is to be preferred.

Completely knocked-out deciduous teeth are not replanted.

Periodontal Diseases.—This term includes diseases of the attachment apparatus of the dentition or periodontium which includes the periodontal membrane, the cementum, the alveolar bone, and marginal gingiva. The cause of periodontal diseases is not yet clear. It is generally accepted that there is a combination of a dystrophic and an inflammatory component, either taking a major role. Sometimes the dystrophic part is dominating, in which case there is periodont*osis*; when the inflammatory component is dominating the picture may resemble an inflammation and there is a tendency to call the disease periodont*itis*. Little is known as yet about the dystrophic component; disturbances in general health, combined with a bad peripheral circulation with a diminished resistance to inflammations (e.g., diabetes), may stimulate periodontosis, while the picture is also seen in children with hyperkeratosis palmaris et plantaris. Racial factors seem to play a part too. The inflammatory component is due to an apical extension of the bacterial plaque and tartar between gingiva and root surface. This is promoted by a poor hygienic condition of the mouth. Local irritating factors, such as projecting fillings and crowns and bad contact points, where food is impacted between the teeth, play a part too.

The *clinical* picture is characterized by retraction of the gingiva and/or detachment of the gingiva from the teeth. The gingiva is bluish-red in colour, is slightly oedematous, and has a chronically inflamed character; a deep fissure (gingiva pocket) exists between root and gingiva, from which pus can often be massaged (*Fig.* 18 a). The gingiva bleeds easily and there is a marked foetor oris. In most cases of easy bleeding of the gingiva this is caused by periodontal disease. Sometimes the teeth seem to be overerupted and tiltings or tippings may occur without any distinct mechanical reason. The marginal alveolar bone is resorbed and finally the teeth come loose (*Fig.* 18 c).

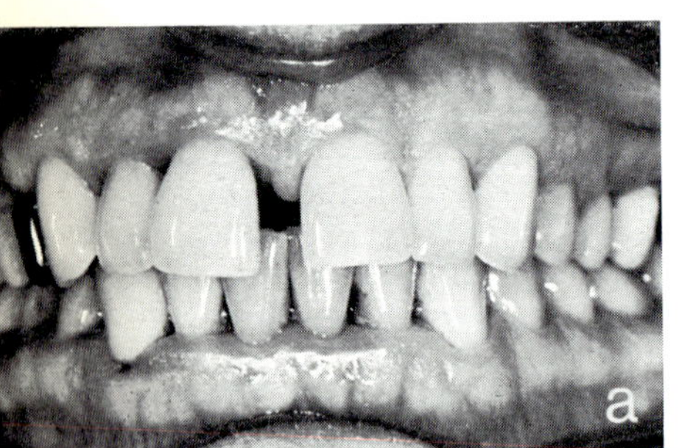

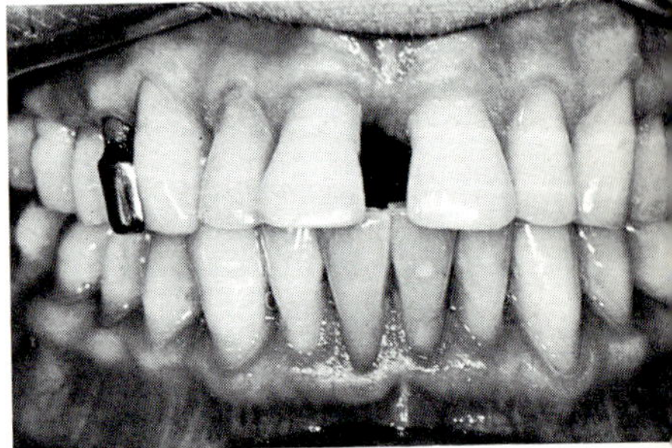

Fig. 18.—a, Periodontal disease of lower and upper dentition with deep pockets and migration of teeth in the right upper jaw. b, Same dentition about 1½ years after gingivectomy in lower and upper jaw. Marked improvement of the gingival aspect. No foetor oris. c, Complete set of dental radiographs showing distinct resorption of the alveolar margins, especially in the areas indicated by arrows (a=upper dentition; b=lower dentition).

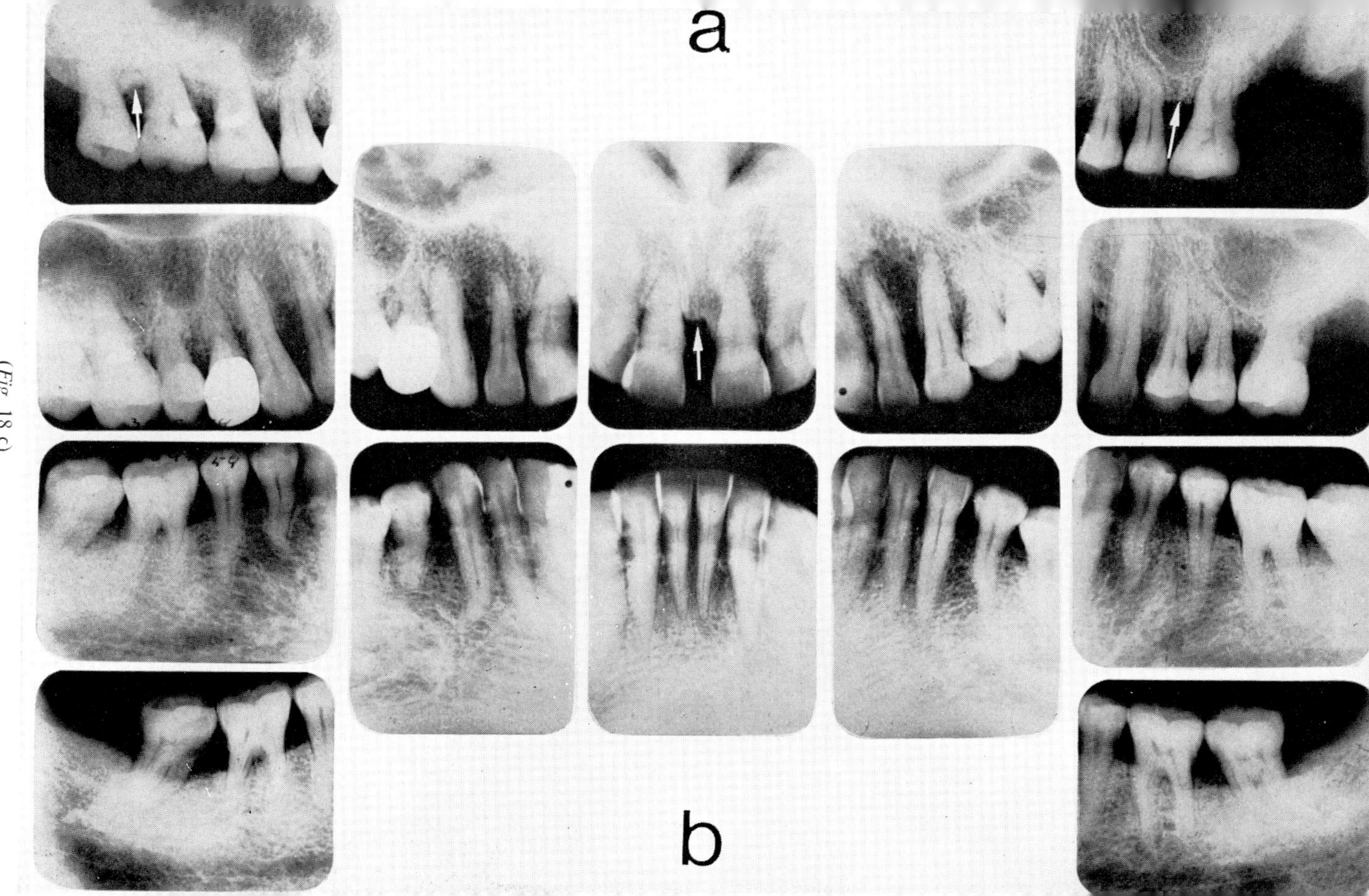

(*Fig.* 18 c)

The disease is of very common occurrence and nearly as many teeth get lost owing to periodontal diseases as by dental caries. A *causal therapy* and a *reparatio ad integrum* are mostly impossible. Treatment, aimed at arresting the progress of the disease, consists of thorough periodical cleaning by a dentist and the patient has to observe an extremely good oral hygiene. Reduction of the sugar consumption between meals and limited smoking promote the hygienic condition of the oral cavity. In cases of deep gingival pockets the loose gingiva can be excised (gingivectomy). Then the teeth can be thoroughly freed of subgingival calculus, so that the patient can keep them clean more easily. Toothpicks and electric toothbrushes may be of considerable help. If the teeth have come loose the interdigitation of the teeth can be diminished by corrective grinding, thus limiting the horizontal forces during masticatory function. It is also possible to anchor the teeth *en bloc* by a vitallium splint. A disadvantage of all the above-mentioned methods of treatment is that the aesthetic aspect of the dentition does not improve and the exposed necks of teeth may be very sensitive (*Fig.* 18 b).

Vitamin-C administration or rinsing with hydrogen peroxide or antiseptics is of no value in the treatment of periodontal disease.

CHAPTER 2

THE JAWS

CONGENITAL ANOMALIES

Cleft Lip and Palate.—The majority of this group is formed by patients with a cleft lip and a cleft upper jaw and/or palate. The anomaly occurs in all kinds of gradations and may be either unilateral or bilateral. About 1 out of 1000 newborn babies have a hare-lip or cleft palate in one form or another. In about 30 per cent of all cases the anomaly is familial.

Treatment is performed by a team which includes a plastic surgeon, a paediatrician, an anaesthetist, an ear, nose, and throat specialist, a speech therapist, an orthodontist, an oral surgeon, and a prosthodontist. Although not directly involved in the treatment, but nevertheless other important members of the team, are a psychiatrist, a psychologist, and finally a geneticist and an embryologist. It is not the intention to enter extensively into discussion of treatment of these patients, but some important points will be mentioned.

The lip is closed when the child is 2 or 3 months old, whereas closure of the palate will be performed before the child starts speaking—at about 6 months to $1\frac{1}{2}$ years. In order not to disturb the development of the upper jaw some specialists do not start treatment before the child is about 8–12 years of age. Most palate surgeons, however, believe in an early closure. Constant control during growth of the child is of major importance.

When the soft palate is too short or has insufficient muscular function the closure between nasopharynx and oropharynx can be insufficient during speaking or swallowing. Correction can be made for instance by pharyngoplasty during which a connexion is made between the dorsal pharyngeal wall and the soft palate by suturing a pedicled mucous flap of the dorsal pharyngeal wall to the soft palate. The flap may have its base either cranially (Sanvenero Roselli flap) or caudally (Rosenthal flap). On either side of the flap remains a small opening for nose breathing and drainage of nasal secretion (*Fig.* 19).

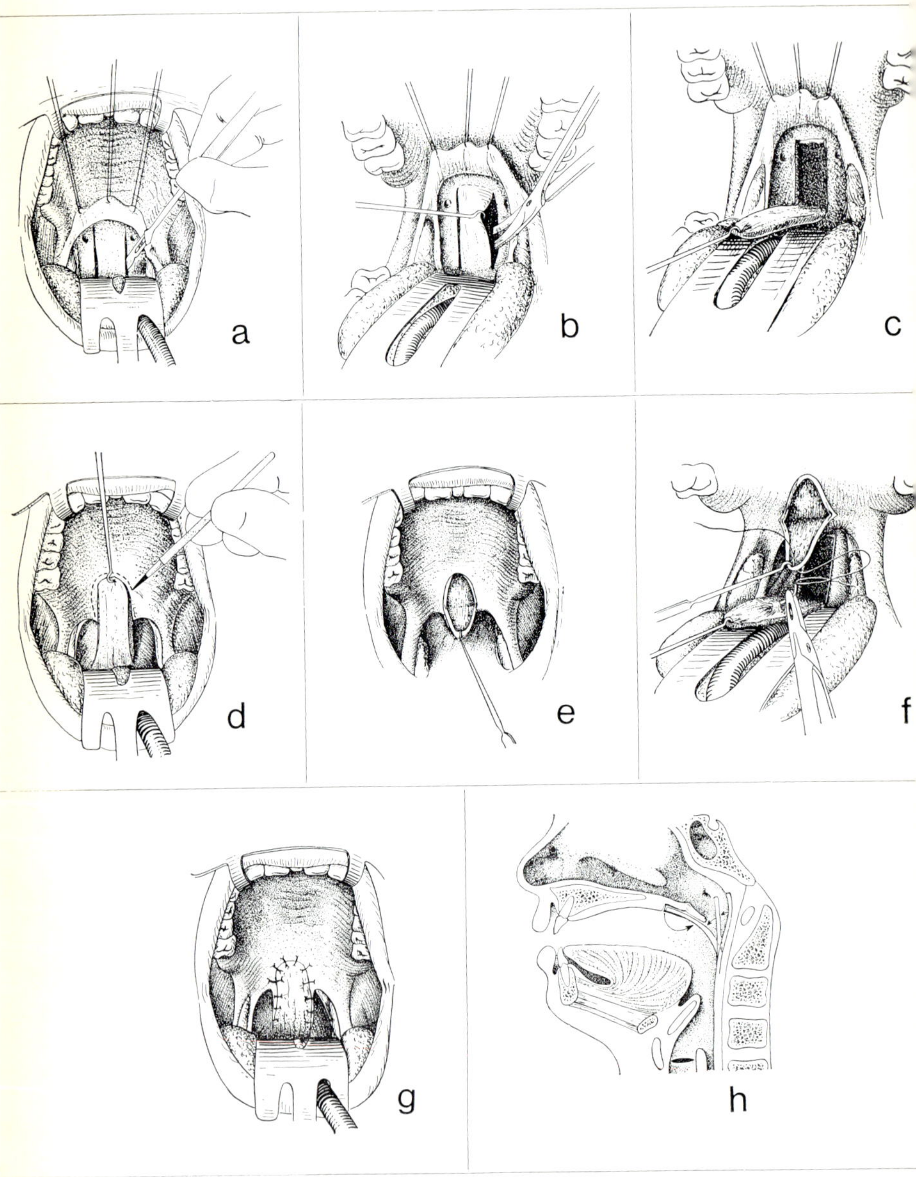

Fig. 19.—Principles of pharyngoplasty.

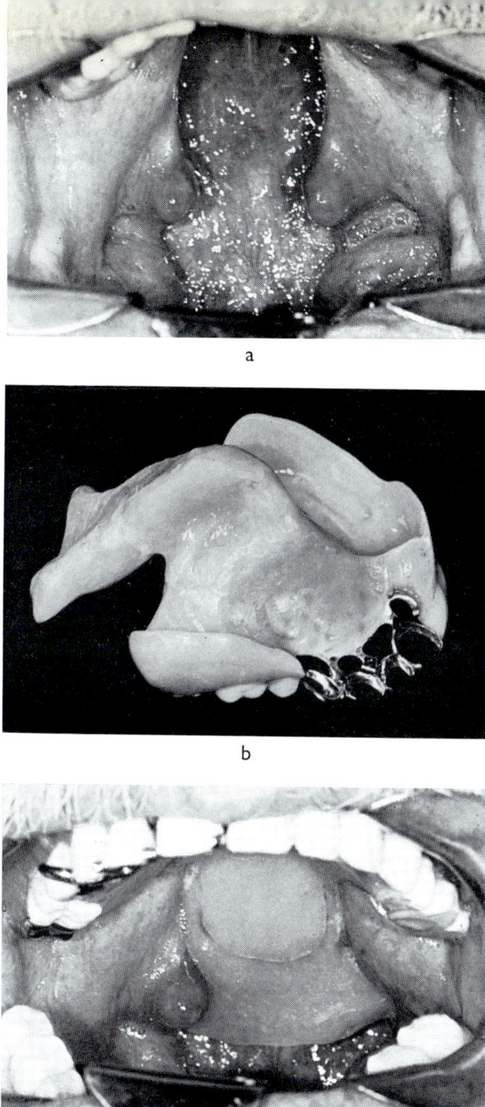

Fig. 20.—a, Unoperated cleft palate. b, Obturator consisting of a partial prosthesis and obturator body, which is so shaped that during speaking, together with the action of velum and pharynx muscle, a closure between oro- and nasopharynx can be effected. c, Obturator in situ. The dorsal end is situated just clear of the pharyngeal wall in the place where, when speaking, Passavant's bar can be observed.

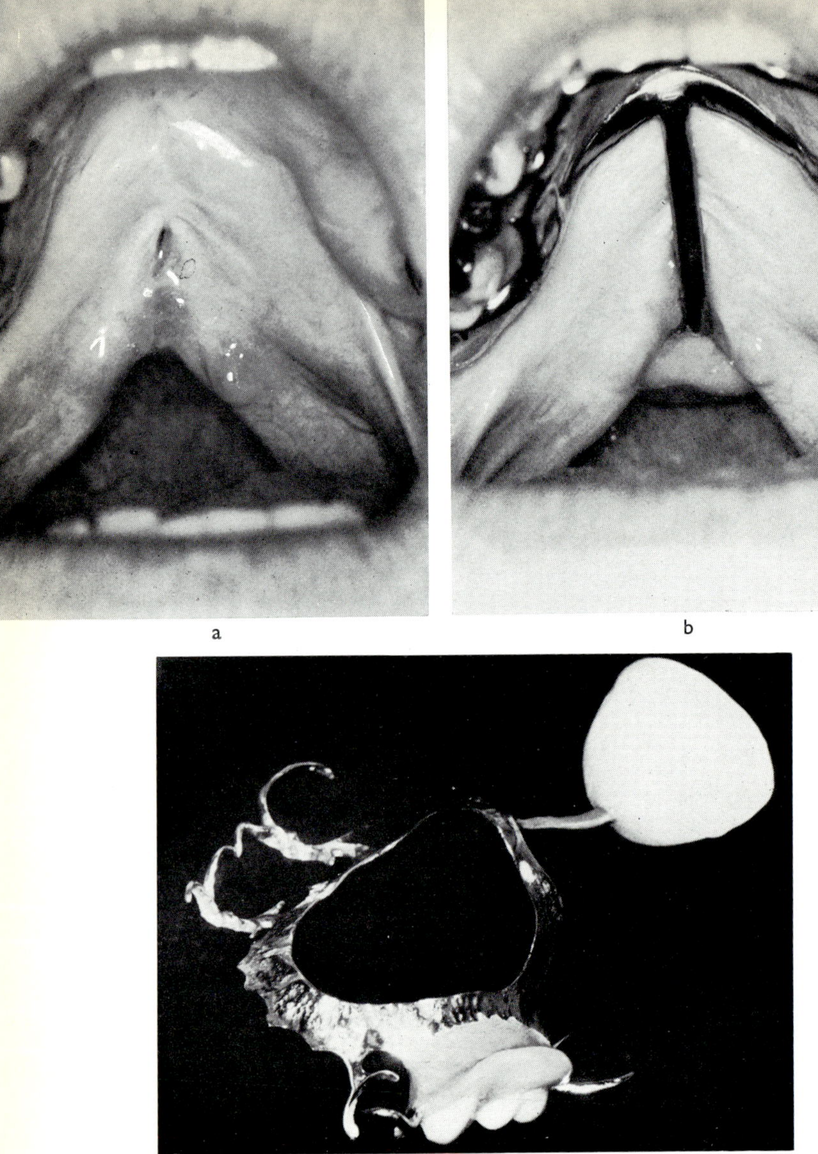

Fig. 21.—a, Operated cleft palate. The soft palate has remained too short. b, In the pharynx an obturator is introduced, enabling a closure of the nasopharynx. c, The obturator consists of a metal frame for fixation to the natural dentition, a narrow connective part, and a triangular acrylic obturator body.

The prosthodontist cares for those patients whose anomalies cannot be treated surgically or orthodontically or in the case of very extensive defects in which these methods of treatment are not desirable. When the palate cannot be closed owing to lack of tissue or when the palate is too short to enable good speech, an obturator can be made to close the cleft or, in the form of a triangular mould in the pharynx, to make a closure possible between naso- and oro-pharynx during speech (*Figs.* 20 and 21). An optimal result is only obtained after speech therapy; the patient has to learn how to handle the inserted apparatus.

When the maxilla is underdeveloped, especially in a ventral direction, a reversed lip relation is the result, resembling a mandibular prognathism (the difference is, however, that in this case the anomaly is localized in the upper jaw) (*Fig.* 22 a). Sometimes corrections can be made by orthodontic treatment. If, however, orthodontic treatment is contra-indicated, or if the result of such treatment is insufficient, aesthetic or functional help may be achieved by a so-called 'cover prosthesis'. This prosthesis is made over the remaining and abnormally positioned teeth and supports the upper lip in a ventral position, resulting in a much better profile (*Fig.* 22 a, b, c). Before inserting this cover prosthesis, it is necessary to provide the teeth covered by this prosthesis with metal crowns to prevent early decay (*Fig.* 22 d, e, f, g, and h). When the upper lip is too short or when it is connected with the jaw, it is necessary that it is first elongated and mobilized by plastic surgery.

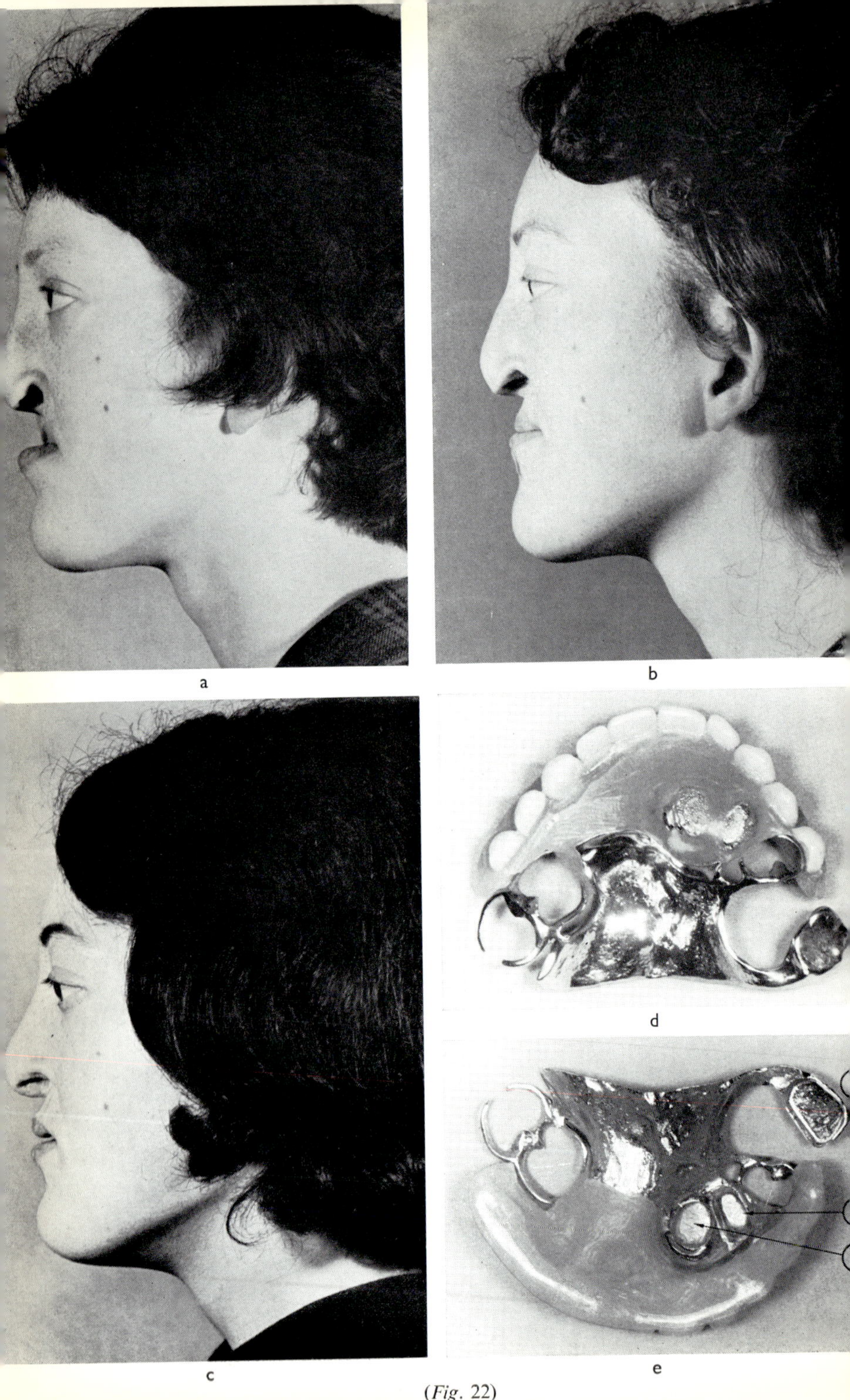

a

b

c

d

e

(*Fig.* 22)

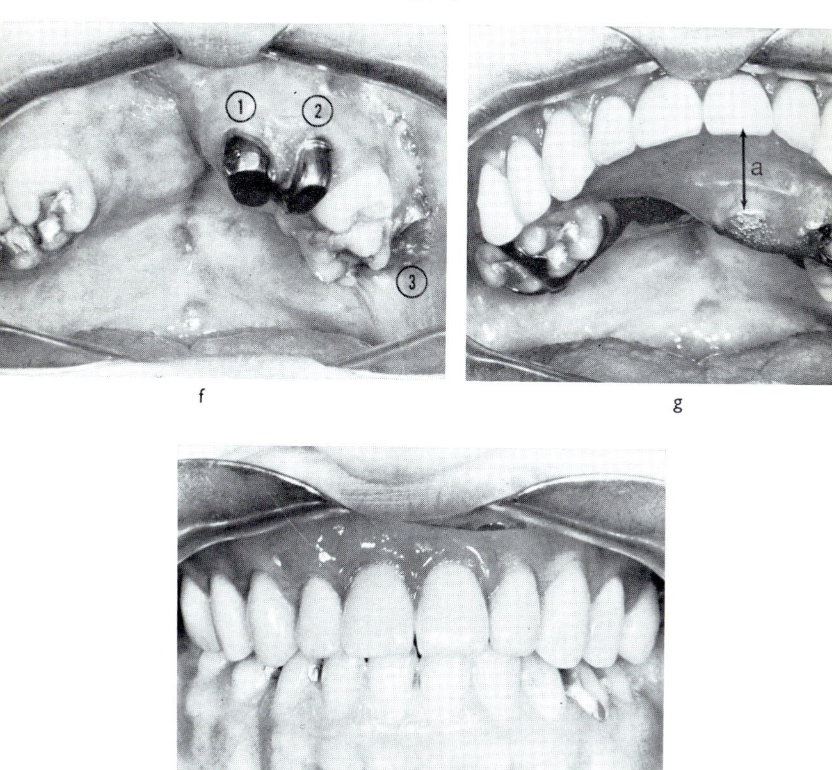

Fig. 22.—a, Bilateral hare-lip and cleft palate in a 17-year-old girl. Marked retroposition of the upper lip and deformation of the nose. b, The upper lip is elongated in a transverse direction by a plastic surgeon (*Professor Dr. A. J. C. Huffstadt*) by means of a triangular pedicled graft from the hypertrophic lower lip (*Abbe* flap). c, The nose is corrected by a plastic surgeon and the upper lip brought into a more ventral position by means of a cover prosthesis. d, Example of a cover prosthesis (lingual side). e, Cavities in the palatal side (1, 2, and 3) fitting on the crowned teeth (*see* f). f, The teeth, covered by the prosthesis, are provided with metal crowns (1, 2, and 3). g, Prosthesis in situ. The anterior position of the artificial teeth (a) provides that the upper lip is sufficiently supported in a forward position. h, There is a normal occlusion with the natural lower dentition.

Mandibulofacial Dysostosis.—This rather rare congenital anomaly is characterized by an underdeveloped mandible and middle third of the face. Bilateral anomaly (Treacher Collins's syndrome) is

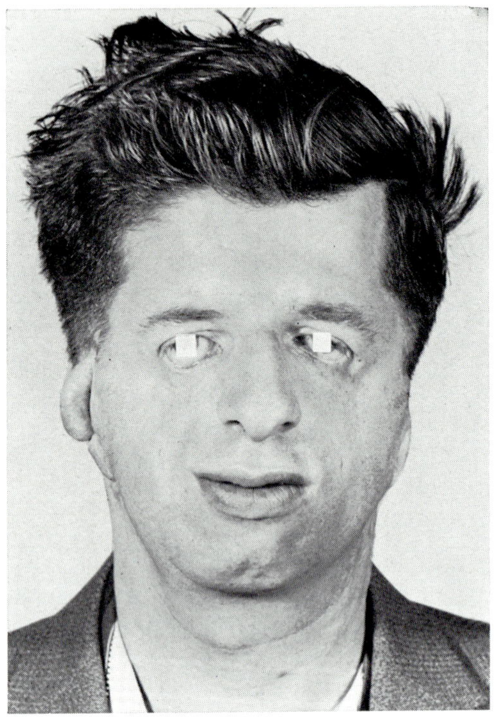

Fig. 23.—Bilateral mandibulofacial dysostosis (Treacher Collins's syndrome; Franceschetti-Zwahlen-Klein syndrome). Anti-mongoloid obliqueness of the eyes, underdeveloped mandible, zygomatic complex, and ears. Often colobomata are seen bilaterally in the outer third part of the lower eyelid.

extremely rare (*Fig.* 23). Unilateral anomaly (*Fig.* 24) is characterized by a conspicuous obliqueness of the face caused by unilateral underdevelopment of the mandible (especially of the ascending ramus), the ear, the maxilla, zygomatic complex, and overlying soft tissues. Sometimes macrostomia is seen, while epibulbar dermoids also often occur. Presumably the syndrome is due to a developmental disturbance in the first and second branchial arch area. Surgical treatment can start at an early age and is mainly masking. In children the growth of the underdeveloped jaw and soft tissues may be stimulated by inserting two

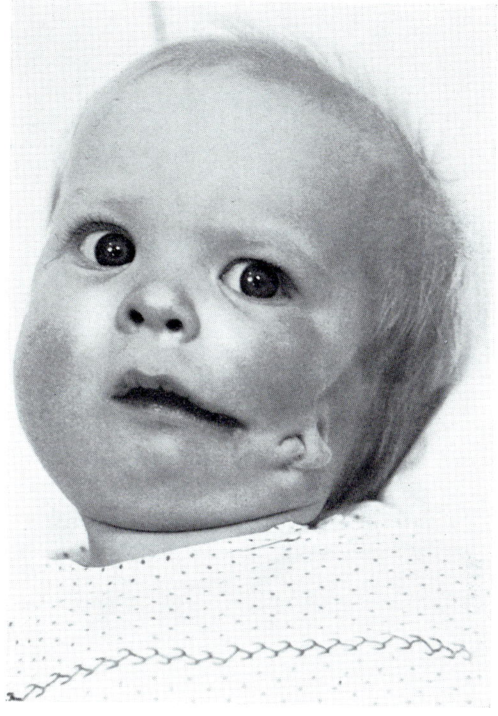

Fig. 24.—Unilateral mandibulofacial dysostosis with marked macrostomia, distinct hypoplasia of the ear, and underdeveloped left half of the face, becoming more and more conspicuous as the child grows older. The left mandibular ramus is missing. No anti-mongoloid obliqueness of the eyes.

or three times (with long intervals) a split-rib graft on the jaw during the growth period. In adults the asymmetry can be masked by inserting a dermal fat graft (*Fig.* 25). The generally very irregular position of the teeth makes orthodontic treatment almost always necessary.

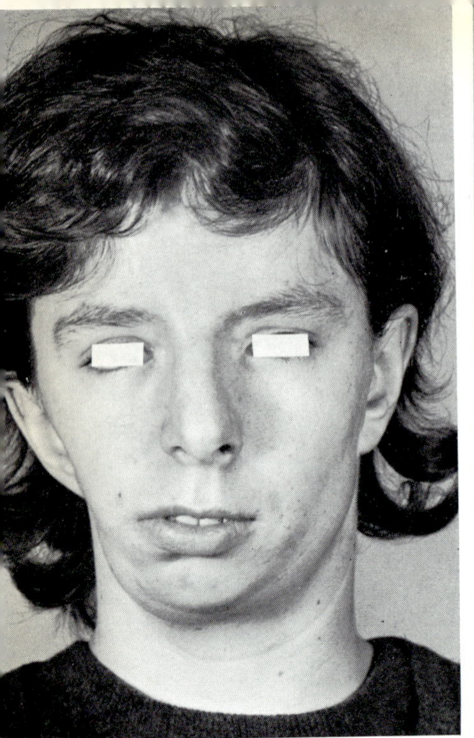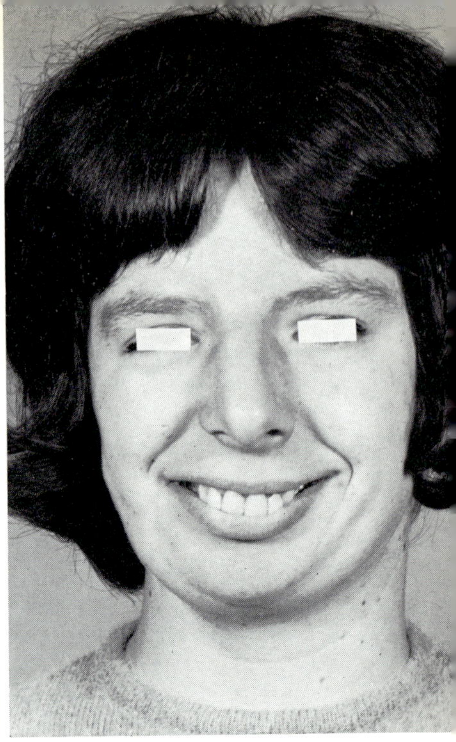

a   b

Fig. 25.—a, Serious unilateral mandibulofacial dysostosis in a 19-year-old patient. b, The same patient 1 year after correction of the cheek by a dermal fat graft (*Professor Dr. A. J. C. Huffstadt*). The irregular position of the teeth was treated orthodontically at an early age (*C. Booy*).

In the case of hypoplasia or aplasia of the external ear surgical treatment rarely gives a good result. A well-constructed plastic auricle is more satisfying. An auricle of soft acrylic would be ideal, but the quality of this material is not yet sufficient. Hard acrylic is still to be preferred. Fixation of the plastic auricle is usually achieved by means of a spectacle frame, while an extension in the external auditory canal prevents shifting in a caudal direction. When the external auditory canal is absent a skin tunnel can be made in which an extension of the artificial auricle can find a hold (*Fig.* 26). A disadvantage of this fixation is that when the patient takes off his spectacles (for instance when they are fogged) he also 'takes off' his ear. Spectacles can be prevented from misting by

42

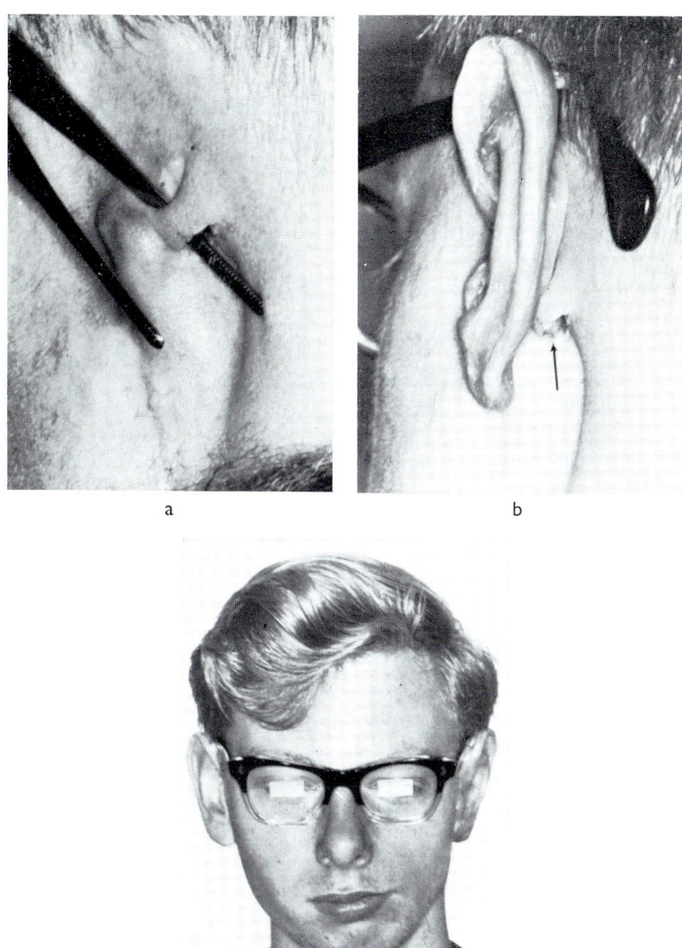

a

b

c

Fig. 26.—Aplasia of the external ear in a 17-year-old patient with unilateral mandibulofacial dysostosis. a, A skin tunnel is made, lined by a free skin-graft (*Professor Dr. A. J. C. Huffstadt*). b, An extension of the acrylic artificial ear fits into the tunnel. Extra fixation by a spectacle frame. c, After treatment. Control period: nearly 10 years.

smearing the glasses with a surface-tension-reducing agent. It is possible to glue the ear with a skin adhesive and to support it with a spectacle frame, but some patients cannot bear the use of this adhesive on their skin for many years at a stretch.

For these patients, too, it is necessary to control them during the growth period and close co-operation of the attending specialists is desirable.

Craniofacial Dysostosis.—This anomaly is of rare occurrence too. Generally the middle third of the face and the neurocranium are involved. There is a premature closure of the sutures of the skull. Furthermore, there is exophthalmos, hypertelorism, and marked hypoplasia of the maxilla (*Fig.* 27). The skull is brachycephalic, whereas there is a shortening in the anteroposterior direction. The forehead is steep and the occiput is flattened. Regarding the dentition the maxillary arch is V-shaped, thus causing lack of space for

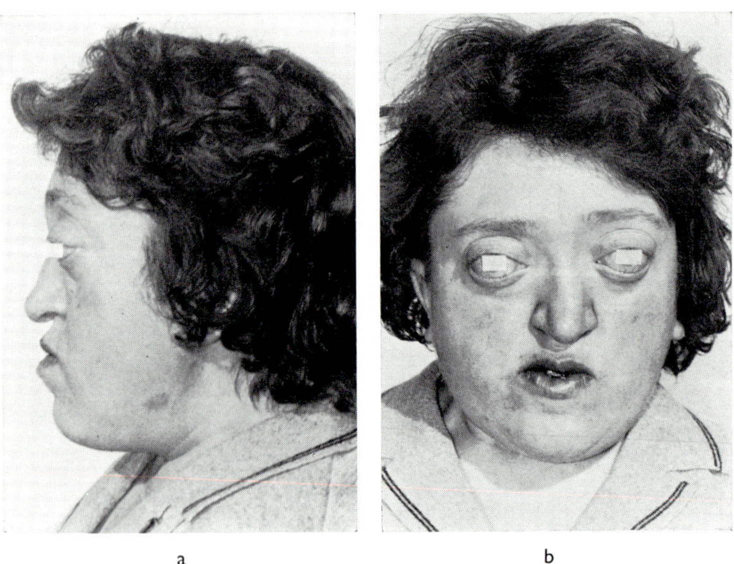

a   b

Fig. 27.—a, b, Craniofacial dysostosis (Crouzon's disease). Distinct exophthalmus and hypertelorism, pronounced underdeveloped middle third of the face, and retruding upper lip.

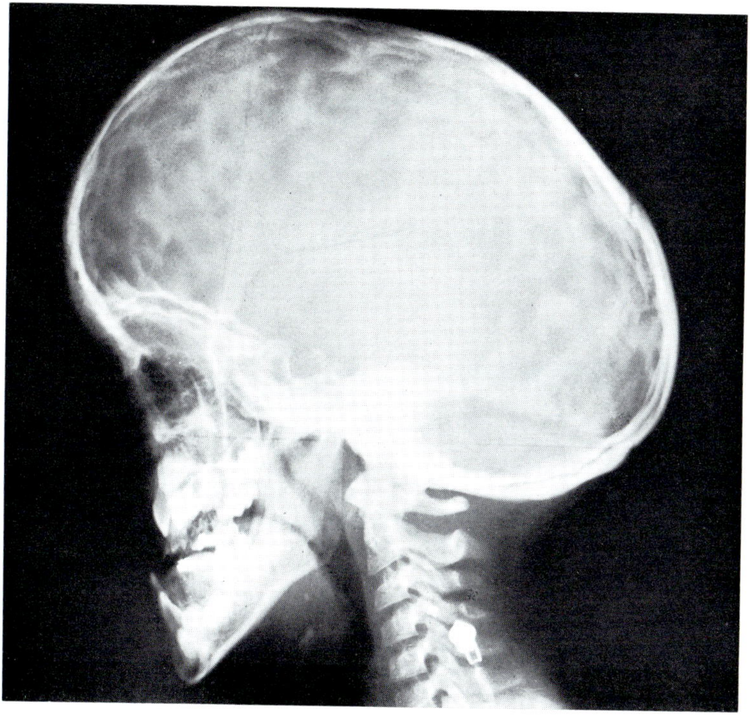

Fig. 28.—Teleradiograph of a boy with craniofacial dysostosis. Steep forehead, flattened back of the head, underdeveloped maxillary complex, and digital impressions.

the teeth. The underdeveloped maxilla is the cause of a prognathic overbite. In the radiograph marked digital impressions are visible (*Fig.* 28). Therapeutic possibilities are limited.

Cleidocranial Dysostosis.—Owing to total or partial aplasia of the clavicles (mostly the acromial part) patients have drooping shoulders which can easily be approximated (*Fig.* 29 a, b). The skull is brachycephalic and the eyes are wide apart. There is marked frontal and parietal bossing. The palate is very high. Eruption of teeth is delayed while failure of eruption may also occur (*Fig.* 29 c). In case of non-eruption the impacted teeth may cause cyst formation.

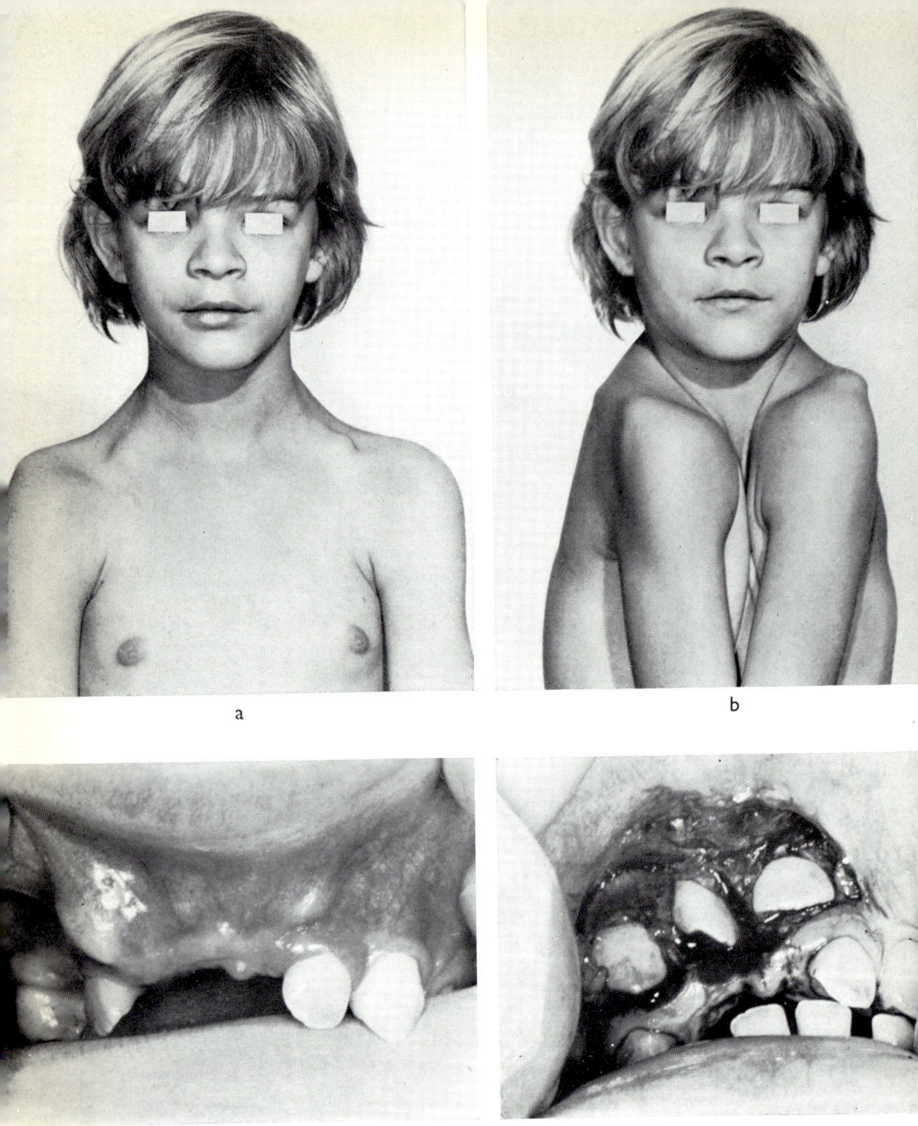

Fig. 29.—a, Cleidocranial dysostosis in a 12-year-old girl. Distinct hypertelorism. b, The shoulders can easily be brought together, because the acromial parts of the clavicles are missing. c, Excessive delayed eruption; the teeth are visible through the mucosa. Many supernumerary teeth. d, The crowns have been exposed to enable orthodontic treatment to be carried out.

Numerous supernumerary teeth may occur, removal of which as early as possible is indicated in order not to disturb the eruption of the permanent teeth too much. When the permanent teeth do not erupt spontaneously, the crowns of these teeth can be exposed, provided with ligatures or orthodontic bands, and regulated into their right position by means of an orthodontic apparatus (*Fig.* 29 d, and *Fig.* 4, p. 15). Cleidocranial dysotosis is also of rare occurrence.

INFLAMMATIONS OF THE JAWS

In general osteomyelitis is more common in the mandible than in the maxilla.

Acute Osteomyelitis.—Acute osteomyelitis is usually caused by exacerbation and extension into the bone of a chronic odontogenic inflammation. Sometimes the odontogenic cause cannot be demonstrated; in such cases a haematogenous spread of infection is assumed.

In babies a very severe acute form of osteomyelitis may occur, especially in the maxilla, with a gross swelling of the soft tissues, and oedema of the lower and upper eyelids, without any apparent cause. Sometimes the picture resembles orbital cellulitis (*Fig.* 30).

There are indications that in some cases the mother's mastitis is responsible for the severe inflammation of the jaw in the baby. Probably the bacteria penetrate via an oral mucosal lesion. It is also possible that the inflammation begins in the maxillary sinus or is connected with tooth eruption.

The correct diagnosis becomes evident when fistulae occur in the buccal sulcus or on the palate or when, after some weeks, sequestration becomes visible on the radiograph (*Fig.* 31).

Treatment (in close co-operation with a paediatrician) consists of immediate administration of very high doses of antibiotics continued for a long period, of incision of the developing abscesses (with culture), and of removal of sequestra as soon as they are visible on the radiograph. With regard to the tooth germs and the uninvolved jaw bone a conservative attitude is indicated. The tooth germs have a high resistance against infection. Aggressive treatment may result in serious disturbances in the dentition and the growth of the involved part of the jaw. Prolonged hospitalization and radiographic control are necessary.

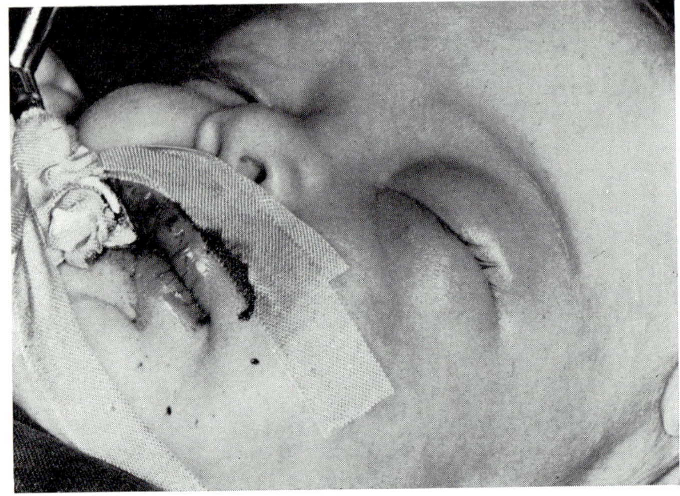

Fig. 30.—Acute osteomyelitis of the maxilla in a baby. Oedema of the left upper and lower eyelids.

In children with a deciduous or a transitional dentition (*Fig.* 32) an odontogenic cause responsible for the osteomyelitis is often found. In these cases, also, the germs of the permanent teeth, lying in the jaw, make removal of sequestra a difficult task. A conservative attitude is indicated. The causal tooth can best be extracted as early as possible, while the infection can be cured by administration of high doses of a (specific) antibiotic.

The prognoses for both types of acute osteomyelitis are generally rather favourable. Often, however, a number of permanent teeth are lost and there may be a slight growth disturbance. If, however,

Fig. 31.—a, Acute osteomyelitis of the left half of the mandible in a 3-month-old baby. The serious acute inflammatory symptoms are depressed by antibiotics. b, Removed sequestra. c, Extensive destruction of the left half of the mandible. Pathological fractures, for instance of the neck of the mandible (k=molar germ; t=tracheal cannula for intratracheal anaesthesia). d, Good healing of the mandible $4\frac{1}{2}$ years after treatment. It is, however, likely that a growth disturbance will occur (k=germ of permanent molar).

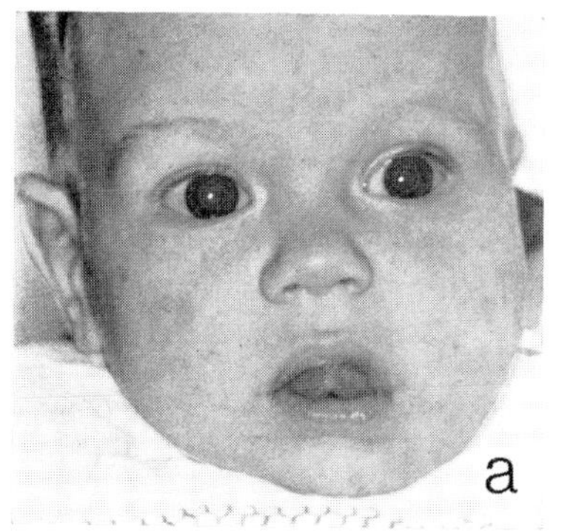
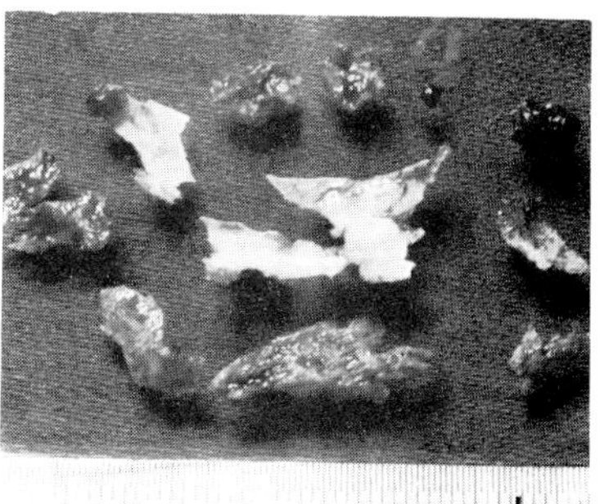
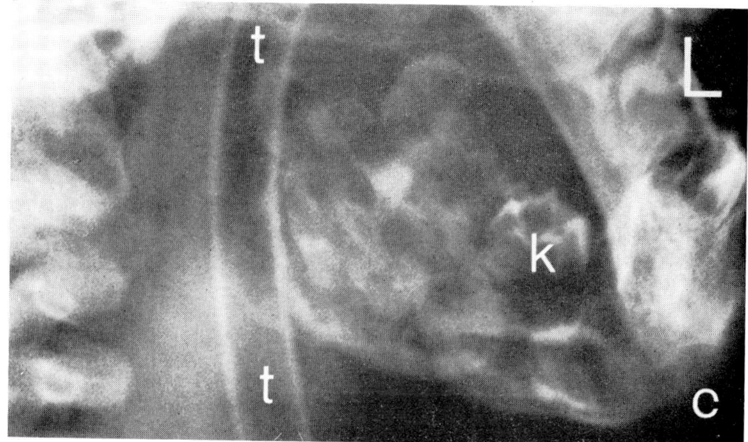
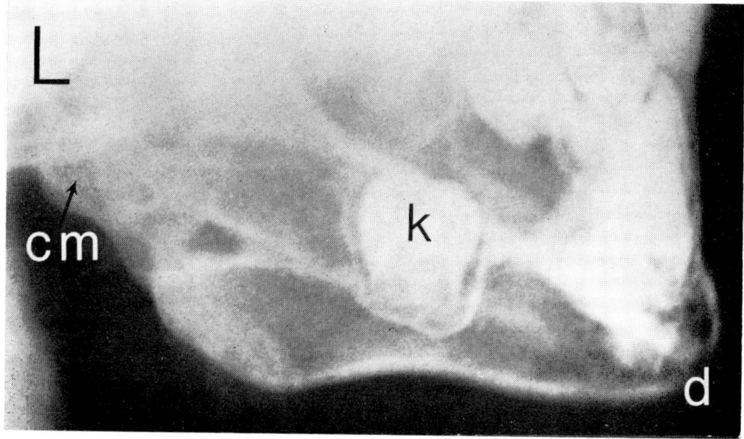

(*Fig.* 31)

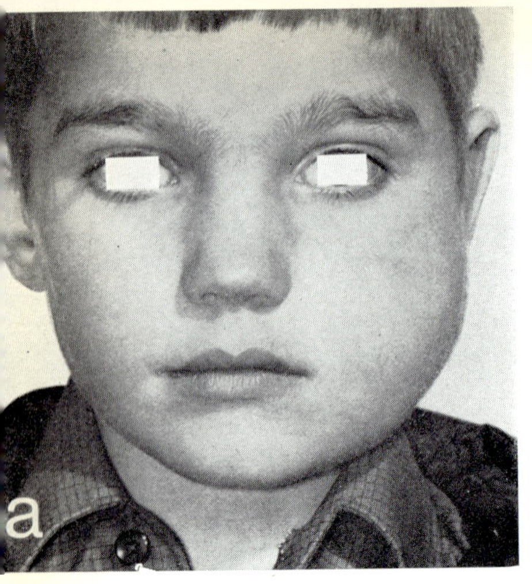
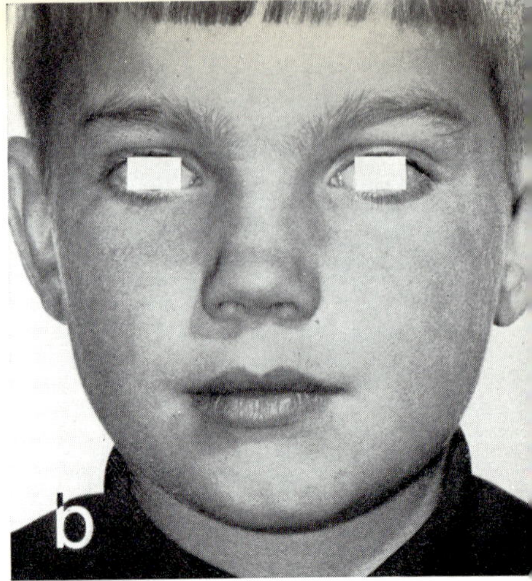

Fig. 32.—a, Acute osteomyelitis of the left part of the mandible in a 6-year-old boy. The acute symptoms have been depressed by a broad-spectrum antibiotic. b, After 1½ years. Complete healing. No growth disturbance. c, The mandibular ascending ramus shows marked sequestra 1 month after the beginning of the inflammation. The head of the mandible seems to be involved too, so that a growth disturbance is to be expected. It is necessary to splint the mandible to prevent spontaneous fractures (k = molar germ; s = sequestrum). d, Good healing of the mandible after 1½ years.

the head of the mandible is involved as well, an ankylosis may occur, resulting in a very serious growth disturbance (*Fig.* 91, p. 113).

Acute osteomyelitis in adults is characterized, apart from the acute inflammatory symptoms, by pain on percussion in many teeth and by the fact that adjacent teeth may come loose. In most cases the cause is odontogenic; a haematogenous cause is rare. Treatment consists of the administration of antibiotics, extraction or endodontic treatment of the causal tooth, and sequestromy. The loose teeth need not be removed and may often be preserved by splinting.

Chronic Osteomyelitis.—Secondary chronic osteomyelitis may remain after the acute type. Periodically, fistulae occur, which may intermittently close again, resulting in many scars on the skin, for instance along the lower border of the mandible. On the

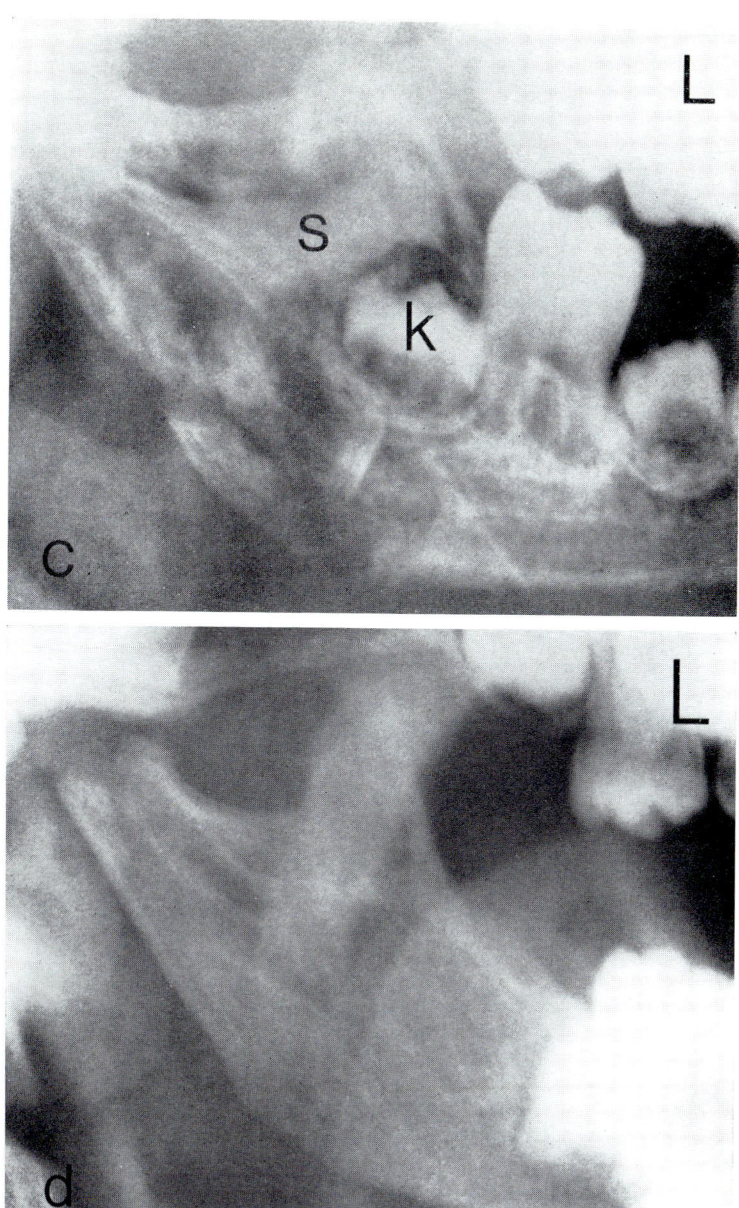

(*Fig.* 32)

radiograph radiolucent foci can be seen and areas of dense bone. Periosteal bone apposition is a common feature.

The affection may last for months or years and both patient and therapist have to exercise much patience.

In general, primary chronic osteomyelitis of the jaw does not cause many clinical symptoms. It is mainly the radiographic picture on which the diagnosis is based. The less extensive form is the localized sclerosing osteomyelitis (condensing osteitis) (*see* p. 177), which is sometimes seen as dense bone at the root of a tooth with chronic pulpitis or a necrotic pulp. Therapy consists of endodontic treatment or extraction of the causal tooth.

In differential diagnosis, other localized bone densities, which are seen in the jaw and are of unknown origin and having no relation to any tooth (enostoses), have to be considered.

Diffuse sclerosing osteomyelitis is a very chronic form also, which is accompanied by very compact bone over a larger area. As a rule symptoms are few; sometimes there may be a gnawing pain.

In older persons a form of osteomyelitis is occasionally seen characterized by a more marked periosteal reaction and more inflammatory symptoms; there may be pain and sometimes anaesthesia or paraesthesia of the mental nerve. Radiographically there is a diffuse, very dense, and fine trabecular bone structure, showing local radiolucencies.

Treatment of the latter two forms is only indicated if there are marked symptoms and exacerbations occur repeatedly. Removal by curette or bur of the pathologically changed area may result in healing.

Taking a biopsy is necessary to verify the diagnosis. Periodical radiographical control is desirable.

Fig. 33.—Osteomyelitis sicca (Garré's osteomyelitis) of the left half of the mandible, starting at the age of 10. a, Acute exacerbation at the age of 11. b, At the age of 17 healing is not yet complete. c, Radiograph of the left half of the mandible at the age of 12. Marked thickening by periosteal bone formation. Fine-meshed bone structure; there are densified areas and areas of greater radiolucency (r). The cortex and mandibular canal can hardly be distinguished. d, At the age of nearly 14 the mandibular contour is almost normal again. The bone structure is still very fine-meshed.

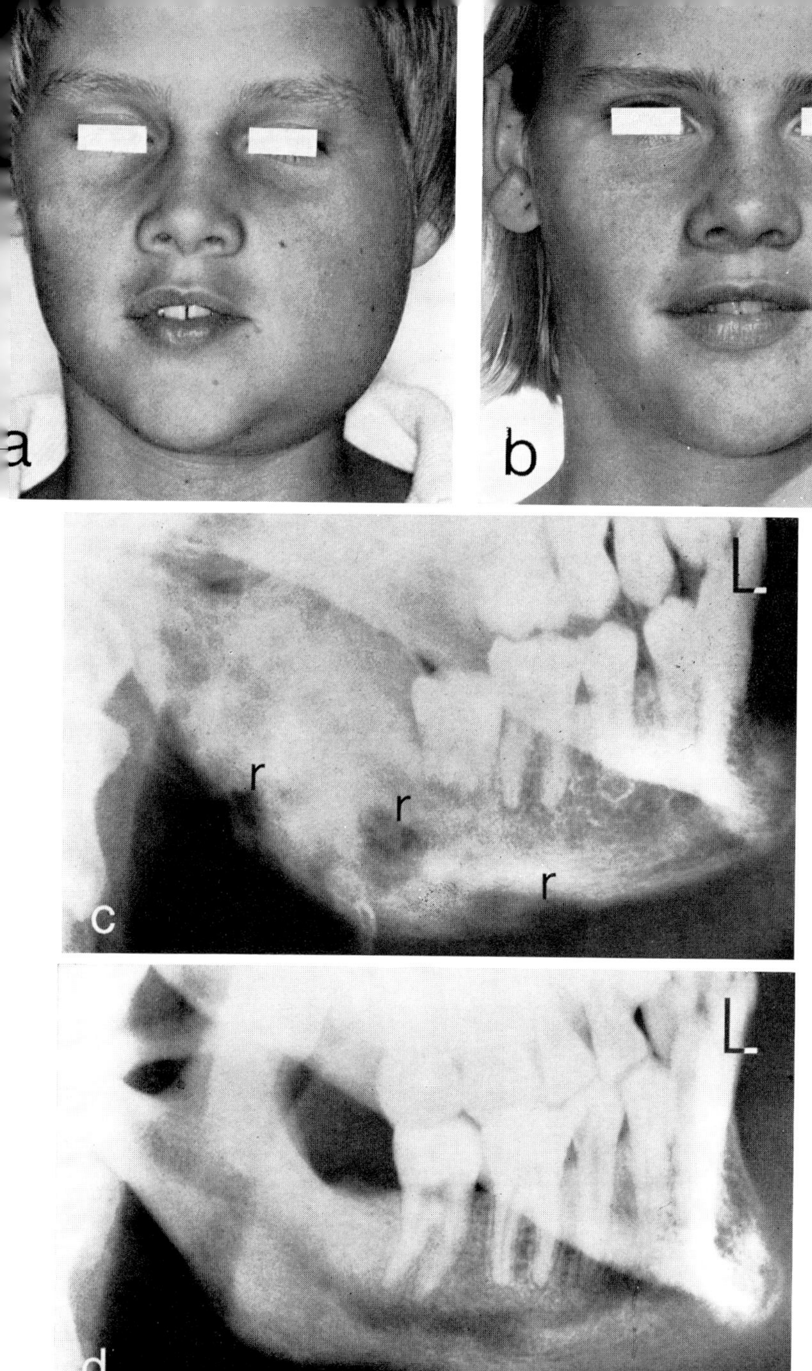

(*Fig.* 33)

Osteomyelitis sicca (Garré's osteomyelitis) is a rare form of a very chronic osteomyelitis, occurring in the mandible, as well as elsewhere in the skeleton, and is characterized by marked periosteal bone apposition and a very fine-meshed bone structure. Periodically, acute exacerbations occur, never resulting in pus formation or distinct sequestration. Its aetiology is unknown, bacteria cannot usually be demonstrated. The process may last for many years. The disease occurs predominantly in children and adolescents (*Fig.* 33).

Little can be done therapeutically. Tetracycline, lincomycine (Lincocin), and irradiation (inflammatory dose) in the acute phase are sometimes recommended. In the long run the prognosis is good. The lesions may heal spontaneously after many years, during which process the jaw regains its original contours.

Osteomyelitis following irradiation is also chronic. Large sequestra may be formed in this process. Reduced vitality or necrosis of bone is primary, so that there is little or no resistance against bacterial infection. The inflammation may originate from exacerbation of a chronic inflammation of a tooth or after tooth extraction in an irradiated area. Fortunately this lesion is very rare at present. It is advisable to treat or extract beforehand all suspect teeth in that part of the jaw which is to be irradiated, in this way preventing an often mutilating osteomyelitis. Irradiation can be started as soon as the epithelium over the extraction wounds has healed.

FRACTURES

Trauma to the Facial Skeleton is of common occurrence owing to modern high-speed traffic. Not only does the number of fractures increase, but also their severity. Respiratory difficulties and lung complications may occur when these patients lie unconscious on their backs for a long time or when they are transported lying on their backs.

If possible, it is advisable to move them lying on their stomachs or on their sides with lowered head (*Fig.* 34). Blood and saliva will then run out of the mouth and not into the respiratory tract. The mouth has to be examined for dentures or fragments of them and for completely dislocated teeth (aspiration danger). In the case of serious fractures tracheostomy, as soon as the patient arrives at the hospital, may be life-saving.

The complexity of the injuries necessitates treatment by a specialized team. The need for an accident centre, where all specialists working in this field are present or can easily be consulted and where the nursing personnel is trained in taking care of these seriously injured patients, makes itself felt more and more. In the case of multiple injuries the director of such a centre will have to decide, after consultation, which treatments are of prime importance to preserve the patient's life and which can be postponed. Afterwards the definitive treatments can be scheduled.

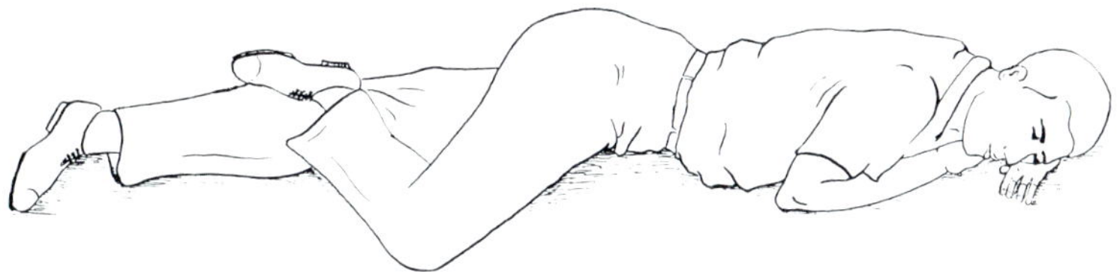

Fig. 34.—Example of a patient with serious facial injuries lying on his side to prevent aspiration.

The simplest fracture of the jaw is that of the *alveolar process*, which is most frequently seen in the front of the maxilla. A group of adjoining teeth can be moved in combination with the attached alveolar process. On the dental radiograph a fracture line is usually visible. Treatment consists of repositioning and immobilization of the detached alveolar process by means of a wire splint fixed to the remaining teeth (*Fig.* 35).

Mandible.—Fractures of the mandible can be classed according to their location (body of the mandible, ascending ramus, the neck, and the head). The dislocation depends on the direction and intensity of the trauma and on muscular forces. The overlying soft tissues are swollen over the fracture site at the place of the fracture. A haematoma is visible subcutaneously and in the buccal sulcus. The fracture is usually not very painful.

In cases of fracture of the *body of the mandible* a step can often be palpated in the lower mandibular border and in the buccal sulcus, while there is an interruption in the dental arch (*Fig.* 36). If the fracture line lies between the foramen mandibulae and the mental foramen, the lower lip is unilaterally numb (disturbance of the inferior alveolar nerve).

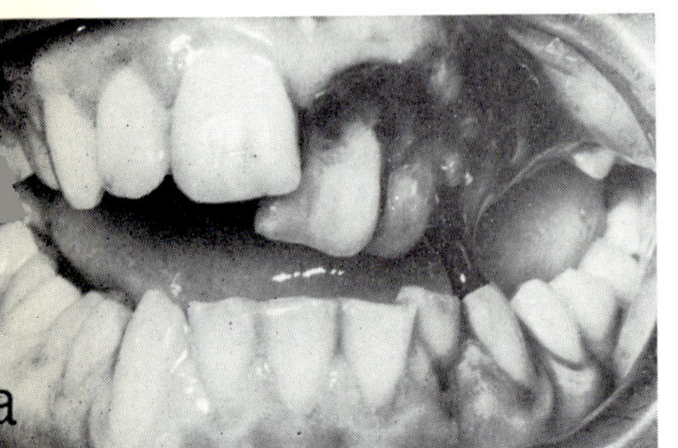
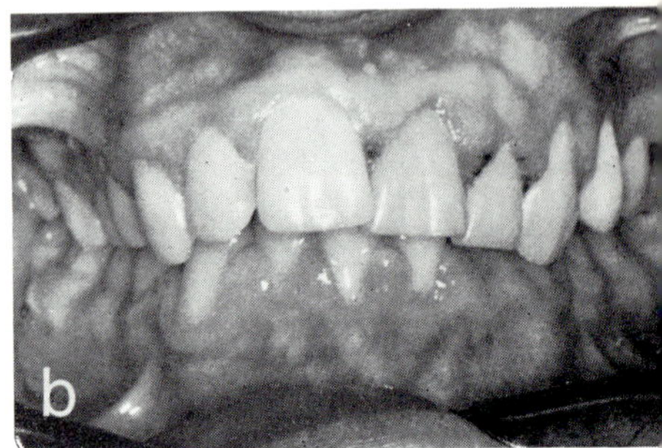

Fig. 35.—a, Fracture of the alveolar process. b, After treatment by means of a metal arch bar.

A fracture in the midline can be detected by exercising pressure on mandibular angles. The result is an elastic mobility and pain in the frontal part of the mandible.

In cases of *bilateral mandibular fracture* in the mental area, the chin may be displaced in a dorsal direction if the fracture line runs unfavourably, thus causing glossoptosis, resulting in respiratory difficulties (*Fig.* 37). Immediate treatment of these fractures is

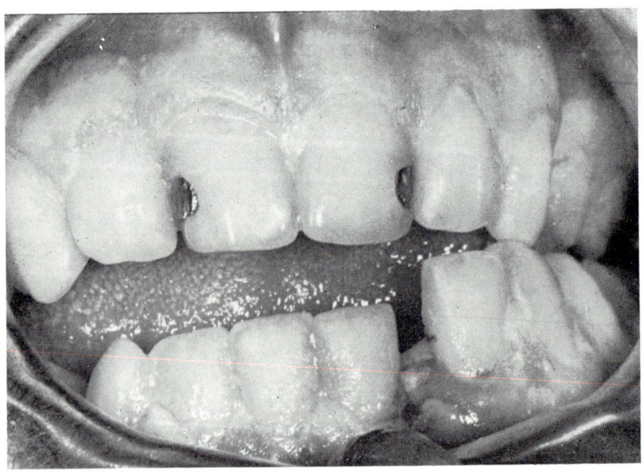

Fig. 36.—Interruption of the dental arch and malocclusion owing to a mandibular fracture in the region of the lower left incisor teeth.

necessary. Utmost care is required with regard to local anaesthesia in the floor of the mouth because there is an increased chance of suffocation due to decreased muscle control.

A fracture of the *neck of the mandible* is caused by a fall or a blow on the chin. There is a deviation of the point of the chin towards the diseased side. There is pain and a swelling anterior to the ear. On palpation, an empty fossa is felt just anterior to the ear. When the mandible is moved, there is no movement in the affected temporomandibular joint area (finger in the external acoustic duct) (*Fig.* 38 b). There is an occlusal disturbance in the dentition; on the contralateral side the teeth of the lower and upper jaws do not contact (open bite), owing to displacement of the lower dental arch towards the affected side (*Fig.* 38 a). Movements towards the affected side are limited owing to disturbed function of the lateral pterygoid muscle, which is inserted into the head and neck of the mandible.

In the case of a *bilateral fracture of the neck of the mandible* (parade-ground fracture) the local symptoms are bilateral, the chin lies back and the teeth cannot be brought in occlusion (frontal open bite). Sometimes there is haemorrhage from the ear, when the head of the mandible is displaced by the blow so far dorsally that the frontal wall of the external auditory meatus is torn also, in which case the picture resembles a basal fracture of the cranium. In very rare cases the head of the mandible penetrates the roof of the mandibular fossa into the middle cranial fossa.

An *intra-articular fracture of the head of the mandible* (rare) may cause ankylosis after organization of the fracture haematoma. In children this ankylosis may be followed by a serious growth disturbance (asymmetrical face in case of a unilateral fracture and a bird-face if the fracture is bilateral).

The most common radiographs for the diagnosis of mandibular fractures are the occlusal radiographs, the lateral oblique projection of the mandible (*Fig.* 37 b and c), and the infracranial contact radiograph (Parma) (*Fig.* 83, p. 104).

Treatment of fractures in the tooth-bearing part of the jaw consists of ligating a stainless-steel splint with small hooks to the teeth after reduction of the fracture. By ligating a similar arch in the upper jaw immobilization in the correct occlusion by the use of intermaxillary stainless-steel wires is possible (*Fig.* 39). Of primary importance is the restoration of a good occlusion of the dentition.

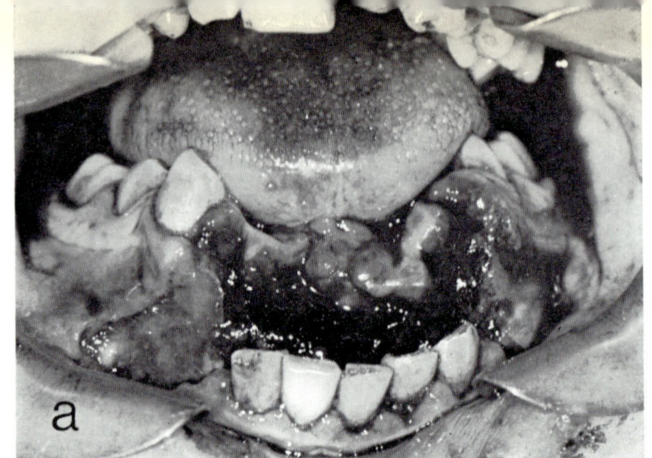

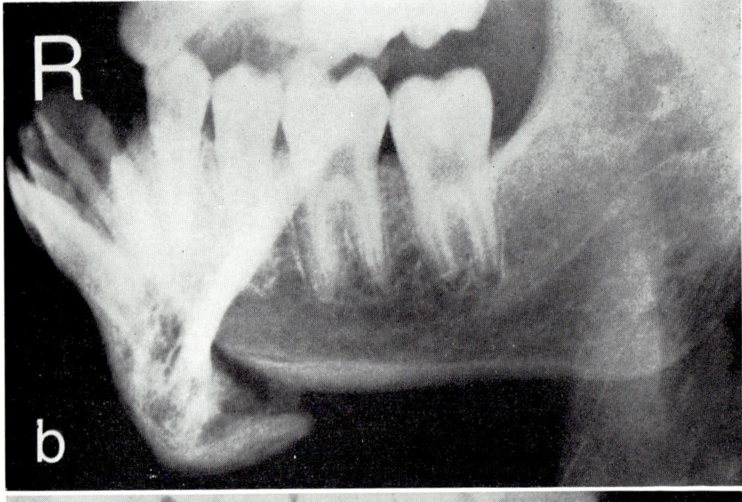

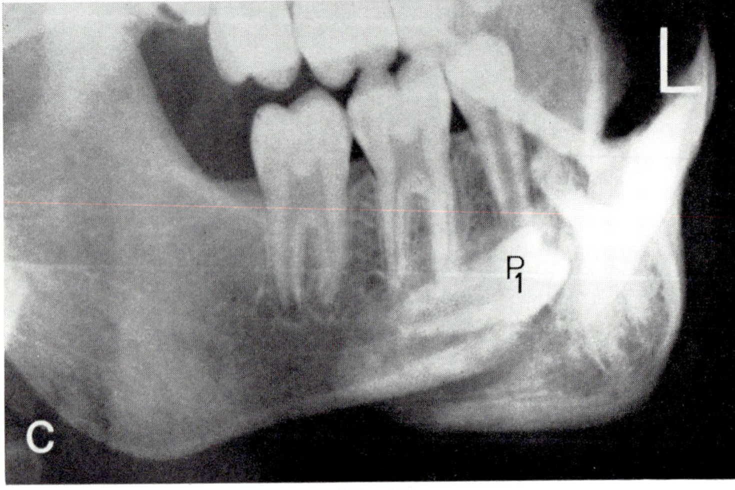

(*Fig.* 37)

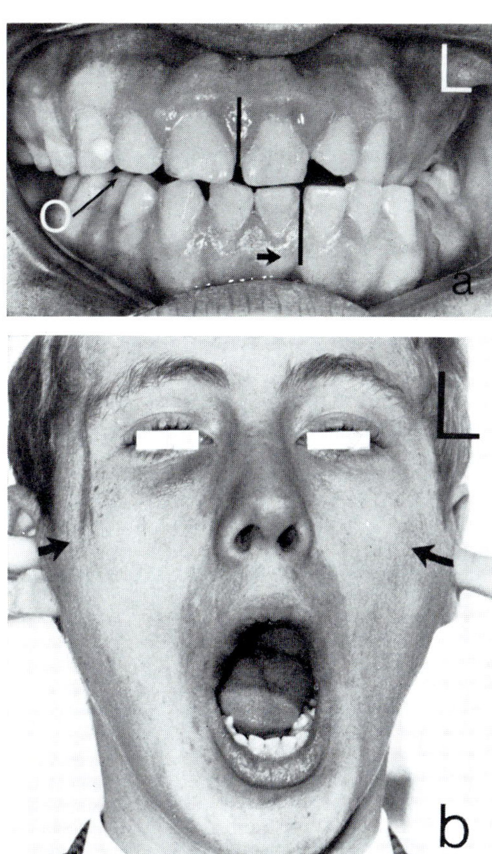

Fig. 38.—a, Occlusal disturbance due to a fracture of the neck of the left mandible. Marked deviation of the mandible towards the affected side (arrow). Open bite (o) on the contralateral side. b, Fracture of the neck of the left mandible. When opening the mouth there is a deviation towards the fractured side. The head of the mandible cannot be palpated in the external acoustic duct, not even when moving the mandible.

Fig. 37.—a, Bilateral mandibular fracture; owing to the musculature of the floor of the mouth the frontal part has swung down. b, c, The radiographs give a good impression of the extreme dislocation. The lower left first premolar (P_1) is wedged into the adjacent soft tissues. Treatment consisted of osteosyntheses on either side in the lower mandibular border, metal splints fixed to lower and upper dentition, and intermaxillary fixation.

During this 6 weeks' immobilization the patient is dependent on liquid or semi-solid food. It is difficult to keep the mouth in a good hygienic condition, but this is of major importance (use an electric toothbrush).

In the case of *fractures of an edentulous jaw* or in an edentulous part of the jaw with marked dislocation a stable osteosynthesis with stainless-steel wire is necessary or, if the edentulous jaw is very thin, with a metal plate with screws. Moreover, intermaxillary fixation is sometimes also necessary. In completely edentulous patients this can be done by means of dentures or acrylic splints (Gunning's splints) wired to the jaws (*Fig.* 40). The lower denture is fixed by means of perimandibular wires. Fixation of the upper denture can be obtained by means of extra-oral extensions to a plaster-of-Paris headcap (*Fig.* 48, p. 68), by means of peralveolar wires (wires through the alveolar process), or by suspension to the zygomatic arch.

In the case of a *fracture of the neck of the mandible*, immediate mobilization aimed at a good occlusion is the most simple form of treatment; sometimes elastic traction is helpful (bilateral cases) (*Fig.* 39). This is a functional treatment. In children very early movement of the joint is necessary; adapted movement exercises are prescribed to prevent ankylosis and growth disturbances. Anatomical reposition by means of open reduction is indicated when the bone fragments have lost contact (*Fig.* 41).

When the general condition of the patient does not permit immediate treatment of a mandibular fracture, repositioning may be postponed for maximally 1 week, except when the fracture is open towards the skin.

Administration of antibiotics is advisable when the fracture is open to the oral cavity. In most cases it is not necessary to remove a tooth standing in the fracture fissure.

Maxilla.—The simplest fracture of the maxilla is a *low-level horizontal fracture* (*Fig.* 42), just above the floor of the maxillary sinus and the floor of the nose (Le Fort type I fracture). The whole maxilla is movable in relation to the rest of the skull if the maxilla is held by the frontal teeth. A haematoma is visible in the buccal sulcus. In the region of the first permanent molars a step can be felt in the zygomatic process. Sometimes the upper jaw is displaced dorsally by the blow (no displacement by muscular action), causing

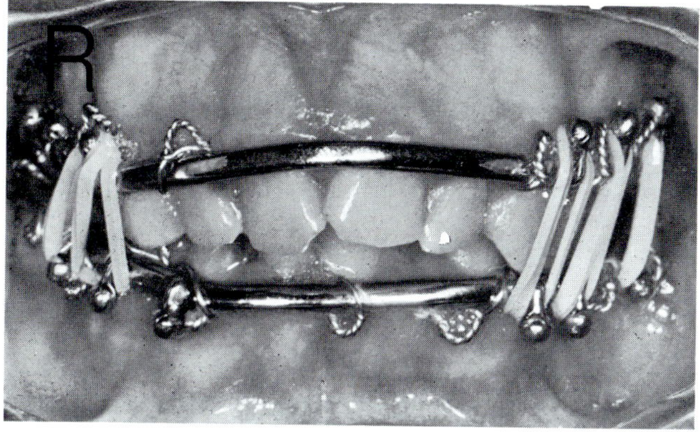

Fig. 39.—Metal arch bar with extensions (Jelenko's splint) and inter-maxillary elastics in treating a fracture of the neck of the right mandible. Direction of traction is opposite to the tendency of the mandible to deviate to the right.

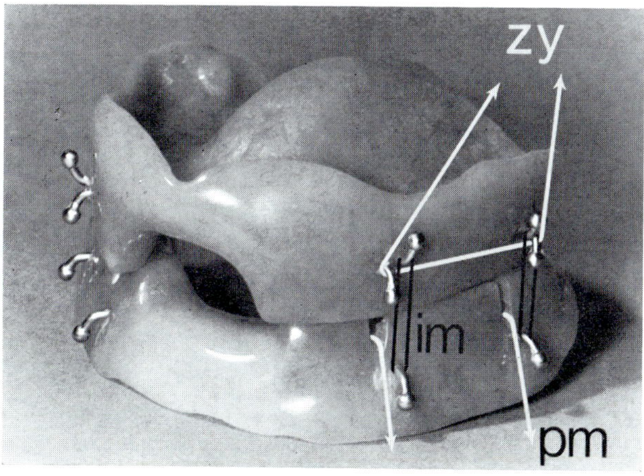

Fig. 40.—Lower and upper acrylic splints (Gunning's splints), fixed by means of stainless-steel wires to lower and upper jaw (pm=perimandibular wire; zy=perizygomatic wire). By providing the extensions with inter-maxillary ligatures (im) good fixation is obtained. The opening in the front between the splints permits the ingestion of food.

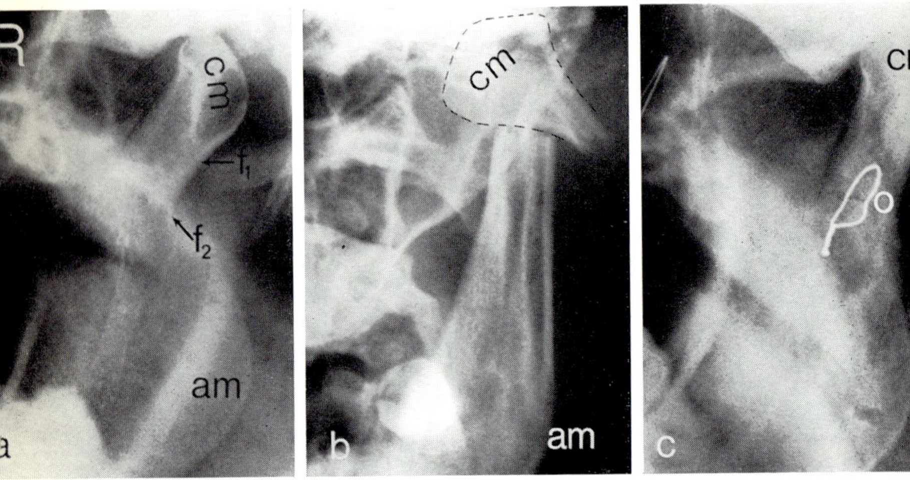

Fig. 41.—a, Lateral contact radiograph (Parma) of a low-level fracture of the neck of the mandible. The fracture ends (f_1 and f_2) seem to lie next to each other (cm=head of mandible; am=angle of mandible). b, Antero-posterior projection of the same fracture. The head of the mandible is strongly tilted medially. There is no contact between the fracture ends. c, Via an incision under and behind the mandibular angle an osteosynthesis (o) was performed by means of stainless-steel wire.

an anterior open bite (*Fig.* 47 a). When the upper jaw is very loose and is floating on the tongue, respiratory difficulties may occur, the more so if the nasal airway is obliterated by a coagulum following epistaxis.

Generally, fractures are far more complicated. The whole facial skeleton may be detached from the rest of the skull, for instance in the case of a pyramidal fracture of upper jaw and nose area and especially in the case of a high-level horizontal fracture through both orbits (*Fig.* 42).

In both types, which seldom occur in pure form, there is an oedematous swelling of the facial soft tissues, and unilateral or bilateral circumorbital and subconjunctival ecchymoses (*Fig.* 43). Serious injuries of soft tissues occur (*Fig.* 45 a), but in most cases they are strikingly few and bear no relation to the extensive destructions of the skeleton (*Figs.* 43 and 44). There is nasal bleeding, while

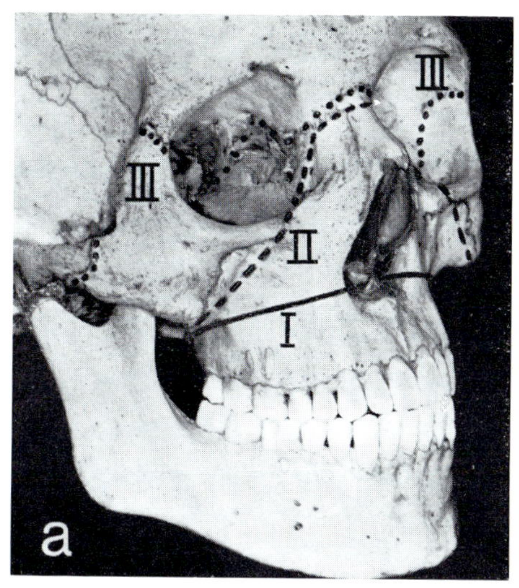

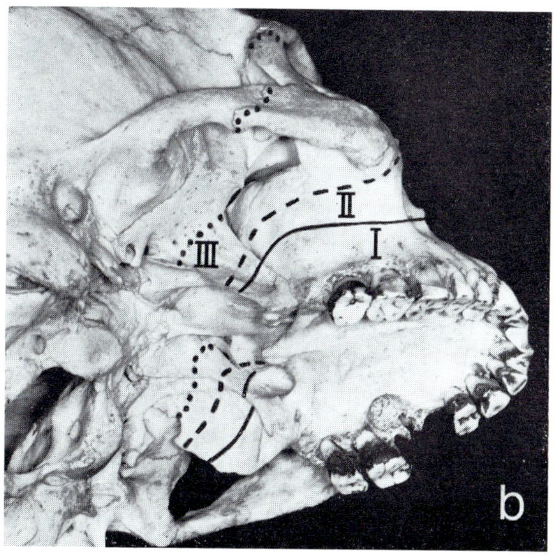

Fig. 42.—a, b, Classification of fractures of the facial skeleton according to Le Fort. The fracture lines extend through the weakest places of the facial skeleton. Le Fort type I: low-level horizontal fracture just above the palate; Le Fort type II: pyramidal fracture having its top in the nasal bones; Le Fort type III: high-level fracture through the orbits. Both figures show clearly where in the skeleton the different fractures can be palpated.

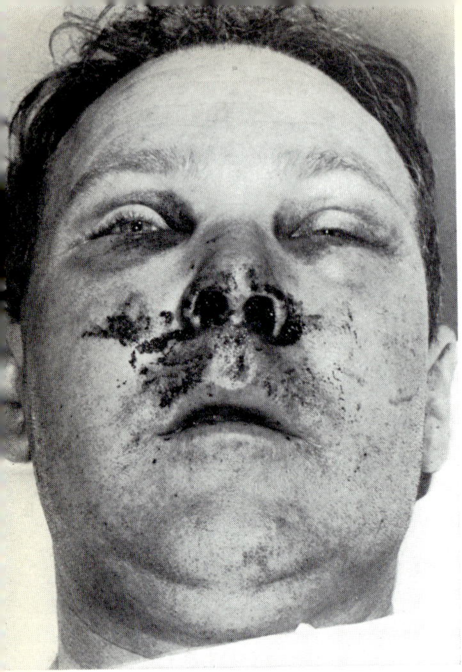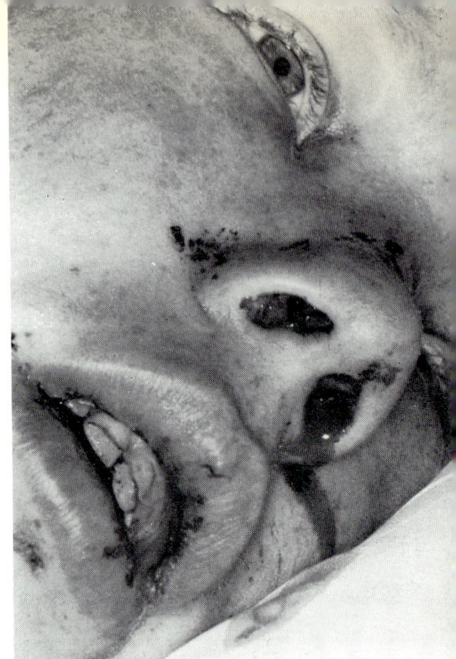

Fig. 43   Fig. 44

Fig. 43.—Le Fort type II fracture in a 35-year-old man 1 day after trauma. Oedematous swelling of the face, bilateral circumorbital haematoma, swollen bridge of the nose, haemorrhage from both nostrils, bilateral subconjunctival bleeding, and disturbance of both infra-orbital nerves.

Fig. 44.—Cerebrospinal rhinorrhoea in a patient with a high-level facial fracture. After the nasal haemorrhage has stopped the liquor is still running. Treatment by team of specialists.

sometimes leakage of cerebrospinal fluid is encountered (fracture of the cribriform plate of the ethmoid bone) (*Fig.* 44).

In the case of a *pyramidal fracture* (Le Fort type II) (*Fig.* 42) steps can be felt on either side in the infra-orbital margin laterally of the infra-orbital foramen. Often there is anaesthesia of the infra-orbital nerves. In the oral cavity the crista zygomatico-alveolare shows an interruption in the buccal sulcus in the upper first molar region. The upper jaw is often displaced dorsally (dish-face), thus causing occlusal disturbance. When holding the upper jaw by the frontal teeth, the bridge of the nose and the medial part of the orbits can be moved.

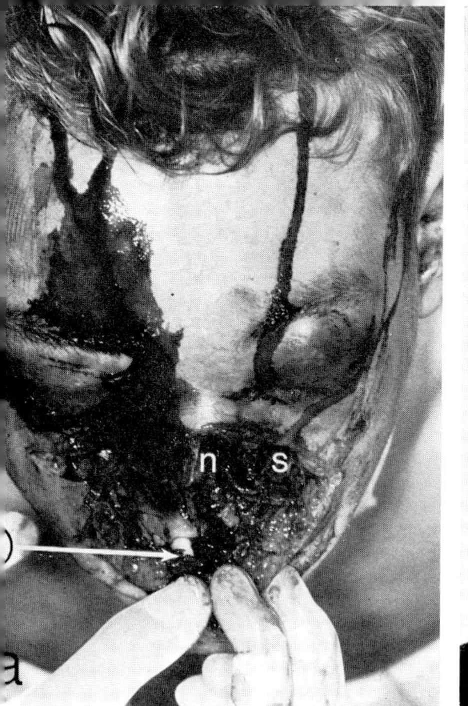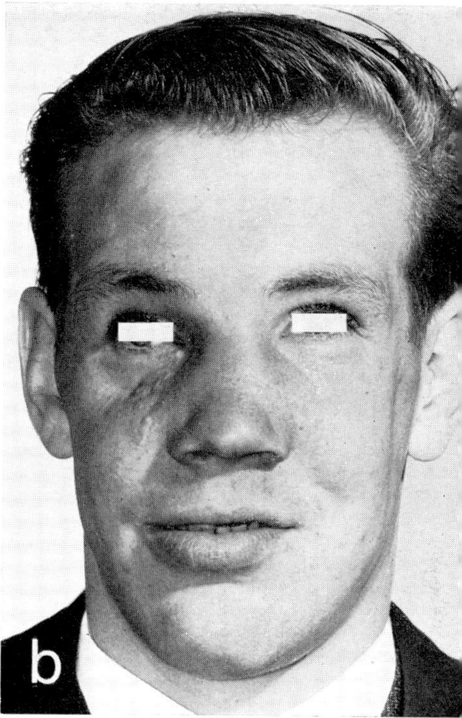

Fig. 45.—a, Multiple maxillofacial fractures (resembling Le Fort types I, II, and III). Comminuted fractures of left and right zygomas, inclusive of the orbital floor. Complicated mandibular fracture at the level of the lower left second premolar and first molar. Fracture of the frontal bone. Nasal fracture. Extensive lesions of the soft tissues. Almost the whole nose and surrounding soft tissues are torn off (n = nasal skeleton; s = maxillary sinus; t = upper incisor; the nasal part of the face is swung down). Treatment by team of specialists. b, About 1 year later.

In the case of a *high-level horizontal fracture* (Le Fort type III fracture) (*Fig.* 42) steps can be felt on either side in the lateral and medial angles of the eye. The face is grossly swollen and may appear elongated when the upper jaw is lowered. Blood is leaking from the nose and there is a bilateral circumorbital haematoma. The occlusion of the dentition is disturbed. Visual disturbances may occur when the floor of the orbit has dropped.

The *most appropriate radiographs* are the occipitomental projection (according to Water, Lilienfeld) and the lateral projection (*Figs.* 46, 47, and 52). Treatment of maxillary fractures consists of

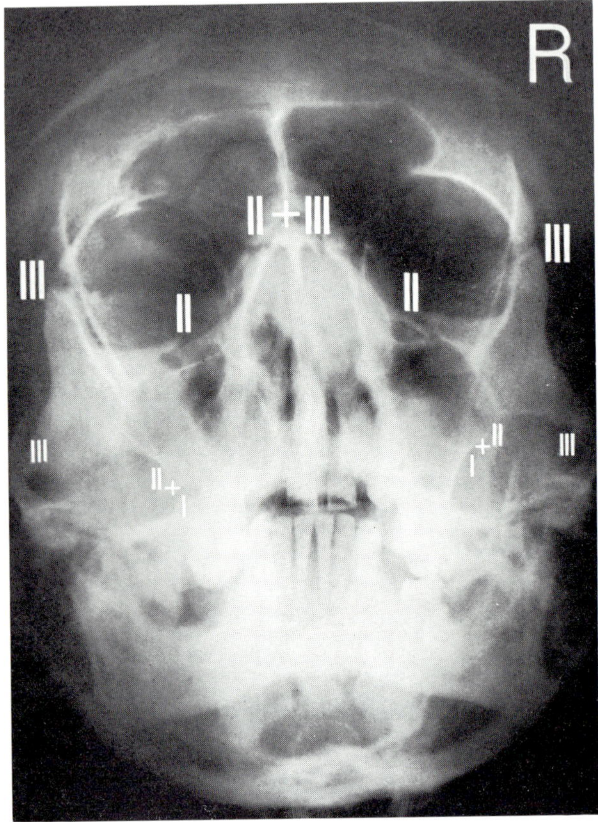

Fig. 46.—Occipitomental projection with multiple fractures of the middle third of the face. The Roman numerals indicate where Le Fort types of fractures are visible or may be expected (*see also Figs.* 52 and 53).

repositioning and fixation of the maxillary bloc against the rest of the skull. This can be done by means of extra-oral extensions on the dentition, which are fixed by means of rods and screws to a plaster-of-Paris head-cap (*Fig.* 48). At present generally internal fixation is applied by suspending the detached jaw by means of stainless-steel ligatures on the zygomatic arch or on the skull in the lateral angle of the eye (*Fig.* 49). As the occlusion of the dentition

66

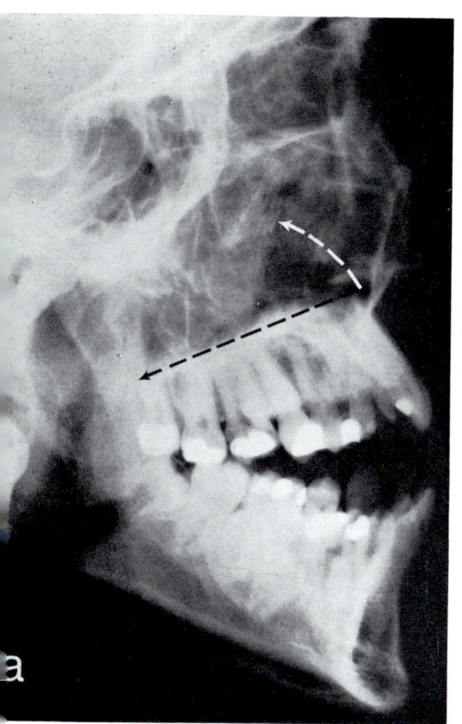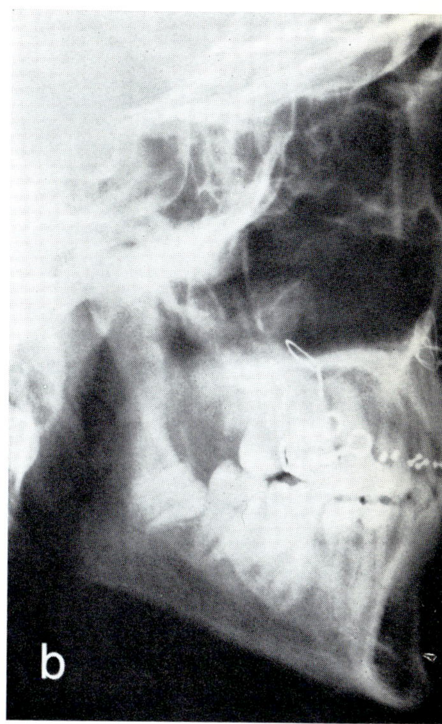

Fig. 47.—a, Lateral view showing clearly the dislocation of the upper jaw cranially and dorsally. b, After treatment. It can be seen from the corrected normal relation of the lower and upper last molars how far the upper jaw in a was dislocated dorsally.

is of guidance, intermaxillary fixation is also necessary in these cases. In extensive comminuted facial fractures and for reduction of orbital fractures many osteosyntheses are sometimes necessary. The extensive injuries caused by modern traffic make teamwork necessary (*Fig.* 45). The order of treatment has to be arranged by mutual agreement. In general it is advisable to restore the skeleton first, before the soft-tissue wounds are closed.

The cerebrospinal fluid rhinorrhoea in high-level facial fractures can be stopped in the majority of cases by careful repositioning and good immobilization of the maxillary complex.

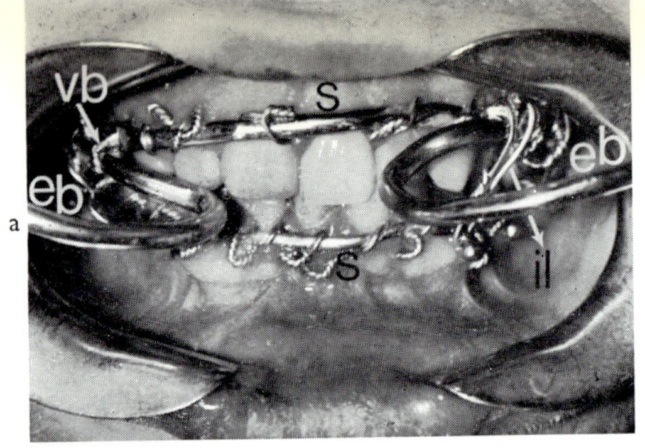

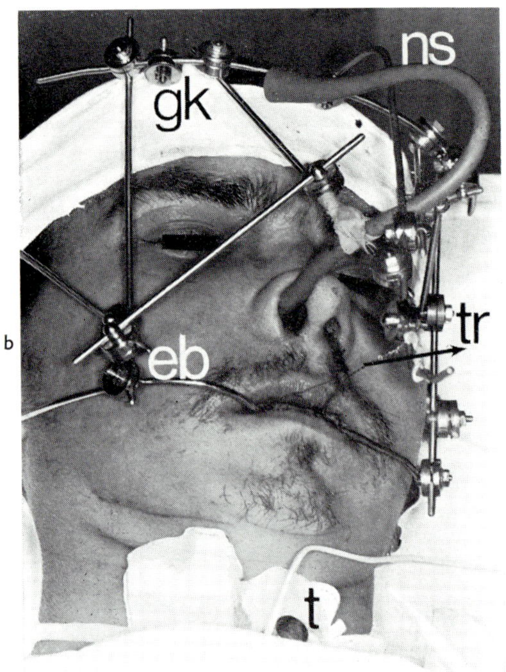

Fig. 48.—a, Intra-oral apparatus for the fixation of a maxillary fracture. Stainless-steel bars (s) provided with extensions are ligated to lower and upper dentition. Around these extensions intermaxillary wires (il) are ligated in order to fix lower and upper jaw in good occlusion. On either side extra-orally the upper splint is provided with small square tubes (vb) in which the square ends of the extra-oral frame (eb) are fitted. b, Extra-oral apparatus for the fixation of a maxillary fracture. By means of an extra-oral frame (eb) fixed to the dentition, the whole mandibulomaxillary bloc is suspended from a plaster-of-Paris head-cap (gk) by means of rods and screws. By means of traction wire (tr) it is possible to keep the maxilla in a somewhat anterior position. A catheter is introduced into the nose (ns) and tracheostomy (t) was done.

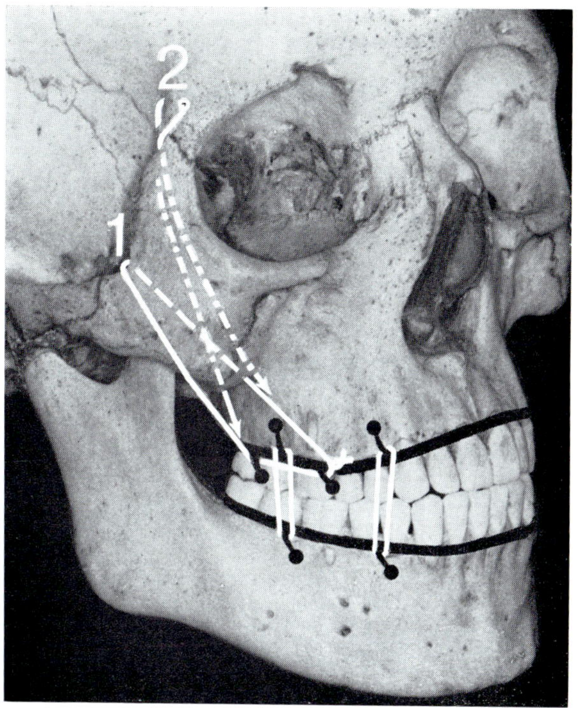

Fig. 49.—Methods of internal fixation for fractures of the maxillary complex. 1. By means of a perizygomatic wire left and right a Le Fort I or Le Fort II fracture can be fixed to the rest of the skull, provided the malar bone has remained intact. 2. In higher level fractures (Le Fort III) a craniomaxillary wire from the lateral corner of the eye may be used. It is sometimes advised to fix the wires 1 and 2 to the maxillary splint; a disadvantage, however, is that for instance for inspection the intermaxillary fixation cannot be loosened without removing the suspension of the maxilla.

For edentulous patients *see also* Fig. 40.

Postponement of treatment in connexion with the patient's general condition for 5 or 7 days at the most is possible provided the fractures are not open to the skin.

Malar Bone.—We have the impression that fractures of the zygomatic bone and the zygomatic arch are often overlooked. A flattening or depression of the prominence of the cheek after a lateral trauma (masked for some time by swelling of the soft tissues),

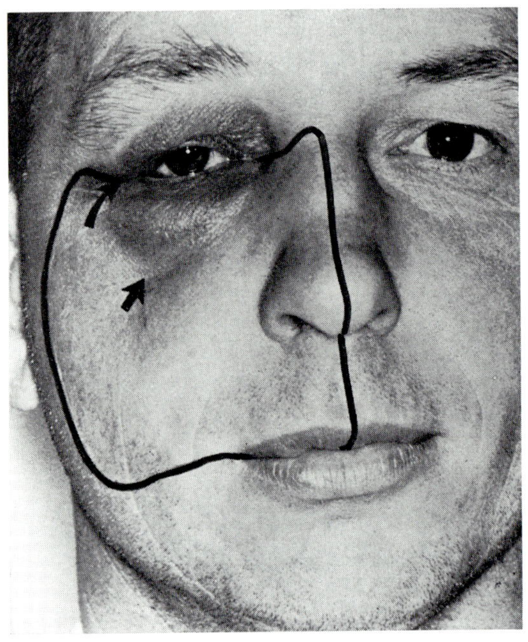

Fig. 50.—Fracture of the right zygomatic bone 8 days after trauma. After reduction of the oedema the impression is clearly visible. Interruptions of the orbital rim are indicated by arrows. Unilateral circumorbital haematoma and subconjunctival haemorrhage. Anaesthesia of the cheek (continuous line) owing to a disturbance of the infra-orbital nerve.

a black eye, a step in the lateral wall of the orbit, and an interruption in the infra-orbital margin characterize a fracture of the malar bone (*Figs*. 50 and 51). Usually there is haemorrhage from one naris.

Anaesthesia or paraesthesia of the infra-orbital nerve is almost always present. Diplopia may occur due to a haematoma in the orbit or a subsidence of the orbital floor. A muscle of the eye, impacted in the fracture fissure, will cause limitation of movement of the eyeball.

Following trauma to the eyeball orbital pressure will be very high for a very short period, resulting in a fracture of the orbital floor in the direction of the maxillary sinus, while the orbital rim may

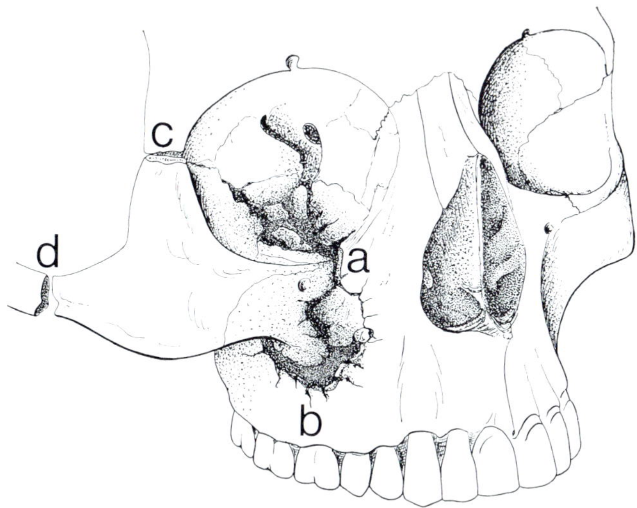

Fig. 51.—Schematic presentation of a zygoma fracture. Comminution of the lateral antral wall and orbital floor is often seen. The fracture is palpable most easily at a and b, whereas sometimes an interruption can be palpated in the c and d regions.

remain intact (orbital 'blow-out' syndrome). This type of fracture can only be recognized by means of tomograms.

Often the mandibular opening movements are impeded because, when opening the mouth, the coronoid process is obstructed by the dorsal side of the displaced malar bone. Intra-oral palpation is painful and there is a step defect in the upper first molar region.

In the case of a *zygomatic arch fracture* there is an obvious depression immediately after the trauma (*Fig.* 54). This depression, however, is masked within a short time owing to post-traumatic

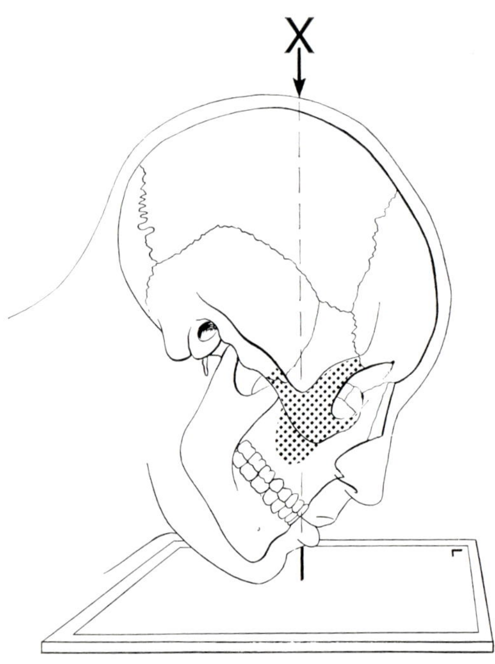

Fig. 52.—The occipitomental projection (Lilienfeld, Water) for the diagnosis of fractures of the maxillary complex (*Fig*. 46) and of the zygoma complex (shaded).

oedema. This fracture may also cause restricted mandibular movements.

The most appropriate radiographs for the diagnosis of fractures of the zygomatic complex are the occipitomental projection (*Figs*. 52, 53) and the submentovertical projection (head tilted backwards as far as possible—plate vertically behind the head—cone under the chin) (*Figs*. 55 and 56 a).

Treatment of malar bone fractures consists of repositioning and supporting the dislocated orbital floor by means of a pack in the maxillary sinus (10 days in situ). In the case of dislocation in the lateral angle of the eye an osteosynthesis on this spot is necessary. Early recognition and treatment of these fractures are of major importance, because only then will undisturbed healing

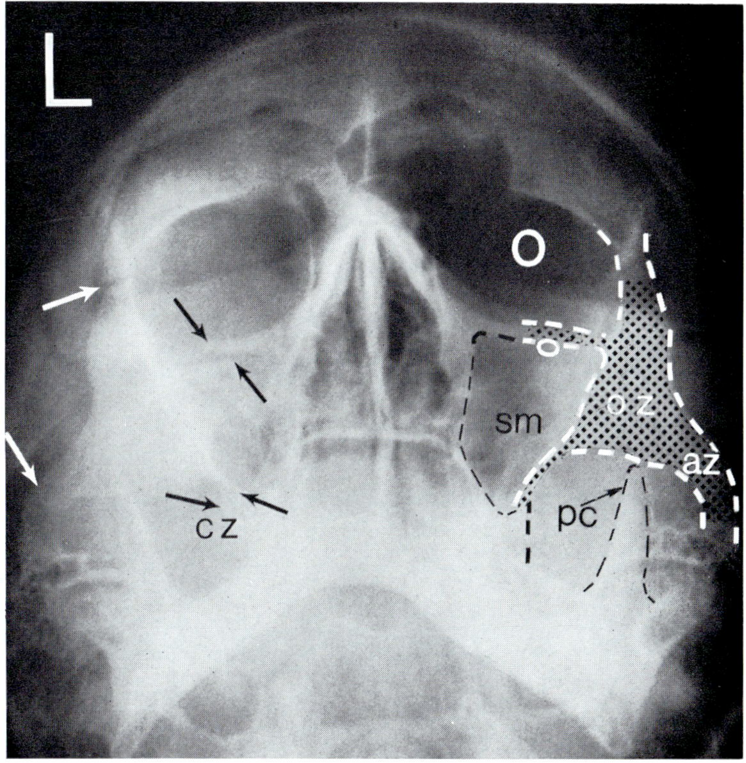

Fig. 53.—Occipitomental projection of left cheekbone fracture. Diffuse fading of the left maxillary sinus (haematoma). Fracture positions are indicated by arrows (infra-orbital margin; crista zygomatico-alveolaris (cz), zygomatic arch and lateral orbital rim) (sm=maxillary sinus; oz= zygomatic bone; az=zygomatic arch; pc=coronoid process of the mandible; o=orbit).

follow. Making corrections later on, because of diplopia or restricted mandibular movements, is extremely difficult.

A fracture of the zygomatic arch may sometimes be repositioned by direct extra-oral elevation of the depressed arch by a sharp, curved hook. In most cases repositioning of the arch fracture will be effected with an elevator via an incision in the buccal sulcus

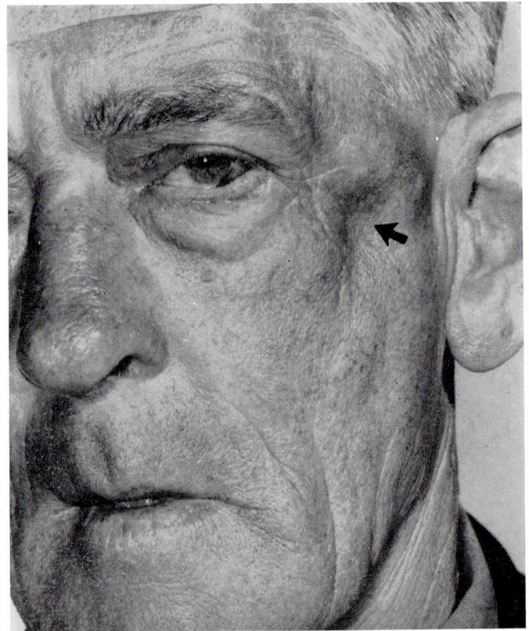

Fig. 54.—Depressed fracture of the left zygomatic arch.

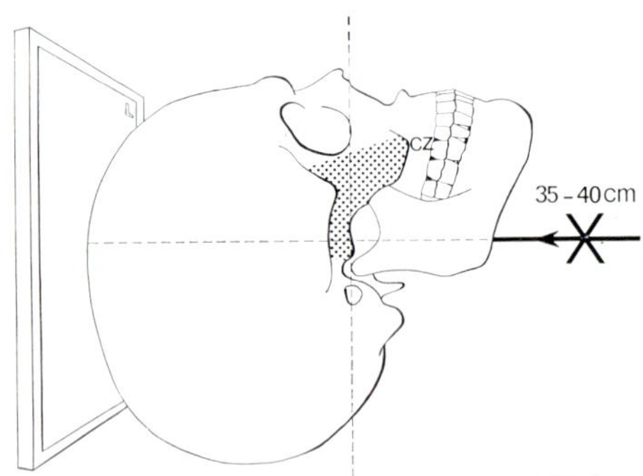

Fig. 55.—Submentovertical projection. The outlines of left and right arch are projected free from the skull. Chin–cone distance = 35–40 cm. The farther the head is tilted backwards the easier the projection (cz = crista zygomatico-alveolaris).

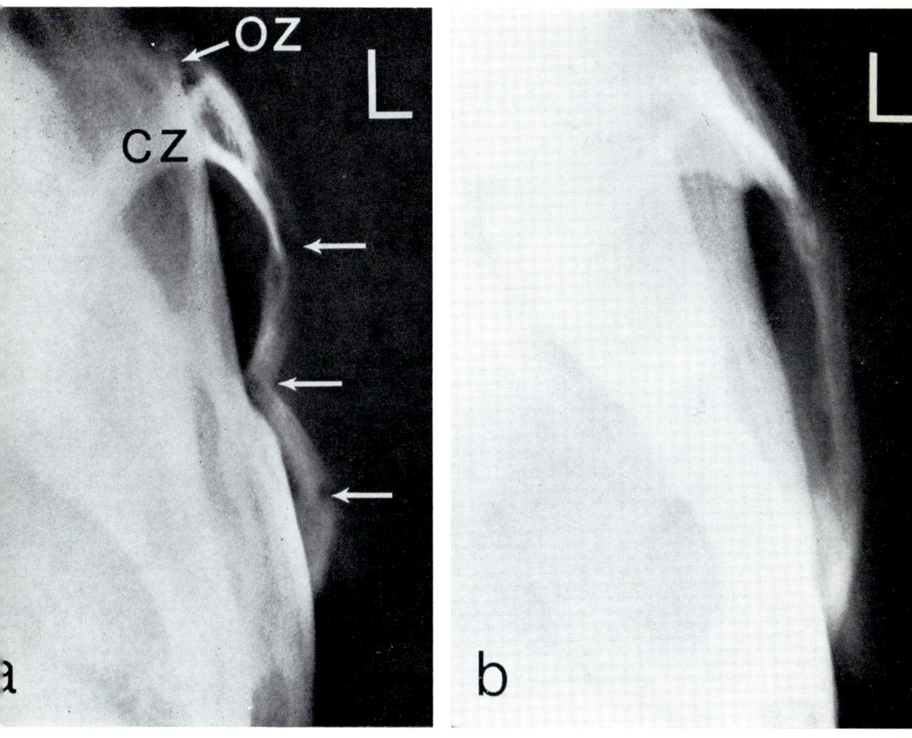

Fig. 56.—a, Part of the submentovertical projection (*Fig.* 55) with a characteristic M-shaped fracture of the left arch (fracture lines indicated by arrows) (oz=zygomatic bone; cz=crista zygomatica). The mouth could be opened only 1·5 cm. b, Reposition of the fracture ends. The mouth could be opened normally 3 weeks later.

dorsally of the zygomatic process. Fixation is seldom required (*Fig.* 56 b).

CYSTS OF THE JAWS

A differentiation can be made between odontogenic and non-odontogenic cysts. The first group includes, amongst others, radicular and follicular cysts and the latter, for instance, fissural cysts. All jaw cysts are lined by epithelium, except some very rare types (aneurysmal bone cyst and traumatic cyst). Clinically, jaw cysts are characterized by a slowly growing swelling of the jaw. At first this thickening is bony hard; if the bony wall becomes thinner crepitation occurs (table tennis ball effect); finally a crater can be felt, in which fluctuation can be elicited. The radiograph shows a clearly demarcated area of radiolucency. The development of a large cyst may take some years. Because these cysts are not painful, if they are not infected, the patient often seeks treatment only at a very late stage.

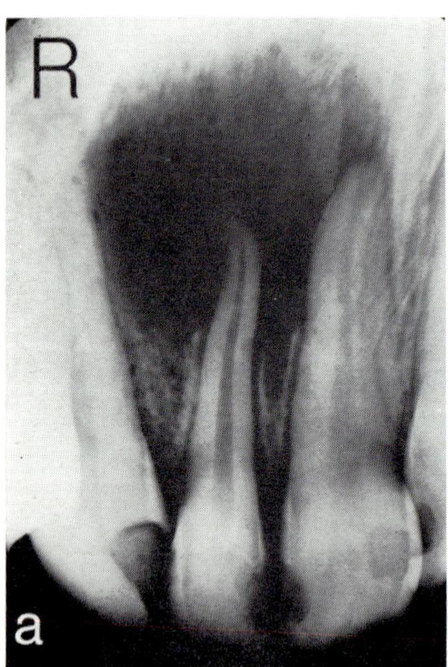
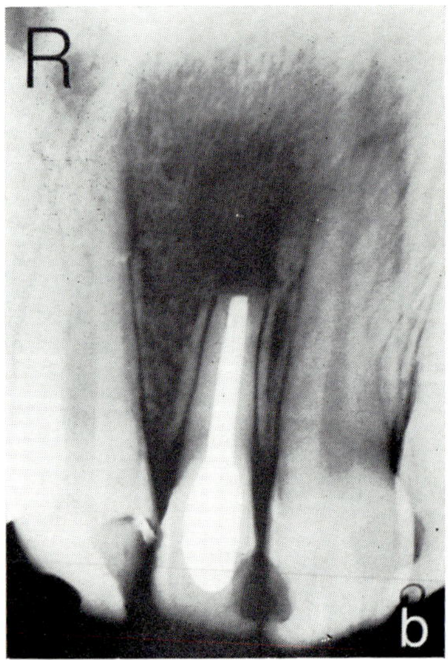

Fig. 57.—a, Radicular cyst of upper left lateral incisor. Pulp is presumably non-vital owing to dental caries. Clinical features: oedematous swelling of the cheek caused by secondary infection. b, Six months after cyst operation and apicectomy good bone healing is visible. The root canal is filled by a radio-opaque gutta-percha point.

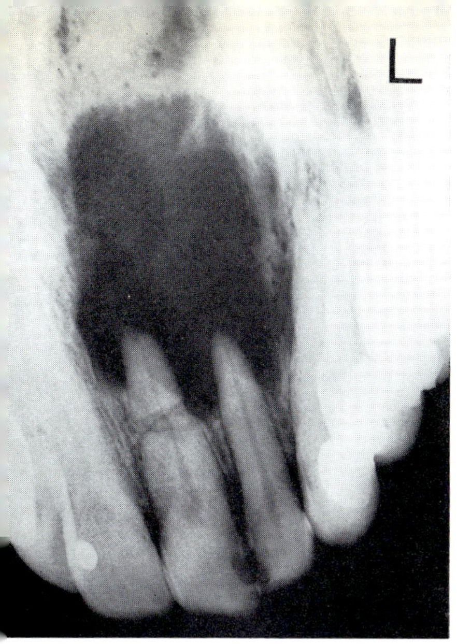
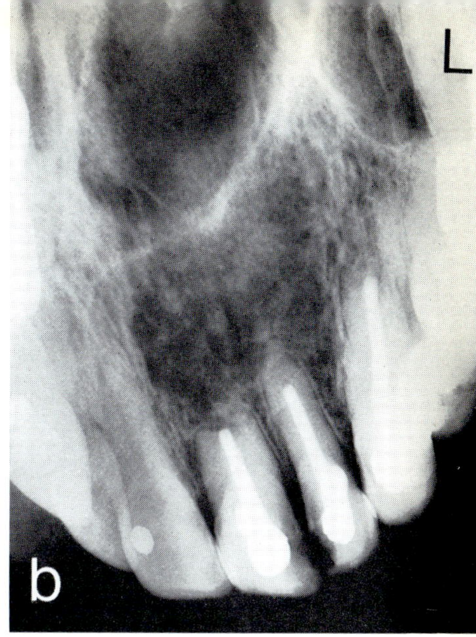

Fig. 58.—a, Large radicular cyst of the upper left central and lateral incisor. Non-vital pulp due to a trauma 3 years before. Fractured root of the upper left central incisor. Clinical features: fluctuating, painless swelling in the buccal sulcus. b, Three and a half years after cyst operation and apicectomy of upper left central and lateral incisor and canine (granuloma). Good bone healing.

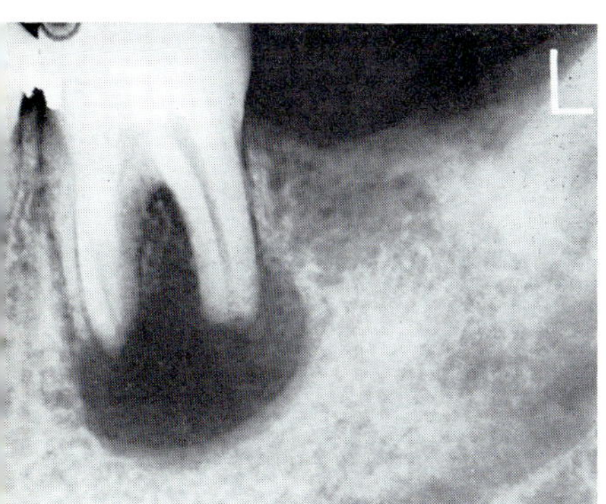
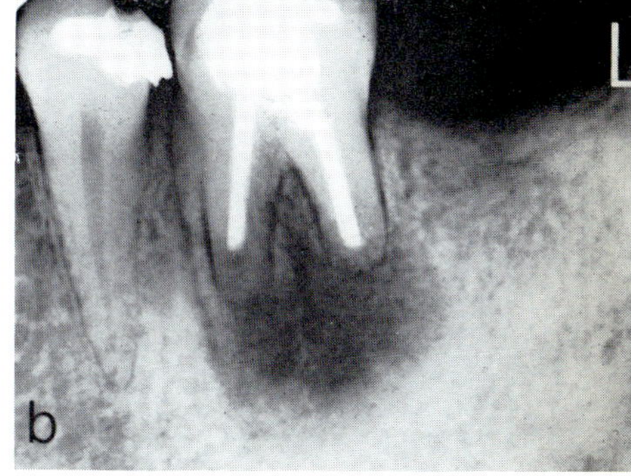

Fig. 59.—a, Putrified radicular cyst of lower left first molar, discovered after secondary infection. b, Good bone healing is visible 6 months after apicectomy and root-canal treatment.

A **radicular cyst** originates in epithelial remnants of Hertwig's sheath (Malassez's rests), which has played a part in root formation. They are located within the periodontal membrane and may proliferate owing to an inflammatory stimulus (dental granuloma), the causative agent being the presence of a tooth with a non-vital pulp. In the radiograph a sharply demarcated, often circular radiolucency can be seen, into which the root tip of the responsible tooth extends. Sometimes this tooth has been extracted at an earlier stage and the cyst has persisted independently (residual cyst, *Fig.* 60).

Treatment consists, in our opinion, of careful extirpation *in toto* of the sac-like cyst, lined on the lumen side by stratified squamous epithelium or (sometimes) of marsupialization and extraction or root-canal treatment of the associated tooth (*Figs.* 57, 58, and 59).

A **follicular cyst** originates from epithelial remnants of a dental follicle of an unerupted tooth. Often a third molar, an impacted upper canine, or a lower premolar, is concerned. In these cases the associated tooth is missing in the dental arch. In the radiograph a well-demarcated radiolucency is visible within the jaw, into which the crown of the responsible tooth extends. Treatment consists generally of surgical removal of the tooth and extirpation of the cyst-wall (*Figs.* 61, 62, 63, and 64).

Fissural cysts (rare) occur almost exclusively in the maxilla. They originate from epithelial rests, left after fusion of several processes, formed during the development of the maxilla. The fissural cysts include nasopalatine cysts (between the upper lateral incisor and canine) and naso-alveolar cysts, occurring in the soft tissues at the base of the nostrils (*Fig.* 67). These cysts may be lined by either squamous, columnar, or respiratory epithelium. Transitional forms occur. Treatment consists of careful extirpation (*Figs.* 65 and 66).

Basal-cell Naevi Syndrome.—This syndrome, which has interested many people in the past few years, comprises, besides basal-cell naevi of the skin, rib, skull, and vertebral deformities, diseases of the eyes and the central nervous system; also in many cases multiple and recurring cysts, lined by keratinizing epithelium.

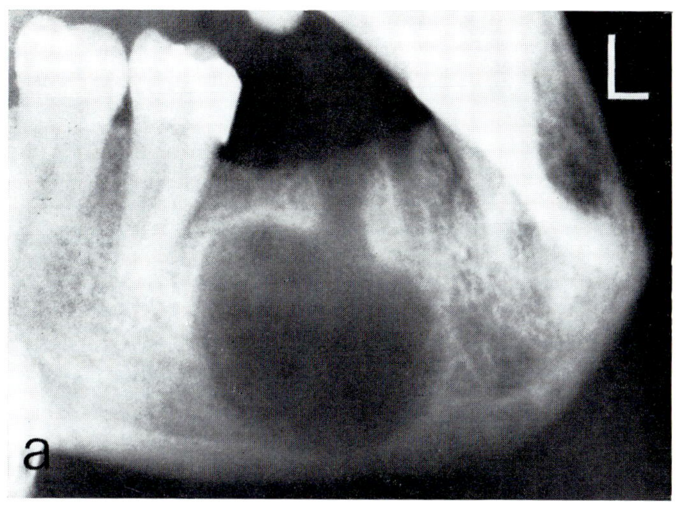

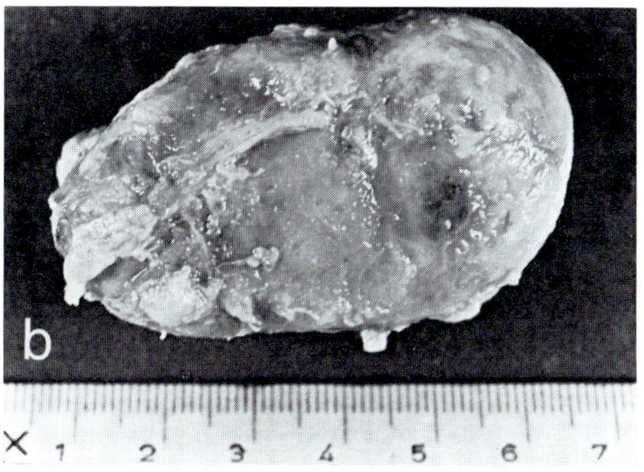

Fig. 60.—a, Residual jaw cyst in the left mandible. Elastic, rather firm swelling in the buccal sulcus. Discovered after secondary inflammation. b, Extirpated residual cyst. Lining: stratified squamous epithelium.

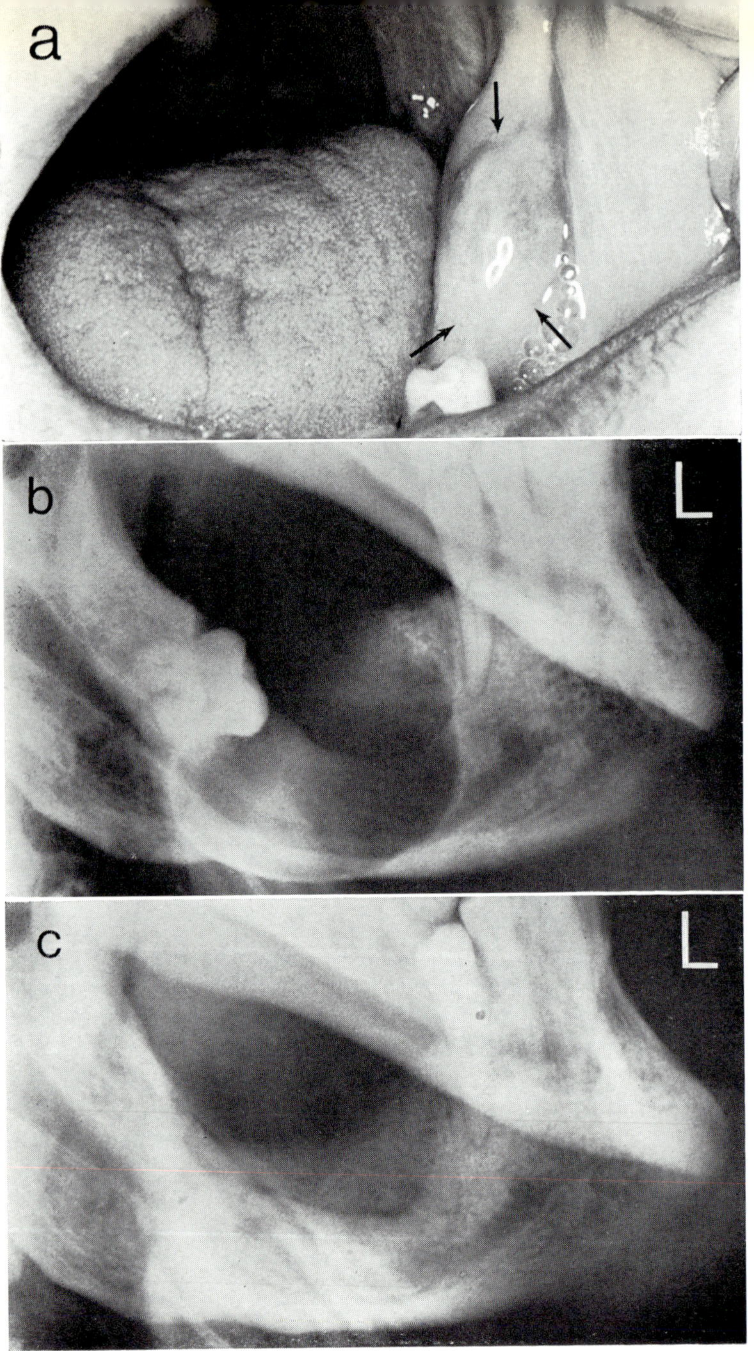

(*Fig.* 61)

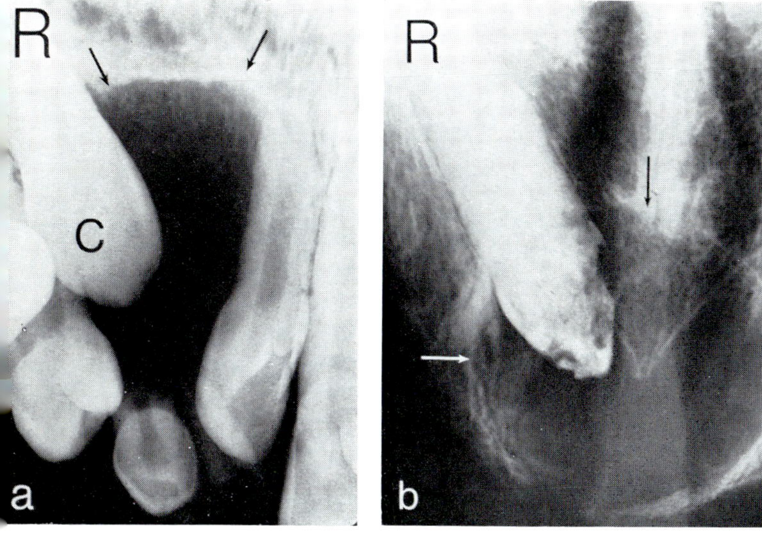

Fig. 62.—a, Infected follicular cyst in a child, arising from an upper canine (c). Discovered after acute inflammation of the involved area. b, Infected follicular cyst, originating from an impacted canine in an edentulous patient. The crown is somewhat resorbed. Nut-sized swelling medially in the upper front. Painful on palpation.

Fig. 61.—a, Fluctuating, bluish, shining, painless, gradually developed swelling about 2 cm. in diameter. Diagnosis: follicular cyst associated with an impacted third molar. b, Radiograph of a large follicular cyst associated with lower left third molar. The crown extends into the cyst. c, Nine months after surgical removal of cyst and tooth good healing of the bone is visible.

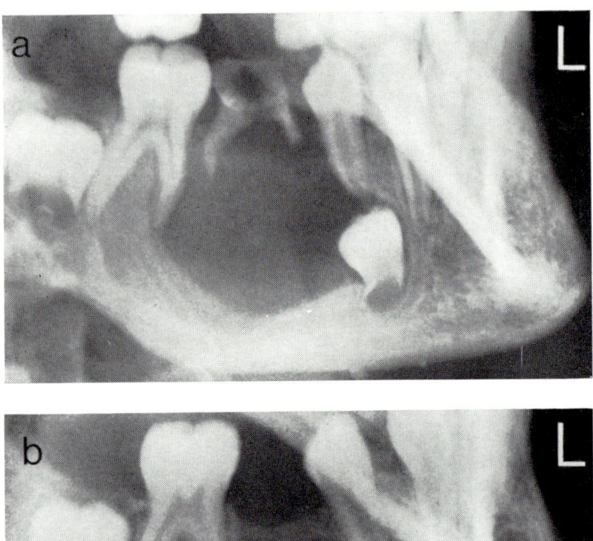

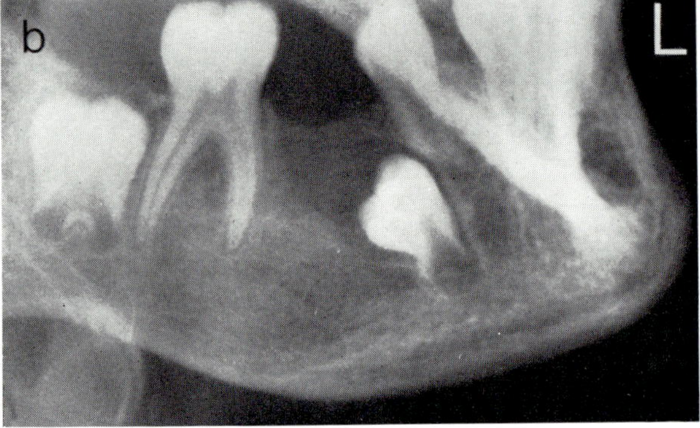

Fig. 63.—a, Follicular cyst arising from a deeply localized lower left second premolar or radicular cyst of the second deciduous molar in an 11-year-old girl. Clinical features: bony-hard painless swelling in the buccal sulcus. b, Six months after operation the bone shows good healing.

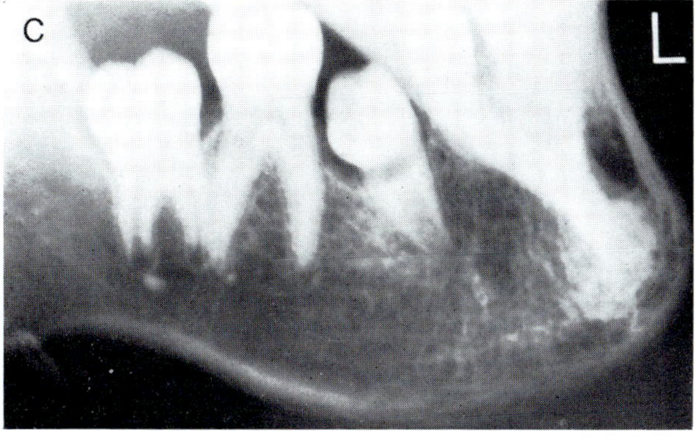

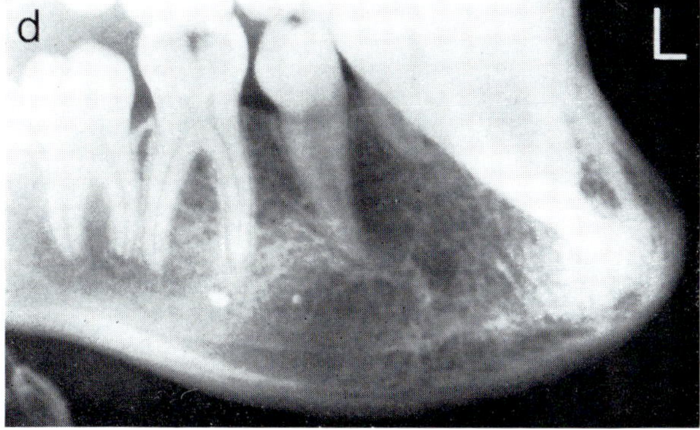

Fig. 63.—c, Two and a half years after operation. Complete healing. Second premolar has nearly erupted. d, Nearly 4 years after operation the second premolar has erupted completely in the dental arch.

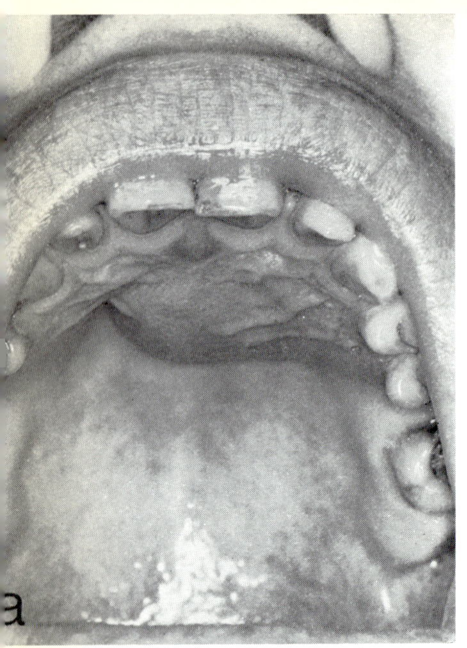

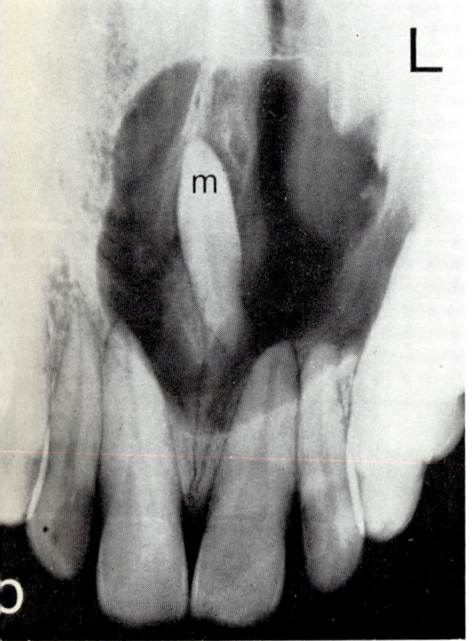

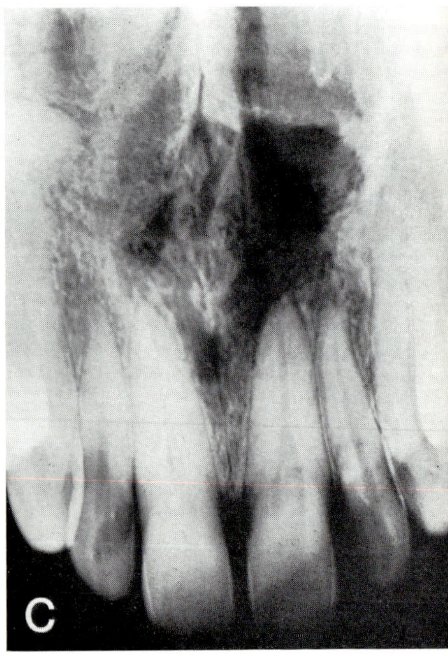

Fig. 64.—a, Painless swelling on the palate of a 30-year-old man. Has existed for some years already. No teeth are missing and all pulps are vital. b, Radiograph of the palate shows a big follicular cyst arising from a supernumerary tooth (m=mesiodens), wedging between the roots of the upper central incisors. c, Two years after removal of cyst and mesiodens good bone healing is visible. The central incisors are somewhat more upright now. Cyst lining: stratified squamous epithelium.

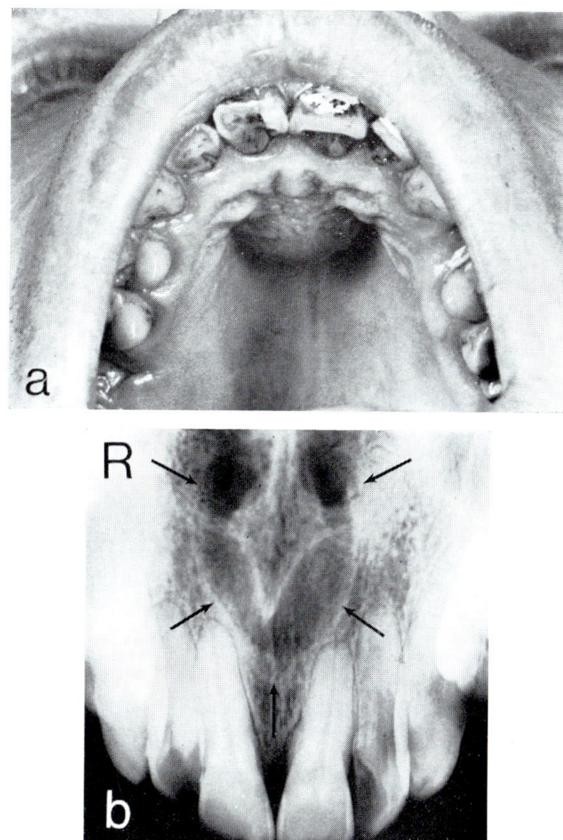

Fig. 65.—a, Painless, bluish, fluctuating swelling in the midline anterior of the palate, caused by a nasopalatine cyst. Lining: stratified squamous epithelium. b, Radiograph of the same cyst. Not associated with any tooth.

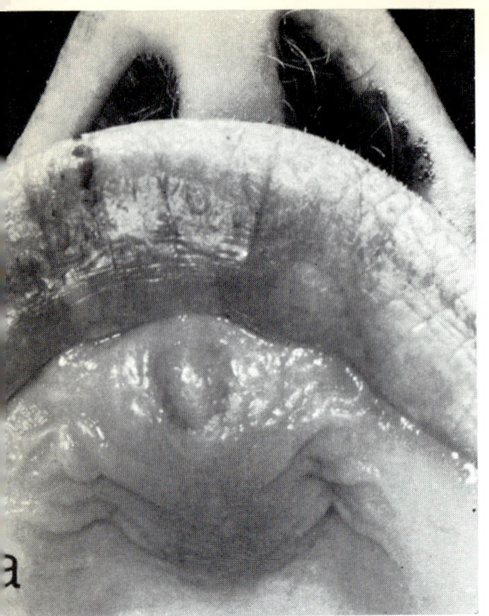
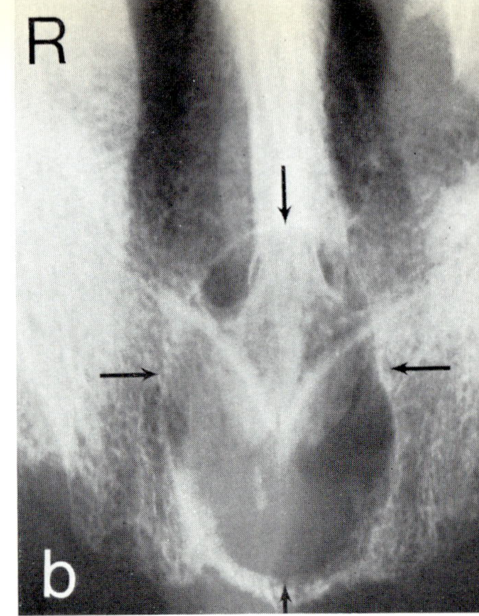

Fig. 66.—a, Nasopalatine cyst in an edentulous 57-year-old man; became manifest after secondary infection. Fluctuating, not very painful. Lining: non-keratinizing stratified squamous epithelium with smaller areas of cylindrical and respiratory epithelium. b, Characteristic radiolucency.

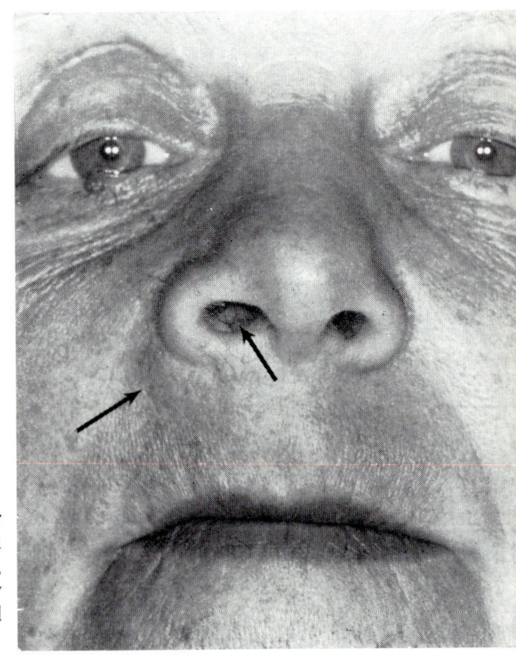

Fig. 67.—Naso-alveolar cyst in a 57-year-old woman. Painless swelling, except after secondary inflammation. Has existed for at least 1 year.

TUMOURS OF THE JAWS

Broadly speaking the same benign and malignant tumours occurring elsewhere in the skeleton may occur in the jaws. This is also applicable to the occurrence of metastases. In addition, there also occur odontogenic tumours.

Benign Odontogenic Tumours.—This group of tumours includes the rather rare *ameloblastoma* (adamantinoma). It is an epithelial tumour, often multicystic, arising from odontogenic epithelial remnants. This benign tumour, most frequently localized close to an impacted mandibular third molar, shows on the radiograph as a multiloculated radiolucency with occasional root resorption of the adjacent teeth. Extensive lesions occur owing to slow and asymptomatic growth. Recurrences are common, probably due to incomplete surgical removal (*Fig.* 68).

An *odontoma* is an odontogenic tumour, showing a higher degree of maturation than the ameloblastoma. This tumour contains both mesenchymal and epithelial dental tissues and may consist of many small crudely formed teeth, or of a conglomeration of hard dental tissues. The lesion is generally asymptomatic; once formed, the tumour remains static for the rest of the patient's life. In contrast with an ameloblastoma there is a radiographic opacity, which may vary in size (*Fig.* 69). Treatment consists of excision. The tumour does not recur.

Finally the *cementoma*, a periapical lesion: it is discovered on a radiograph usually by accident. In the immature stage the radiograph of the (vital) tooth shows a periapical area of radiolucency and in the mature stage the same area is radio-opaque. Presumably it is not a true neoplasm, but a form of dysplasia (periapical fibro-osseous-cementous dysplasia). In general, treatment is not required (*Fig.* 70).

Malignant Tumours.—The most frequently occurring malignant tumours are carcinoma and sarcoma. Clinically both tumours manifest themselves as rather rapidly growing, often painful thickenings of the jaw. Besides these swellings there are often the following clinical features: the *teeth* in the involved side of the jaw *may be loose* and there may be changes in sensation in the area supplied by either the mental nerve (unilateral numbness of the lower lip) or the infra-orbital nerve (unilateral numbness of the upper lip and cheek).

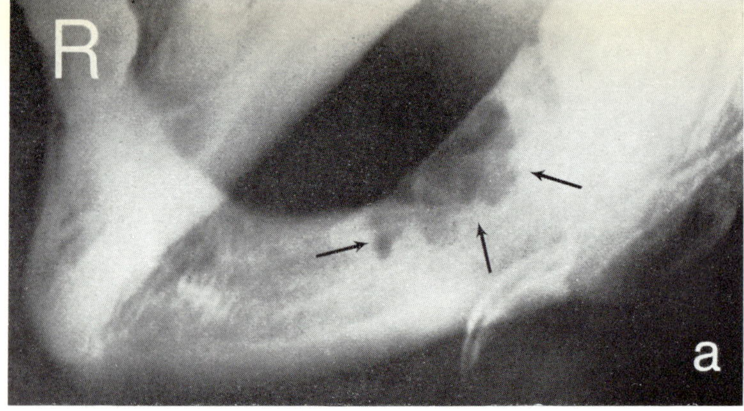

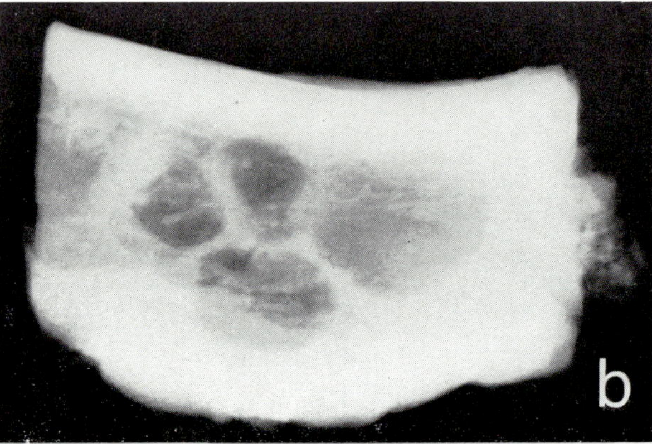

Fig. 68.—a, Ameloblastoma in the mandibular right third molar region in a 41-year-old woman. A large multicystic tumour, also diagnosed as ameloblastoma, was removed in the same area 13 years earlier. Clinical features: no evident symptoms. Treatment: local complete excision into the normal bone. b, Magnified radiograph of the operation specimen. Note the multilocular radiolucency.

Fig. 69.—a, Odontoma in the upper front, surrounded by a distinct capsule in a 13-year-old girl, consisting of a conglomeration of hard dental tissues (complex odontoma). Clinical features: hard, painless swelling palatally of the upper right central incisor. b, Odontoma in the lower right cuspid/first premolar region consisting of small rudimentary teeth (compound odontoma) in a 20-year-old man. The lower left canine is impacted (c).

Fig. 70.—Mature cementoma at the level of the apex of the lower left second premolar (vital pulp). Multiple cementomata were found in this patient. Cementomas may grow together with the roots of the associated teeth (difficult extraction), but as a rule they are separated from the apices by the periodontium. In the latter case the cementoma remains in the jaw when the tooth is extractcd.

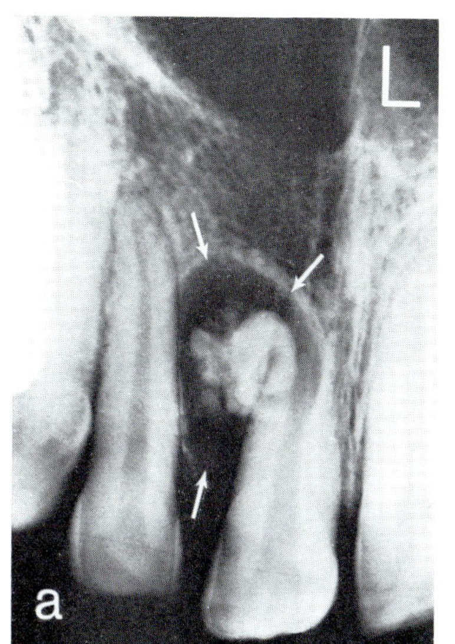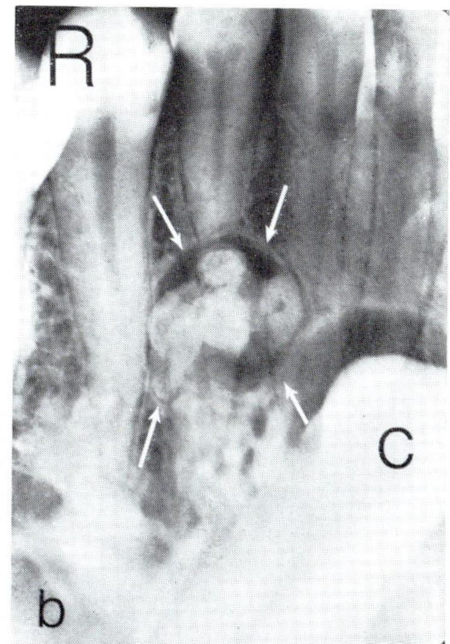

(*Fig.* 69)

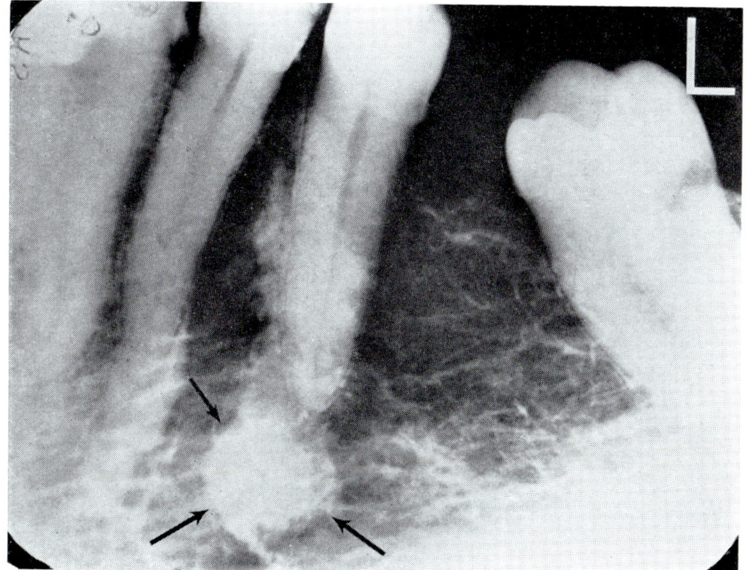

(*Fig.* 70)

89

If the loose teeth are extracted owing to a wrong diagnosis, the sockets fail to heal (danger of metastases), while the swelling is not reduced. The regional, submandibular, and cervical lymph-nodes may be indurated owing to metastases (carcinoma). Sarcomata usually metastasize haematogenously.

Radiographically the initial stage may show only slight alterations. At a further stage of development generally an ill-defined radiolucency becomes visible with irregular destruction of the bone.

The *primary carcinoma of the mandible*, originating from deeply localized odontogenic epithelium or from a cyst, is extremely rare.

The *maxillary carcinoma* usually originates from the maxillary sinus and is, in the majority of cases, a squamous-cell carcinoma. This carcinoma is often erroneously diagnosed as a chronic inflammation. Many patients come for treatment at a very late stage. Early diagnosis is usually difficult. Early symptoms may resemble those of a chronic sinusitis. Sometimes the primary manifestation is an ill-fitting denture (*Figs.* 71 and 72).

When a *sarcoma* occurs in the mandible, the picture, both clinically and radiographically, may resemble osteomyelitis with sequestration and periosteal bone formation (*Fig.* 73).

Be always alert in the case of swellings of the jaws, order a radiograph, and take a biopsy at an early stage!

Treatment of the above-mentioned tumours is performed by an *oncological team.* It is advisable that such a team includes a general surgeon, an ear, nose, and throat specialist, a radiotherapist, a plastic surgeon, an oral surgeon, a prosthodontist, and a pathologist, while other specialists must be available, if needed. Of major importance is that everybody is interested and has much experience in tumour surgery. The often difficult rehabilitation care following the surgical interference is very important for both functional and psychological reasons (*Fig.* 74).

In general it may be said that carcinomata of the jaws, provided they are treated expertly, have a better prognosis than those occurring elsewhere in the body.

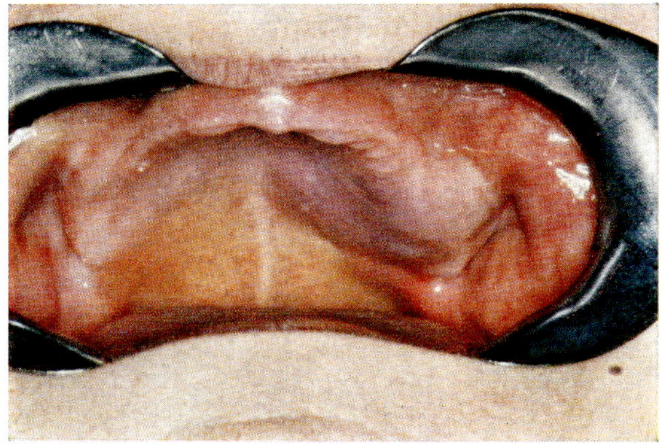

Fig. 71.—Firm-elastic swelling of the maxilla in a 55-year-old woman, causing an ill-fitting prosthesis. For some months there has been a gnawing pain, which has increased in the last 2 weeks. The radiograph shows partial fading of the maxillary sinus and irregular affection of the bone. This may be the initial stage of any malignant maxillary tumour. Diagnosis in this patient: cylindroma.

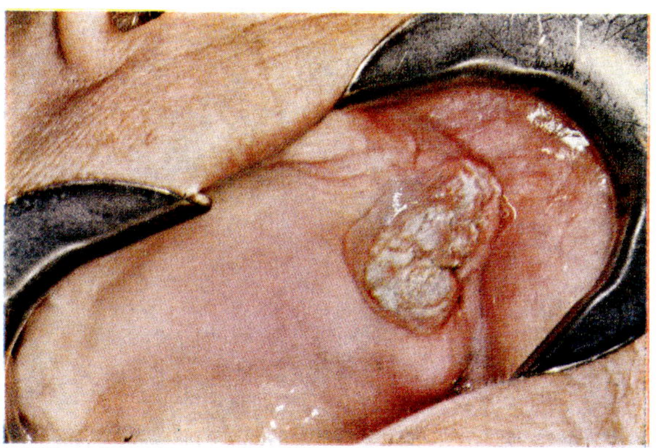

Fig. 72.—The maxillary carcinoma in a 63-year-old woman has penetrated the oral mucosa. The lesion is very painful.

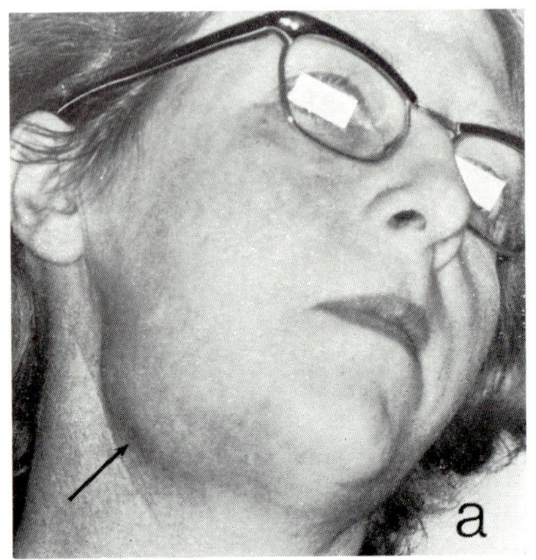

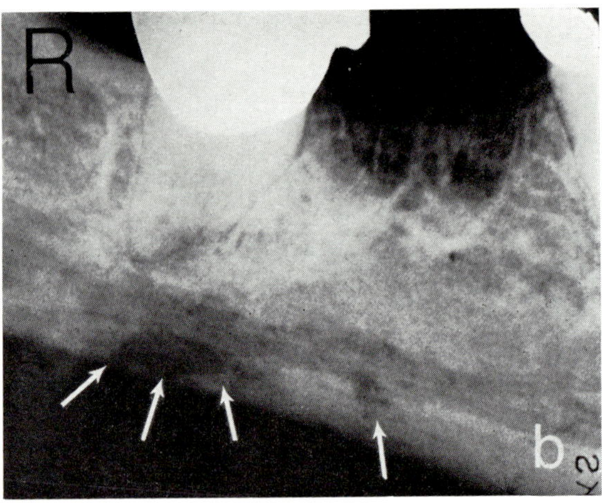

Fig. 73.—a, Rapidly growing swelling at the mandibular angle in a 39-year-old woman. Consistency is that of a hard infiltrate. Numbness of the right half of the lower lip. The dentition gives no complaints. b, The dental radiograph shows irregular destruction of the bone at the level of the mandibular right second molar, especially of the cortex of the lower mandibular border. There is no marked granuloma at the apex of the lower right second molar. c, Eight weeks later. Marked irregular destruction of the bone (the teeth have been extracted in the meantime). Diagnosis: osteosarcoma.

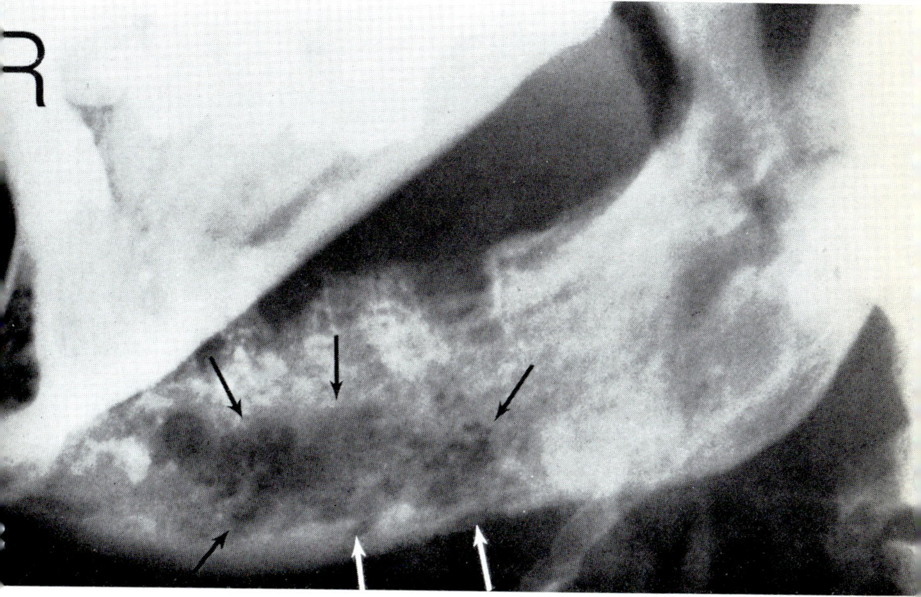

(*Fig.* 73 c)

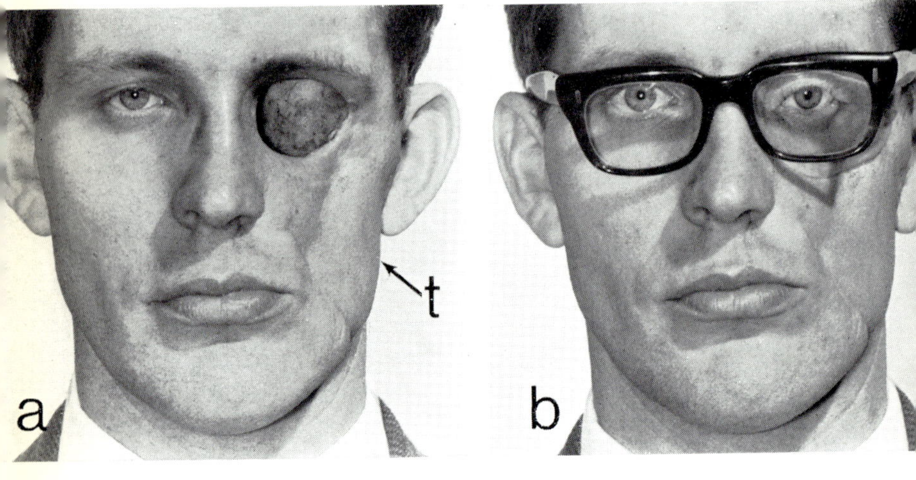

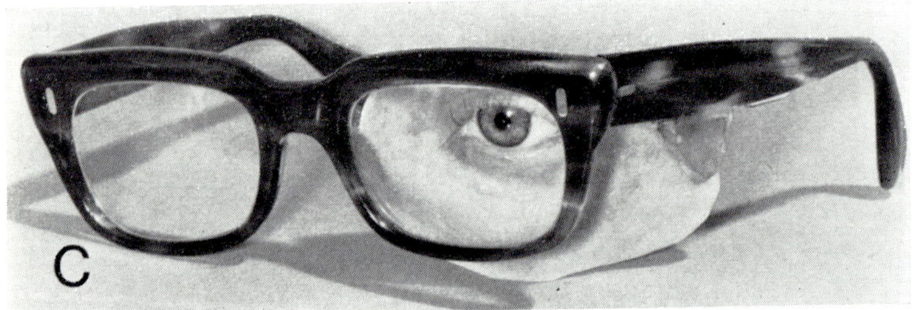

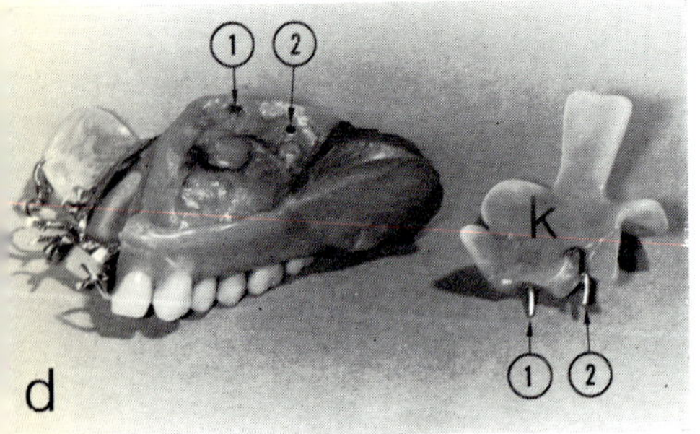

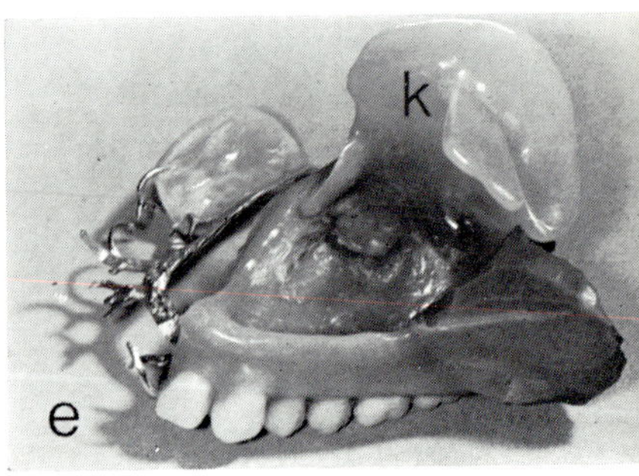

(Fig. 74)

94

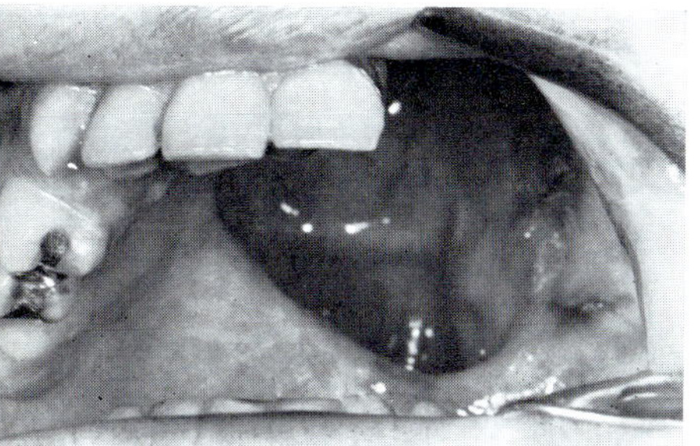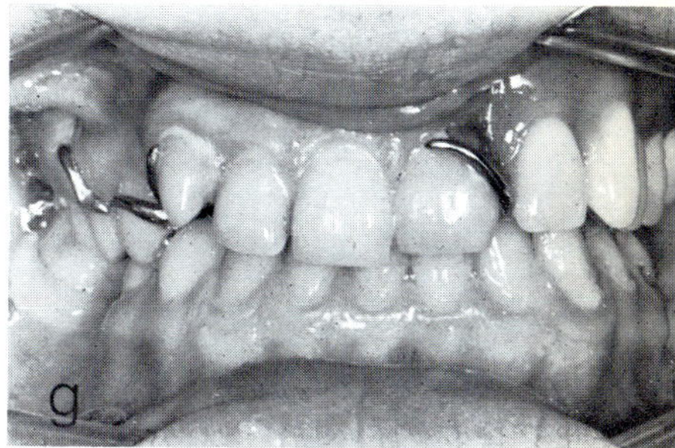

Fig. 74.—a, Resection of maxilla and enucleation of the left eye owing to a malignant neoplasm in the maxilla and two recurrences. The patient was irradiated and methotrexate was administered. The defect of the cheek (t) was closed by means of a tubed pedicle flap after 2 years. b, After operative and prosthetic reconstruction. c, Eye prosthesis with part of the orbit. The spectacle frame is used to support the eye prosthesis. d, e, Surgical prosthesis for closure of the maxillary defect. The 'valve' (k) serves as a sounding-board when speaking. The pins 1 and 2 of the valves are fitting in the tubes 1 and 2 of the prosthesis. f, The maxillary defect. g, Prosthesis in situ.

OTHER LESIONS OF THE JAWS

Torus Palatinus and Torus Mandibularis.—*Torus palatinus* is a bony excrescence, mainly occurring in the midline on the palate. In the majority of cases it is a lobular lesion, covered by a pale muco-periosteum (*Fig.* 75 a).

Torus mandibularis occurs on either side on the lingual surface of the mandible in the premolar area. Often a torus mandibularis seems to consist of a fusion of two or three exostoses (*Fig.* 75b).

In most patients these lesions arise during puberty and do not show any growth afterwards. Hereditary factors seem to be of significance.

From a pathological point of view the lesions are insignificant and should only be removed if they interfere with speech, if the oral cavity cannot be cleaned properly (remains of food under the tori), or if a prosthesis has to be made or readapted.

Dysplasia.—Fibro-osseous-cementous dysplasia includes a series of rather rare lesions, of which the radiographs may vary from radiolucent (fibrous component is dominating) to a very fine-meshed bone density (*Fig.* 77). Sometimes the lesion contains much cementum (cementifying fibroma) (*Fig.* 78). Removal, if practicable, is indicated at an early stage as possible, for some of these lesions may show very rapid growth. In very extensive lesions surgical treatment can be no more than a remodelling operation (*Fig.* 76).

Cherubism.—This intra-osseous lesion mainly occurs in children from 2 to 7 years of age, whereafter growth will subside and finally cease, so that treatment is not required. In its most characteristic form cherubism gives bilateral swelling of the mandible in the mandibular angle region and often of the maxilla too, as a result of which a tension of the skin is effected. The lower eyelids are pulled down. The sclerae become visible so that the patients seem to look upwards (cherubs). On the radiograph the mandible and sometimes the maxilla too show extensive multilocular radiolucencies. Histologically a varying number of giant cells are found in a fibrous stroma. Cherubism is a familial disease.

Central Giant-cell Reparative Granuloma is a slowly growing, painless lesion, which may present in the long term, after resorption of the cortex, as a bluish-red swelling. The radiograph often

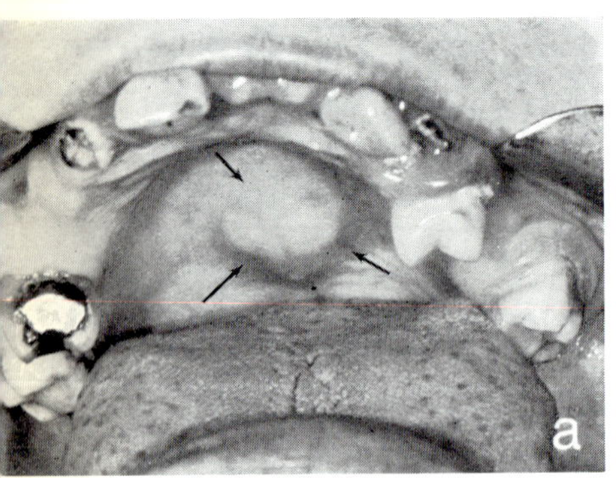
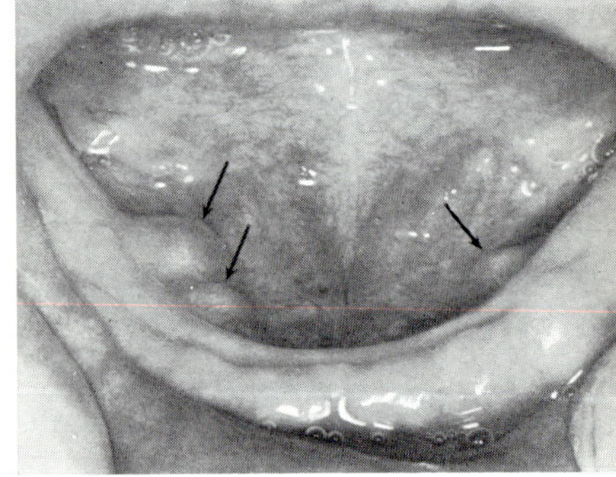

Fig. 75.—a, Torus palatinus. b, Torus mandibularis on either side of the lingual (edentulous) lower alveolar process.

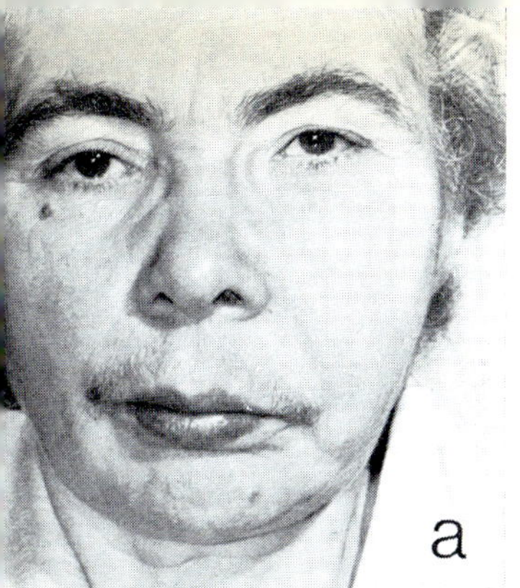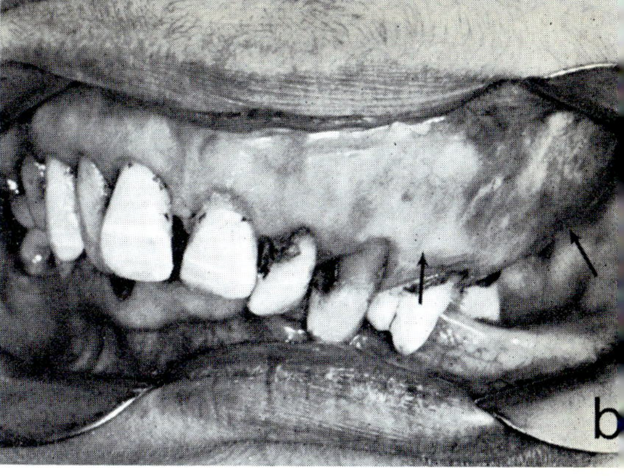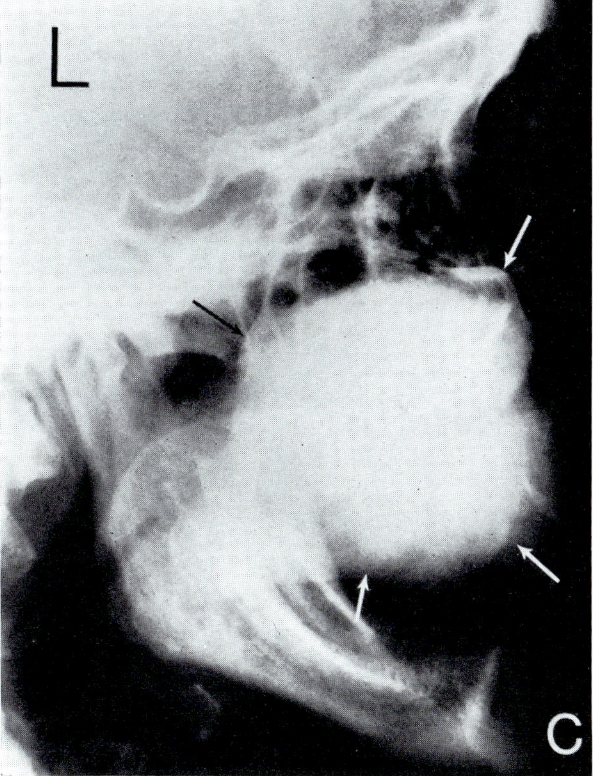

Fig. 76.—a, b, and c, Fibro-osseous-cementous dysplasia of the left maxilla in a 45-year-old woman. Large bone-hard swelling extending into the zygomatic area. Marked displacement of the teeth (b) and deformation (a) of the face. The radiograph (c) shows very dense, fine-meshed spongy bone. Growth has ceased.

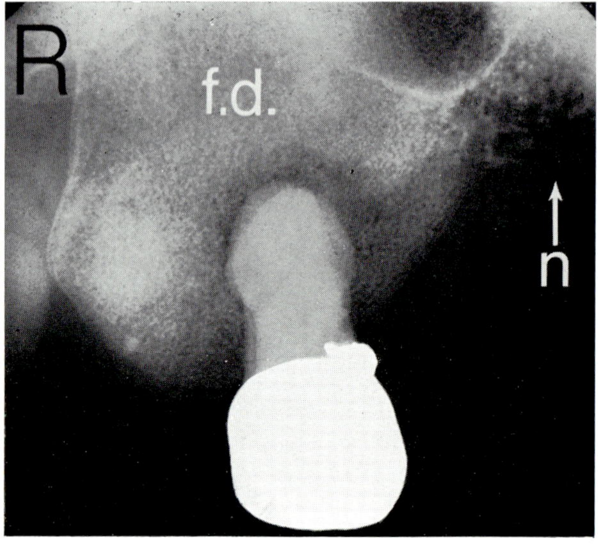

Fig. 77.—Very fine-meshed dense bone due to fibro-osseous-cementous dysplasia (f.d.) of the right maxillary tuberosity (n = normal bone).

shows an ill-defined radiolucency (*Fig.* 79). Migration of teeth and root resorption are common findings. Treatment consists of excision.

Peripheral giant-cell reparative granuloma (epulis gigantocellularis) is described on p. 157.

Giant-cell Tumour is a true neoplasm and is identical to the giant-cell tumour occurring elsewhere in the skeleton. This tumour is of very rare incidence in the jaws.

Aneurysmal Bone Cyst is most frequently seen in the long bones and spine in children and young adults. When occurring in the jaws (rare) the lesion is characterized by an eccentric growth. The radiograph may show a wide-meshed, 'foamy', honeycomb-like radiolucency, bounded on its periphery by a thin bone lamella. The lesion is of unknown origin. The histological picture is characterized by multiple, endothelial-lined cavities, filled with old or

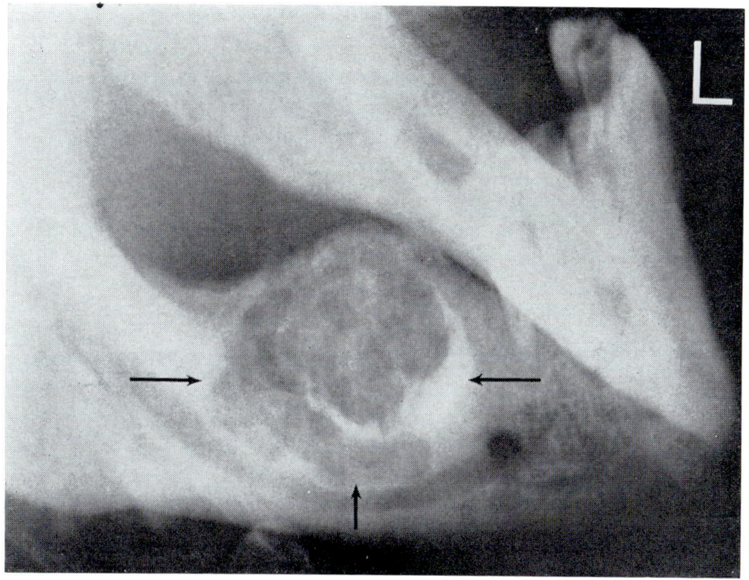

Fig. 78.—Fibro-osseous-cementous dysplasia containing much cementum (cementifying fibroma) (48-year-old man). No dense fine-meshed bone, but a sharply demarcated radiolucency with radio-opaque structures. The lower alveolar nerve is displaced. Treatment consisted of local excision.

fresh blood. In the septa numerous giant cells may be found. If teeth extending into the lesion are extracted, serious haemorrhages may be produced. Treatment consists of total extirpation.

Hyperparathyroidism.—In an advanced stage this rather rare disease may cause the same lesions in the jaws as elsewhere in the skeleton. One of the characteristic features may be loss of lamina dura of the dental alveoli. On the dental radiograph there appears a variable widening of the periodontal fissures. At what stage and frequency resorption of lamina dura occurs is still unknown.

Paget's Disease.—In this disease the normal cancellous bone tissue, with its trabeculae arranged along the lines of stress, is replaced by irregular immature bone. The cortex disappears and the jaw is markedly thickened, because there is, except for bone destruction, far greater bone formation (*Fig.* 80 a and b). Around the teeth large areas of hypercementosis may be found. The latter may make extraction difficult, while the weakened bone may easily fracture (*Fig.* 80 c). The patients are usually over 40 years of age.

Radiographically Paget's disease may resemble fibrous dysplasia (*see* p. 95). Paget's disease, however, generally involves the whole mandible or maxilla, whereas this is not a common finding in fibrous dysplasia. Paget's disease is of rare occurrence in the jaws.

Acromegaly.—This hormonal disturbance may cause marked enlargement of the mandible. The patient's profile becomes prognathic and diastemata appear between the teeth (*Fig.* 81).

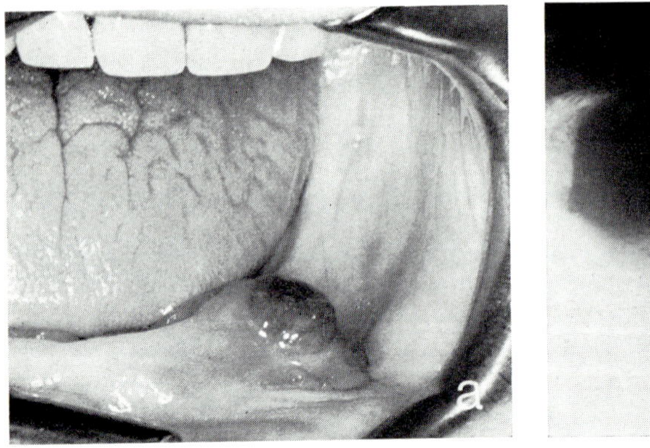
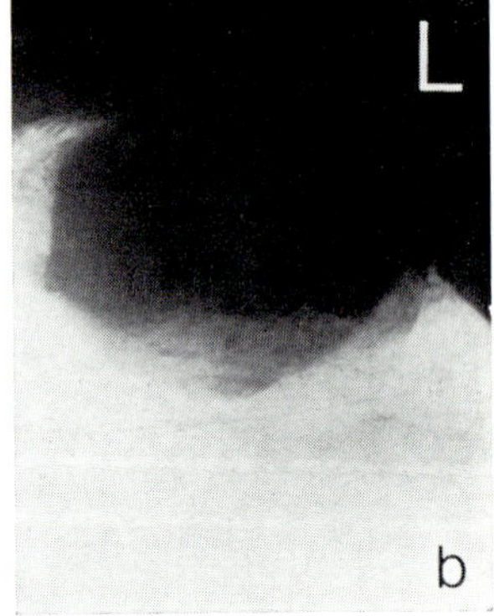

Fig. 79.—Central giant-cell reparative granuloma. a, Reddish-blue, painless, soft, easily bleeding swelling of the mandible in a 54-year-old man. Slow growth. b, Rather extensive, somewhat irregularly demarcated bone-resorption in the mandible.

Fig. 80.—a, b, Paget's disease in the mandible in a 66-year-old woman. The jaw is enlarged and gives a massive impression. No complaints. The lesion was discovered after a fracture following tooth extraction. c, The jaw is markedly thickened, the cortex has disappeared, the spongy bone has altered, and there are strongly radio-opaque areas, owing to hypercementosis (c). Fracture at the level of the socket of the mandibular right second molar (f).

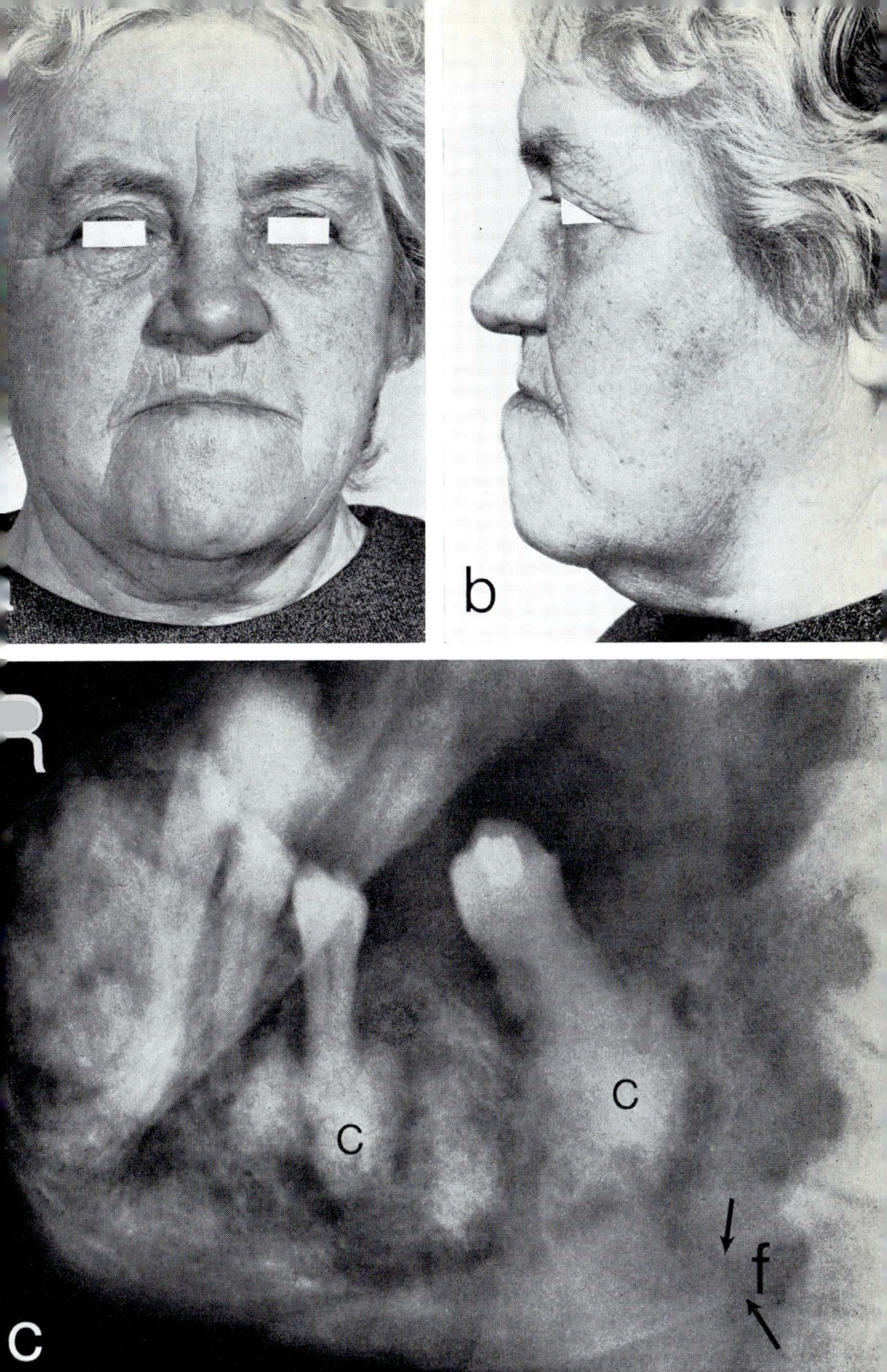

(*Fig.* 80)

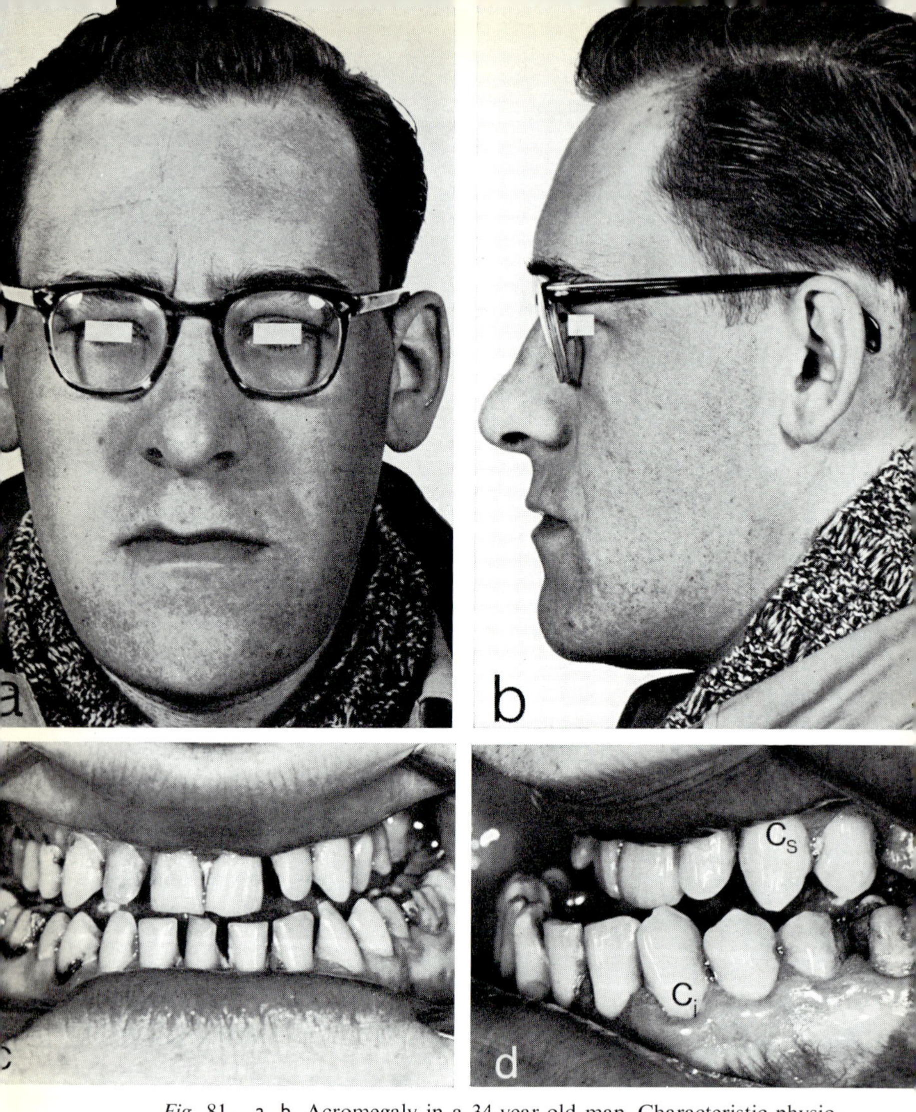

Fig. 81.—a, b, Acromegaly in a 34-year-old man. Characteristic physiognomy. Sturdy nose, lips, and chin. c, When closing the mouth there is only contact between the last molars. Diastemas between the lower incisors. The mandible is grossly enlarged in both ventral and transverse directions, so that the lower dental arch is biting nearly outside the upper arch. d, A prognathic front relation is effected. The lower front is extending far ventrally of the upper front. The lower cuspid (Ci) is situated far ventrally of the upper cuspid (Cs). In a normal dentition Ci is situated dorsally of Cs.

CHAPTER 3

TEMPOROMANDIBULAR JOINT

'Arthrosis Deformans'.—Arthrosis deformans is the most common disease of the temporomandibular joint. The lesion may occur in very young patients, but most patients are women between 20 and 30 years of age. It is not clear why the lesion is predominantly seen in female patients. Clicking of the joint is usually the primary manifestation of the disease. In the course of years clicking may be accompanied by pain and limitation of movement, but may also cease spontaneously. Patients complain of pain when opening the

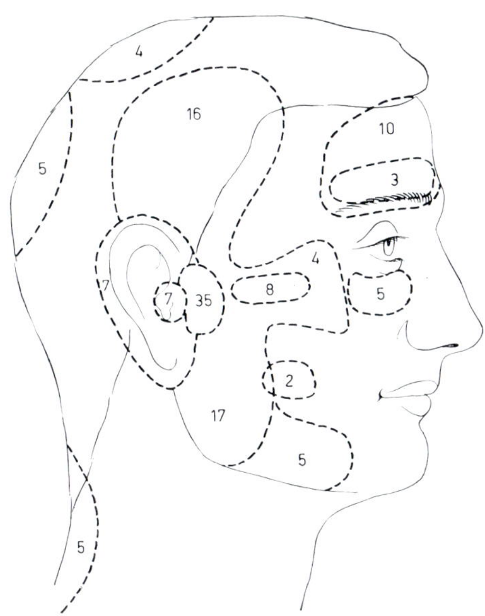

Fig. 82.—Pain areas, as indicated by 50 patients suffering from temporo-mandibular joint arthrosis. Frequencies are indicated by numerals.

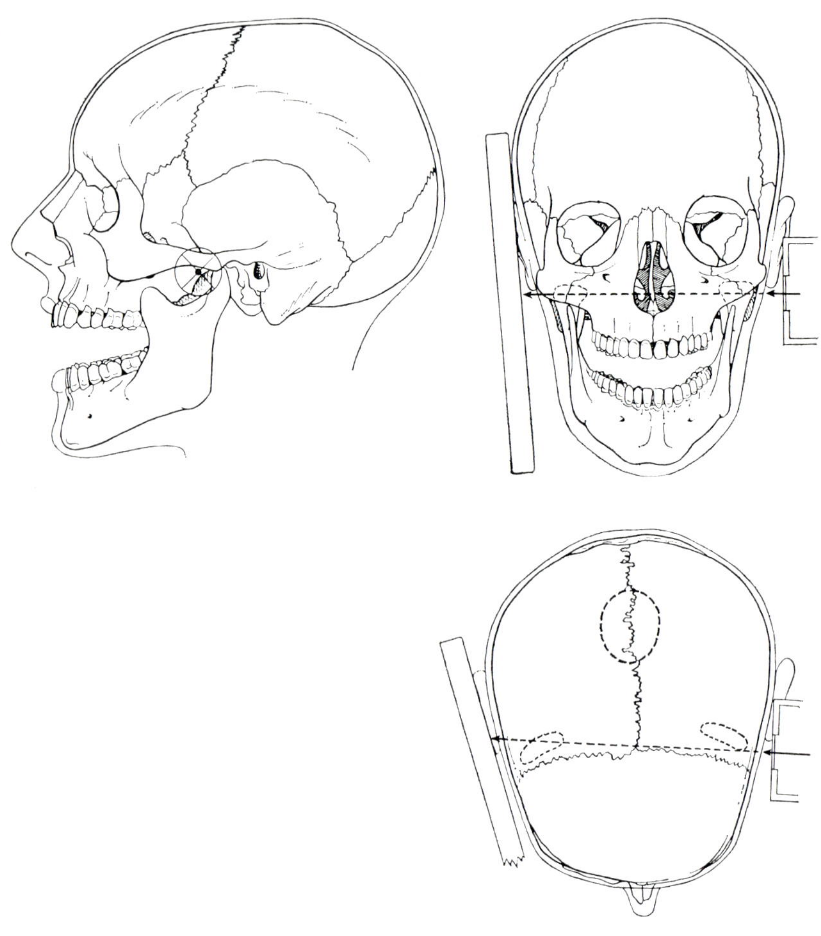

Fig. 83.—Lateral sigmoid infracranial view (Parma). The tube without a cone is placed directly on the skin, in the mandibular notch area. The central ray is directed at the contralateral condylar head. By using an aluminium filter of 2–4 mm., a narrow opening, and purposeful working, too great a dose on the skin can be avoided. The radiograph is taken in the wide-open-mouth position. Outline, structure, and mobility of the condylar head are beautifully projected. A lot of experience is required for good interpretation of these pictures.

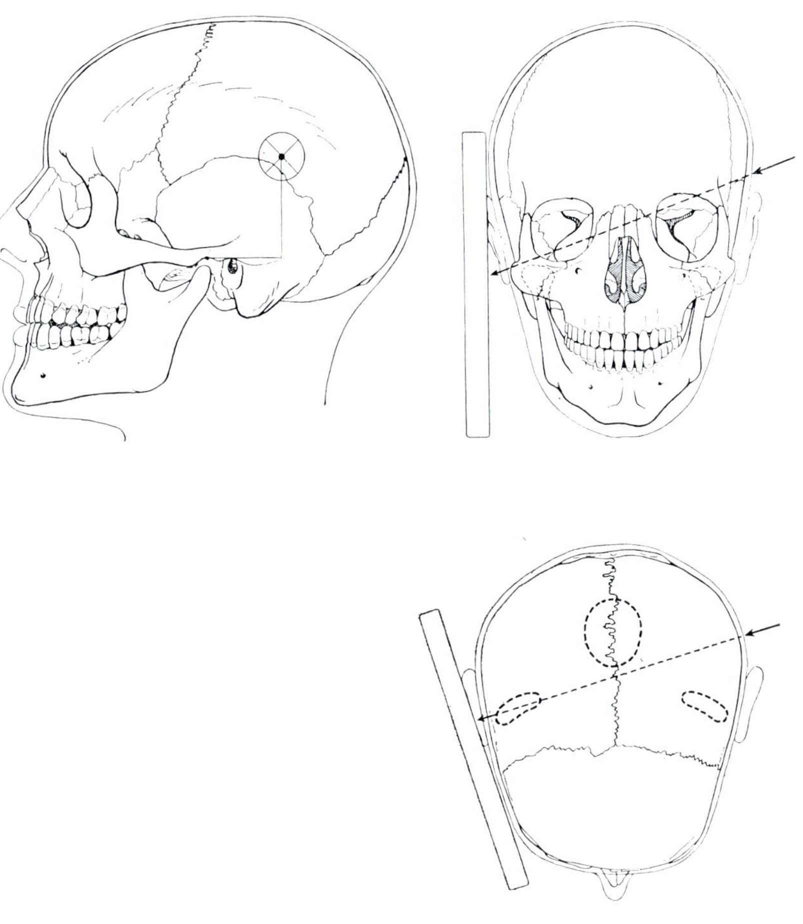

Fig. 84.—Standard lateral temporal view is a modification of Schüller's projection. The central ray is directed at the joint which is to be photographed and reaches the skull at the opposite side somewhat dorsally of and above the ear (angle of 19° with Camper's line and 15° with the frontal plane; focus–film distance 70 cm.). The projection is made with the dentition in habitual occlusion; the width of the joint gap, the tubercle, and relative size of the mandibular head (in relation to the opposite side) are very clearly visible.

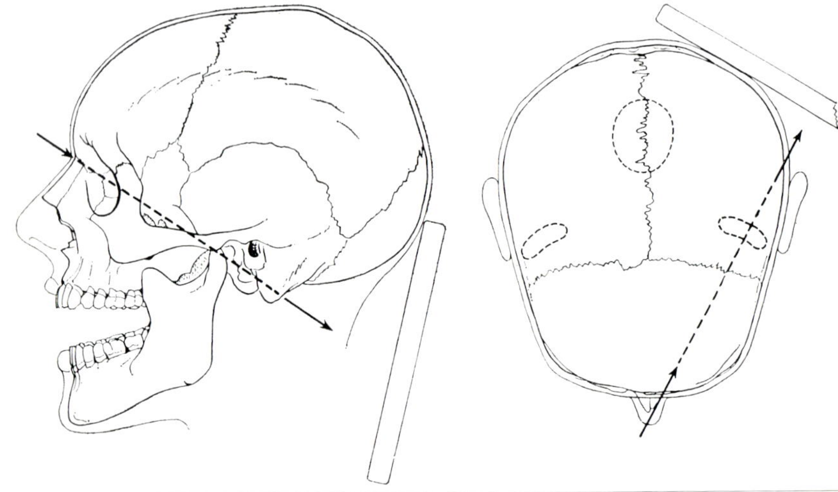

Fig. 85.—Orbitocondylar view of the temporomandibular joint in the wide-open-mouth position shows a frontal view of the condylar head; its structure, outline, and position are plainly visible.

mouth maximally, radiating to the temporoparietal region, to the ear, to the mandible or neck. Sometimes gnawing pain is the only complaint (*Fig.* 82). In the morning the joint feels 'rusted'. Pain and limitation of movements may be very troublesome, especially when they are long-lasting. The lesion is predominantly unilateral.

In the initial stage the radiographs often show no alterations. Generally, radiographic defects are only to be seen after a long period of pain and limitation of movement. It is our experience that for radiographic investigation of the temporomandibular joint a combination of two projections gives the best information, namely the lateral sigmoid infracranial view (Parma) in wide-open-mouth position, combined with the standard lateral temporal view (Schüller) in closed-mouth position (dentition in habitual occlusion) (*Figs.* 83 and 84). It is always necessary to take radiographs of both joints in order to make comparison. In case of doubt an additional orbitocondylar view may be made (*Fig.* 85) or a tomogram.

In serious cases the defects seen in the radiograph are: disappearance of the superficial cortical layer, flattening of the condylar head,

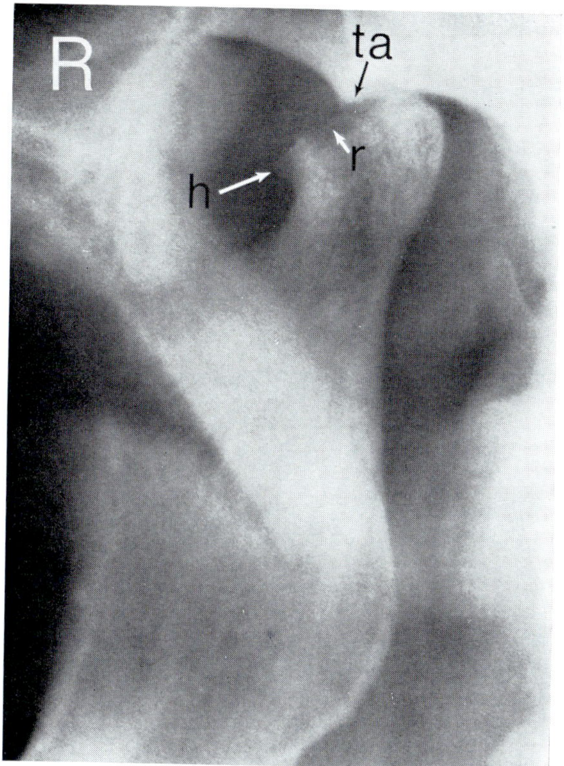

Fig. 86.—Marked arthrosis deformans of the right temporomandibular joint (Parma's projection). The head, being normally rounded and showing a superficial cortical layer and an even density of the spongy bone (*see Fig.* 93), is flattened, the cortical layer has disappeared, there is a small area of resorption (r) and an exophytic margin (h). Mobility is limited (the condylar head does not reach the summit of the articular eminence) and the tubercle (ta) is flattened. Often the ascending ramus as a whole is shortened.

exostoses at the ventral margin, and flattening of the tubercle (*Fig.* 86).

The cause of the lesion is, besides a certain predisposition, presumably a unilateral chewing habit; sometimes patients are forced to chew on one side due to the condition of their dentition. Probably bad masticatory habits (clamping or grinding, mostly in bed by

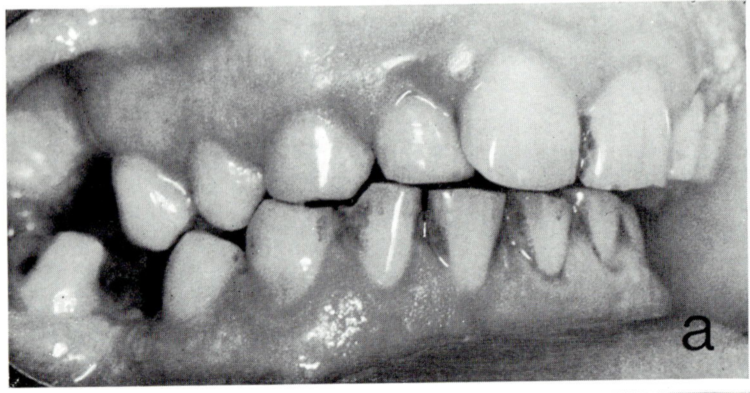

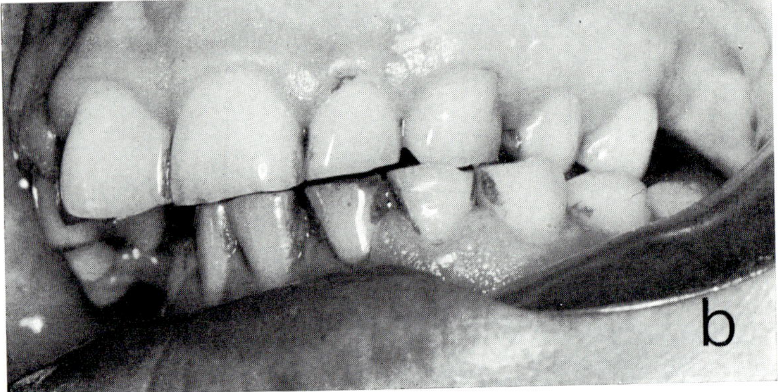

Fig. 87.—a, b, Distinct abrasions due to grinding.

psychically stressed patients) play a part. The dentitions of these patients show marked attritions (*Fig.* 87). During the period when clicking is the predominant symptom, therapy consists of avoiding clicking to prevent further damage of the intra-articular disk ('Do not open the mouth too wide when yawning; do not bite off big or hard things'). During the period when pain is the main symptom, this measure may be combined with infra-red irradiation, diathermy, or intra-articular injection of corticosteroids (*Fig.* 88). The most important thing is that the joint gets as much rest as possible (soft food and no use of chewing gum in case of stiffness, as is sometimes prescribed). Furthermore, the patient's dentition has to be restored by a dentist to enable him to chew on both sides. Much attention has to be paid to a good occlusion and articulation. In many cases an occlusal splint between the occlusal planes of the lower and upper jaw may afford relief from the complaints (*Fig.* 89).

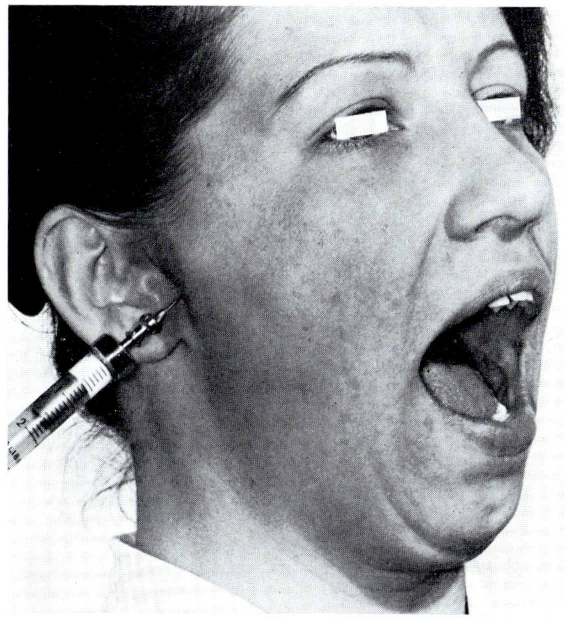

Fig. 88.—Intra- or periarticular injection of corticosteroids. The mouth is maximally opened. The needle has to proceed in a forward and upward direction until there is a bony contact with the tubercle. Local anaesthesia is given beforehand.

As far as the clinical symptoms are concerned the prognosis is generally favourable in the long run; in the end there is only slight crepitation or limitation of movements. Ankylosis is rarely, if ever, the ultimate result.

Surgical treatment is rarely indicated. Disk extirpation is conducive to a progression of the arthrosis and has, therefore, been abandoned as the surgical method of treatment. Extirpation of the mandibular condyle, or condylotomy (in which the neck of the mandible is only sawn through without extirpation of the condyle), may bring relief in

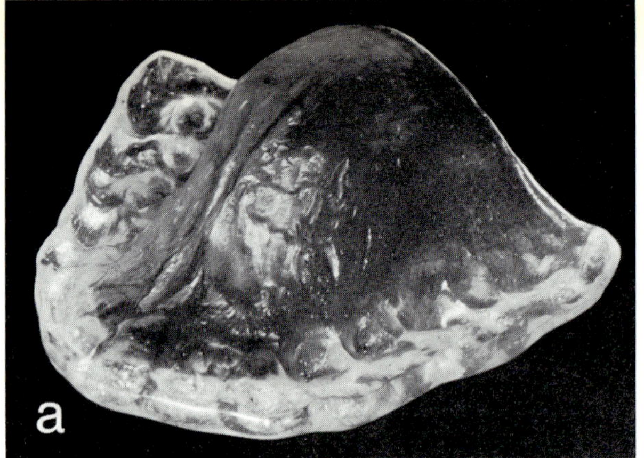

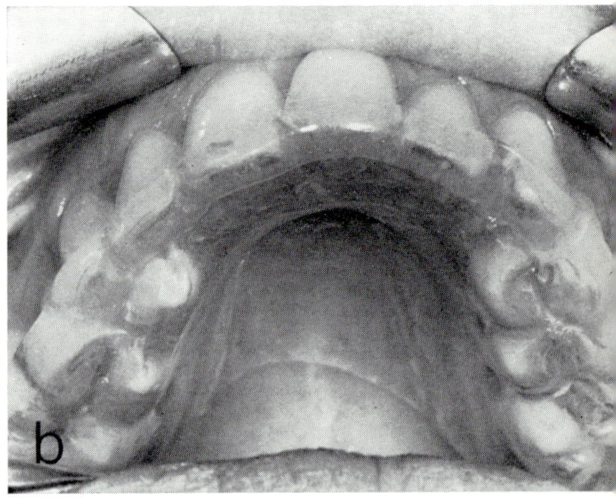

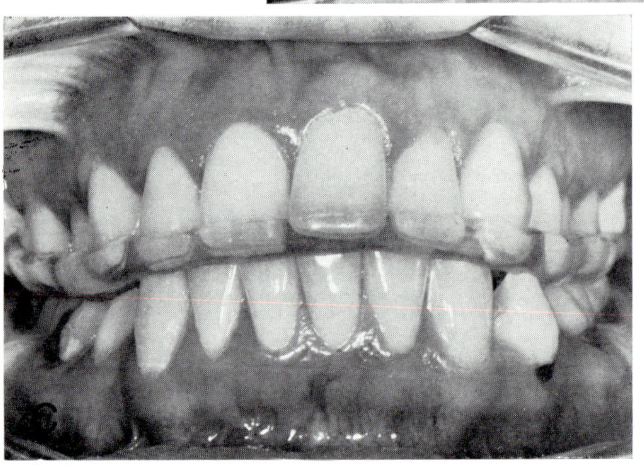

(*Fig.* 89)

very serious cases. Bilateral condylectomy cannot be performed because the lower jaw would be displaced backwards.

Rheumatoid Arthritis.—Rheumatoid arthritis of the temporo-mandibular joint usually occurs only when the disease is already diagnosed in other joints (hands, feet). When both temporomandi-bular joints (pain, stiffness; no clicking) are involved, the symptoms vary simultaneously as those in other joints. The disease is nearly always bilateral. Radiographically the temporomandibular joint may finally show extensive defects (*Fig.* 90). Its function remains good in most cases; ankylosis does not occur. During acute phases, besides the normal general treatment, corticosteroids can be injected intra-articularly. Stiffness may be treated by mouth-opening exercises and the application of heat. It is of great importance to ensure a good occlusion of the dentition as well as adequate rest of the joints (*see above*).

Rheumatoid arthritis occurring at a very young age may cause serious growth disturbance of the mandible, because the articular cartilage, being its growth centre, is destroyed by the rheumatic inflammation. The result may be an underdeveloped mandible with conspicuous retrusion of the chin ('rheumatic bird-face').

Ankylosing Spondylitis.—In very rare cases the first symptoms of Bechterew's disease may be stiffness of both temporomandibular joints. Usually there is no preceding period in which clicking is the main symptom. Within a very short time radiographic alterations occur in both joints. In addition to the general therapy of the disease, treatment should consist of exercises aimed at stretch-ing the mouth as far as possible in order to postpone complete trismus, which may be the ultimate result, as long as possible.

Ankylosis.—Ankylosis of the temporomandibular joint at a young age does not only cause a serious reduction of the masticatory capacity, but also a growth disturbance of the whole facial skeleton on the involved side (*Fig.* 91). As the mouth cannot be opened, keeping the oral cavity in a good hygienic condition causes many

---

Fig. 89.—a, Occlusal splint of clear acrylic in the upper jaw, in order to relieve the temporomandibular joint. b, The upper incisors are just en-veloped. c, Occlusal splint during occlusion.

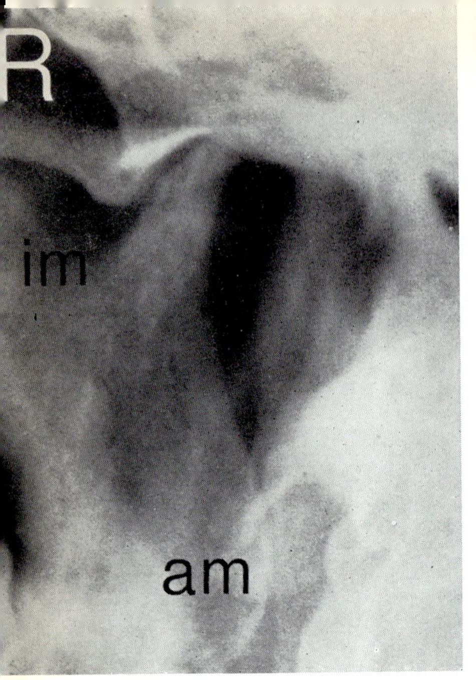
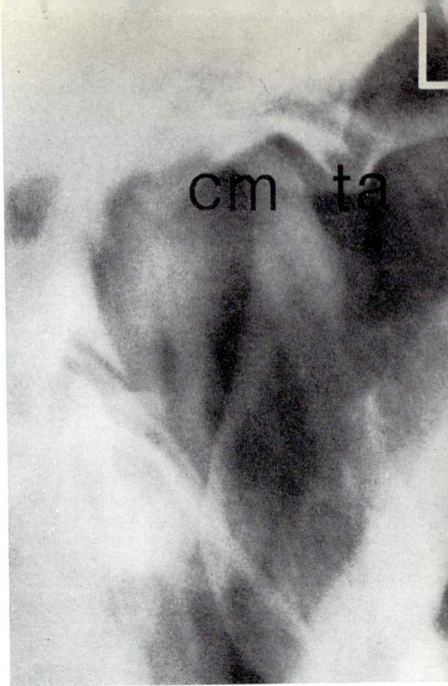

Fig. 90.—Rheumatoid arthritis (Parma's contact radiograph) of both temporomandibular joints in a 39-year-old female patient. Marked flattening of the mandibular heads (cm), shortening of the ascending ramus and stretching of the mandibular hiatus (im). The condylar heads do not reach the top of the articular tubercle when opening the mouth (ta) (am=mandibular angle).

difficulties. Treatment of inflammation, if any, originating from either the dentition or tonsils, is also very difficult. Ankylosis may be caused by trauma of the joint with an intra-articular fracture, osteomyelitis of the mandibular ramus, spreading to the condylar head and the joint, or by an arthritis, following extension of an otitis into the joint.

It may be possible to create a pseudoarthrosis by removing the fused condylar head, the widened mandibular neck, and upper part of the ascending ramus. The distance between the rest of the mandibular ramus and the base of the skull has to be at least 1 cm. to prevent recurrence. Usually this operation is not performed before growth on the affected side has ceased. An active, prolonged after-treatment is very important to prevent recurrence.

Luxation.—Luxation of the mandibular joint may occur in patients with flaccid ligaments or shallow articular fossae when they open the mouth maximally (yawning, vomiting, intubation for

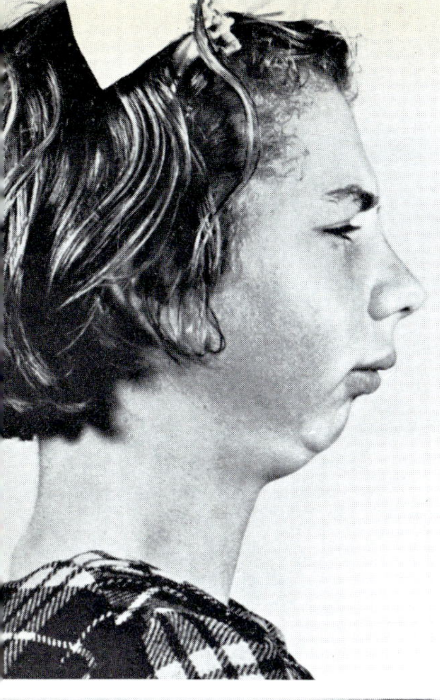

Fig. 91.—a, Ankylosis of the left temporomandibular joint in a 13-year-old girl, originating from an otitis at the age of 12 months. Conspicuous underdeveloped mandible and obliqueness of the face. b, Lateral oblique projection showing a wide ankylosis (*see* black arrows). Just anterior to the mandibular angle (am) is a notch in the lower mandibular border (*see* white arrow); this picture is of common occurrence in a case of under-development.

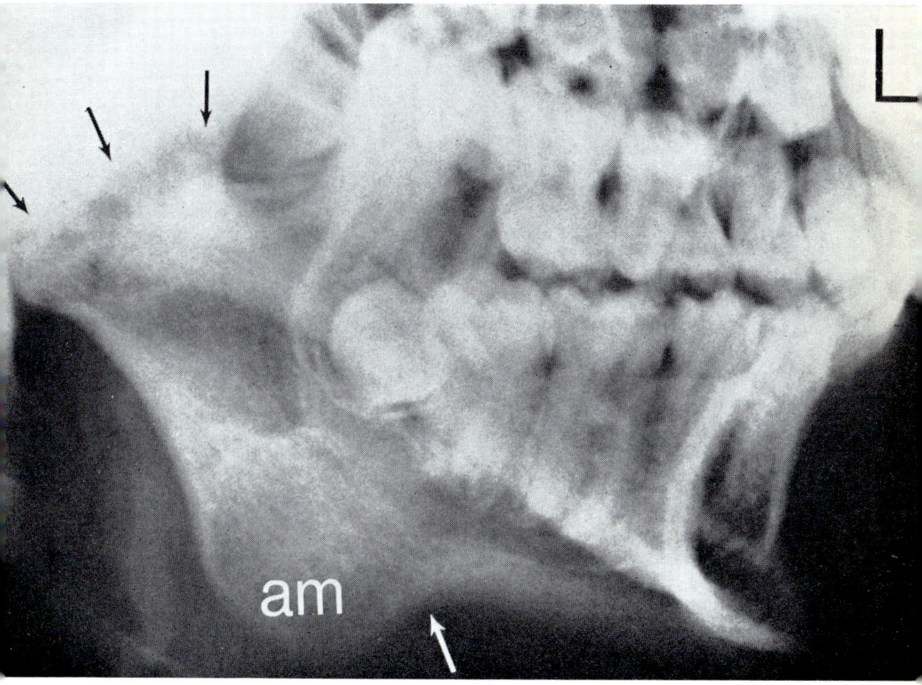

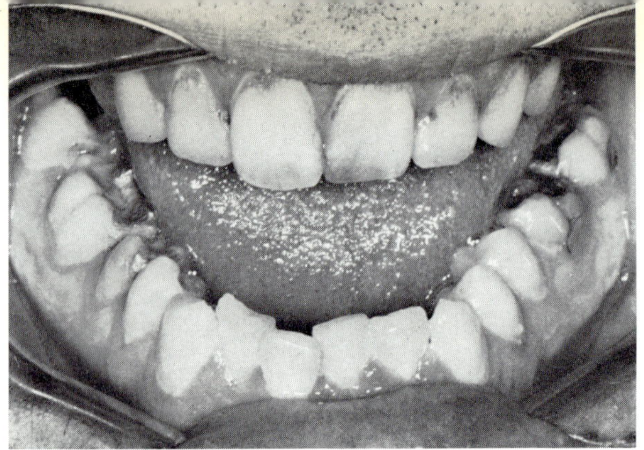

Fig. 92.—Luxation of both temporomandibular joints in a 32-year-old man. Characteristic anterior position of the mandible with open bite. In this patient repositioning was done under general anaesthesia. Fixation by a plaster-of-Paris head-cap.

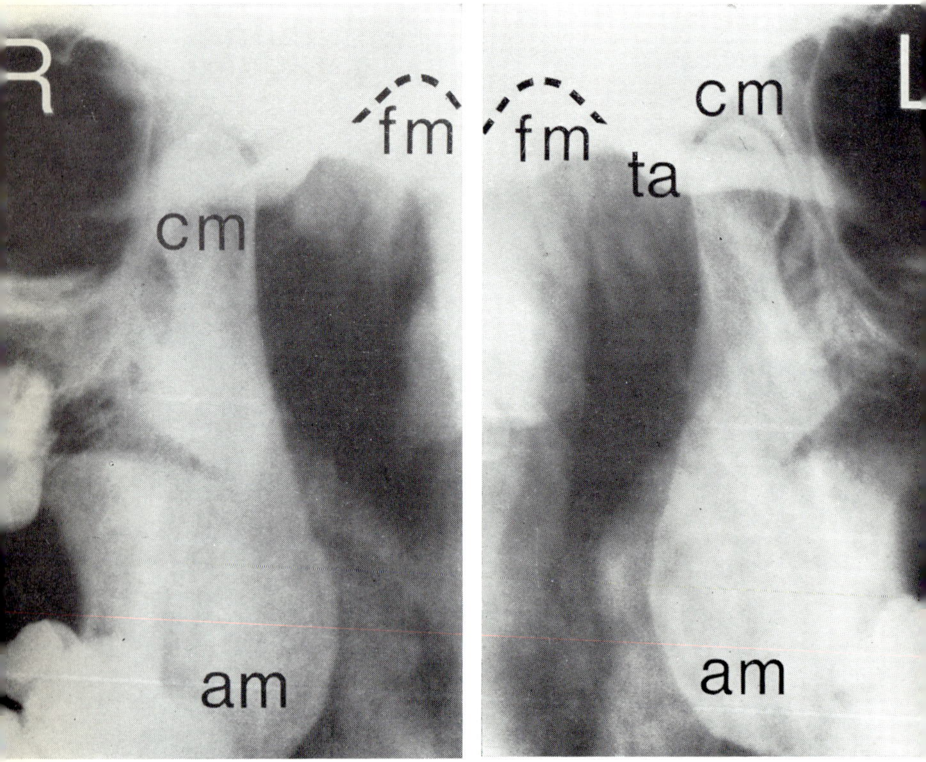

Fig. 93.—Contact radiograph (Parma) of both luxated joints. The condylar heads (cm) are located anterior to the articular tubercle (ta) and are displaced in an upward direction (fm=mandibular fossa).

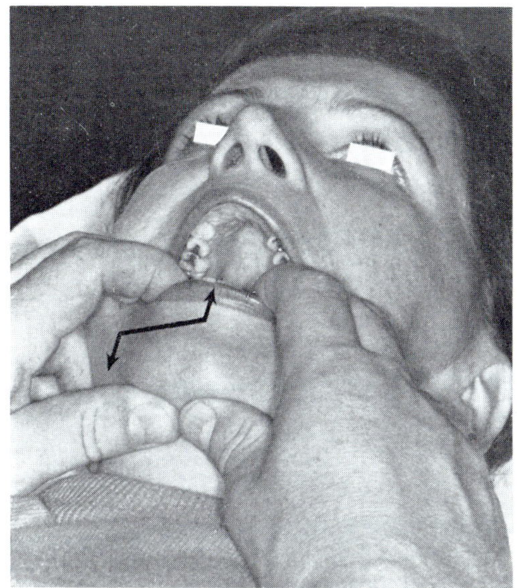

Fig. 94.—Repositioning of a luxation of the mandible.

general anaesthesia, throat inspection, bronchoscopy, dental treatment) (*Figs.* 92 and 93). Repositioning can best be done in the recumbent patient by exerting pressure on either side on the occlusal plane of the lower molars in a caudal direction and pushing the chin with the fingers in a cranial direction (thumbs under the chin) (*Fig.* 94). At the same time the luxated side of the mandible is pushed in a dorsal direction. In the case of bilateral luxation it is advisable to reposition one joint first and the other afterwards. If repositioning is painful periarticular infiltration by a local anaesthetic is advisable (2 ml. 2 per cent lidocaine hydrochloride), after which accompanying muscle spasm is eliminated. After repositioning, the mandible may be immobilized for some time and the patient is given the advice to be very careful for about 1 or 2 months when opening the mouth. Operative treatment is seldom indicated.

Contusion.—If the temporomandibular joint is painful and swollen after trauma and the surrounding tissues swollen, and there are no injuries visible on the radiograph, the lesion is a contusion. Treatment consists of rest (soft food, limited opening) and infra-red application. The prognosis is good.

Congenital Lesions.—*Aplasia of the temporomandibular joint* may occur as part of mandibulofacial dysostosis.

Unilateral hyperplasia of the head of the mandible may lead to obliqueness of the facial skeleton. In most cases this unilateral excessive growth ceases after puberty. Deformation of the face may be prevented by extirpation of the rapidly growing mandibular head (control radiographs).

Unilateral or bilateral hypertrophy of the coronoid process may impede mandibular opening movements, because this process affects almost immediately the facies temporalis of the zygomatic bone and cannot move along the crista zygomatico-alveolaris.

CHAPTER 4

THE ORAL MUCOSA

Introduction.—Variations in colour, such as those occurring in anaemia, cyanosis, and icterus, are often clearly recognizable from inspection of the oral mucosa. Addison's disease can be detected from the presence of spotted and striped melanin pigmentation of the buccal mucous membrane.

The Peutz-Jeghers syndrome is characterized by melanin pigmentation around the mouth and on the mucous membrane of lips and cheeks at birth or shortly afterwards. Later, gastro-intestinal polyposis occurs.

Fordyce Spots.—In many people small, yellowish-grey, granular structures occur under the oral mucosa of the inner side of the lips and under the buccal mucous membrane. The granules are small sebaceous glands, showing the ectodermal origin of the greater part of the epithelium of the oral cavity. The lesions are harmless and they should be left untreated (*Fig.* 95).

Hyperkeratosis.—Local keratosis of the oral mucosa (cheeks, lips, buccal sulcus, floor of the mouth, tongue) causes a superficial, smooth, often rather well-demarcated, white discoloration, which cannot be wiped off.

Hyperkeratosis affecting the inner side of the corner of the mouth is sometimes associated with a superinfection with *Candida albicans*. Treating these yeast-like fungi changes the clinical picture of the disease favourably (*see* p. 126). Local irritating factors originating from the dentition or caused by tobacco chewing or smoking must be eliminated, after which the lesion usually disappears in the course of some months. Clinical control is necessary because the picture may resemble a flat type of leucoplakia; if the lesion does not disappear, a biopsy must be taken (*Figs.* 96 and 97).

Leucoplakia.—By this term is meant local hyperkeratosis of the oral mucosa causing white discoloration, which is painless, cannot be scraped off, and does not belong to a known disease (*see* p. 121). Clinically there is no marked difference with the preceding lesion except that this lesion does not disappear when a suspected local irritation is eliminated.

Clinically three groups can be distinguished:—

First, the flat and mostly very extensive type, which has a smooth surface, is benign, when there are no further alterations (*Fig.* 98).

Secondly, there is the so-called 'speckled-type' leucoplakia, characterized by white speckles of abnormal keratosis on a red ground, resulting from local total or partial lack of epithelium (*Fig.* 99 a). Some authors hold the opinion that this picture may result from a superinfection with *Candida albicans*.

Thirdly, there is the verrucous form of leucoplakia with marked keratosis and an irregular surface with elevations and fissures (*Fig.* 99 b).

The latter two forms are considered to be premalignant (carcinoma planocellulare). Fortunately the lesion is of rather rare incidence (*see also Fig.* 131). Taking a biopsy specimen and maintaining permanent clinical control are necessary. Therapy consists of superficial excision when only a small area is concerned (stripping). Larger areas can be excised in several stages. In very extensive lesions difficulties will arise and treatment has to be limited to the most suspect areas. It stands to reason that these methods of treatment are only permitted if malignancy is excluded. It is impossible to resist the impression that in some patients there is a certain predisposition of the oral mucosa for leucoplakia. They often suffer from xerostomia and the uncornified mucosa is thin, smooth, and atrophic (cf. hypochromic anaemia).

Administration of high doses of vitamin A, if desired in combination with vitamin E, may make a severe keratosis disappear. Local treatment with corticosteroids is sometimes recommended. The initially favourable result unfortunately does not always persist. Local irritating factors (*see above*) should of course be eliminated (smoking!).

Syphilis as a cause of leucoplakia is not so significant as was generally thought in former times.

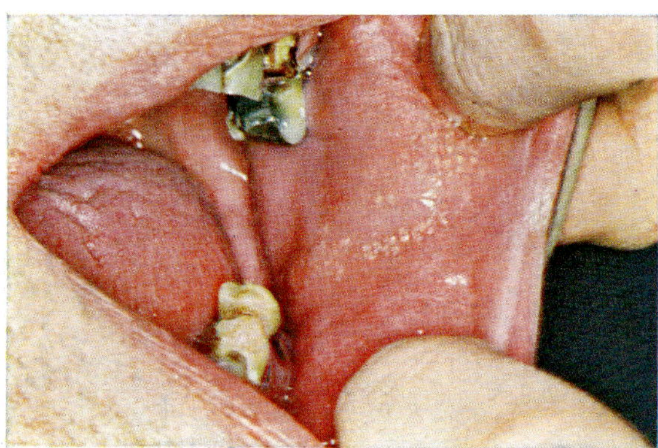

Fig. 95.—Sebaceous glands, visible as yellow spots under the buccal mucosa (Fordyce spots).

Fig. 96.—Retro-angular hyperkeratosis.

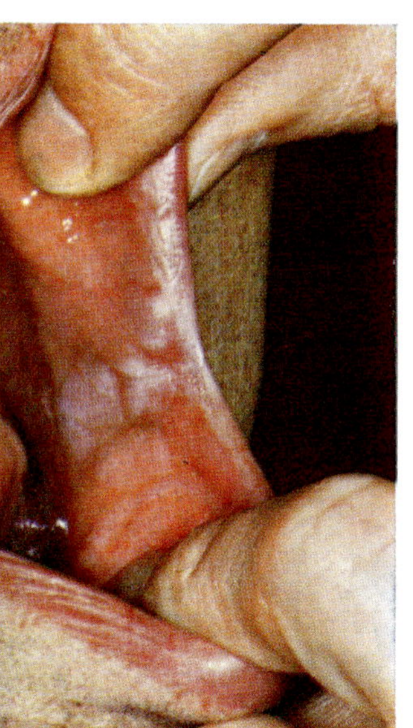

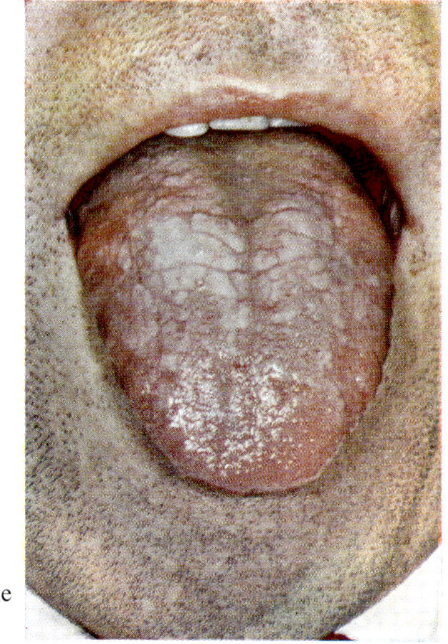

Fig. 97.—Hyperkeratosis of the tongue in a heavy smoker.

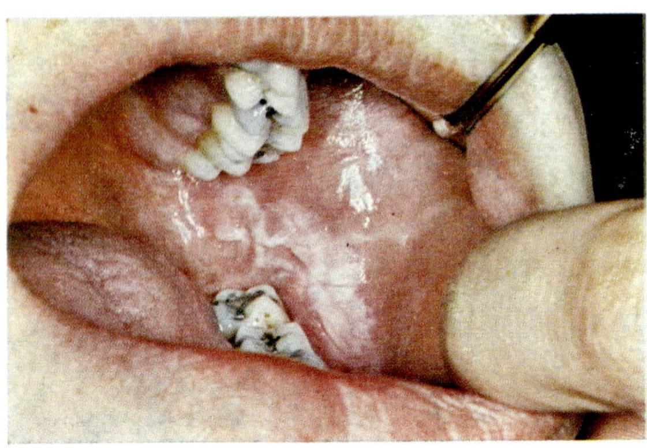

Fig. 98.—Marked hyperkeratosis of the buccal mucosa,
tending to leucoplakia.

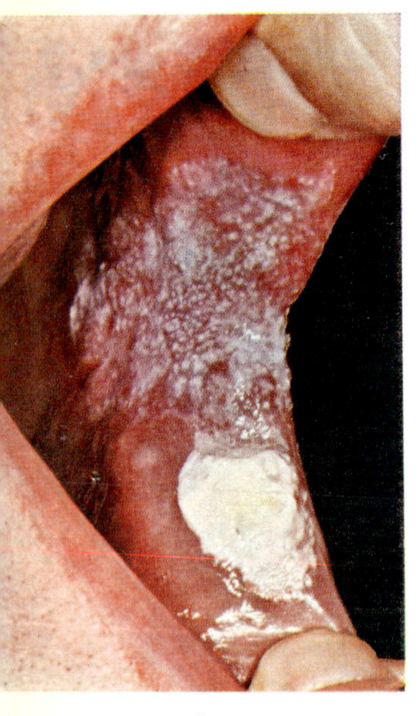

a

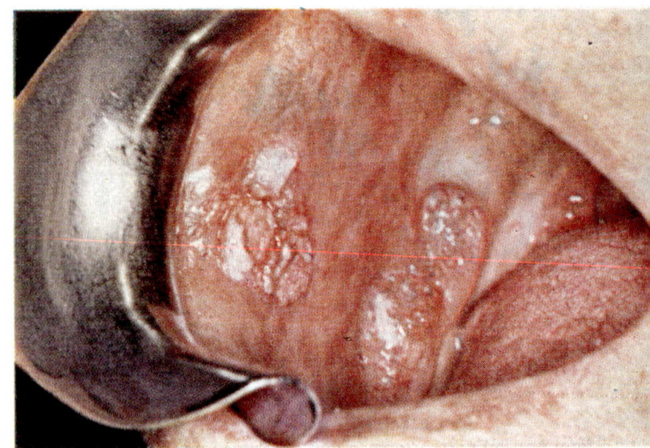

b

Fig. 99.—a, Leucoplakia (speckled type) of the
right buccal mucosa at the level of the corner of
the mouth with a small, strongly keratinized area
at the upper border (58-year-old man). Histopathology: very distinct leucoplakia, much inflammatory infiltrate, a single mitosis, no carcinoma.
Treatment: excision, if desired the wounds can be
covered by a free skin-graft. b, Verrucous leucoplakia
of the buccal mucosa with carcinoma planocellulare.
The lower jaw shows an identical lesion.

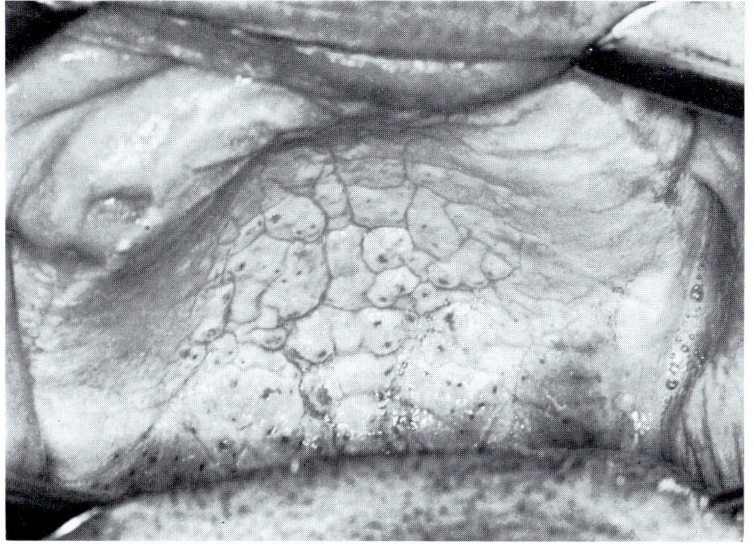

Fig. 100.—Stomatitis nicotina (smoker's palate).

Stomatitis Nicotina.—Excessive smoking may cause hyperkeratosis of the palatal mucosa with swellings of the submucous glands, resulting in a peculiar marbled picture. In the centre of each swelling (inflamed mucous gland) is a red point (inflamed orifice). When passing the edge of a tongue spatula over such a whitish palate, comedo-like plugs of purulent material appear. Though the lesion is classed as leucoplakia, it is not premalignant. Prognosis is generally good if smoking is limited drastically or is completely stopped (*Fig.* 100).

Lichen Planus.—In about 30 per cent of all patients lichen planus occurs alone in the oral cavity, and does not involve the skin. When involving the skin lichen planus appears as salmon-red, polygonal, flat papules with an initially marked predilection for the volar side of the wrists and the adjacent part of the forearm. Other affected sites may be the body (especially abdomen and loins), lower part of the legs, and the penis. Lichen planus is one of the few pure papular lesions of the skin. The lesion is of rather rare

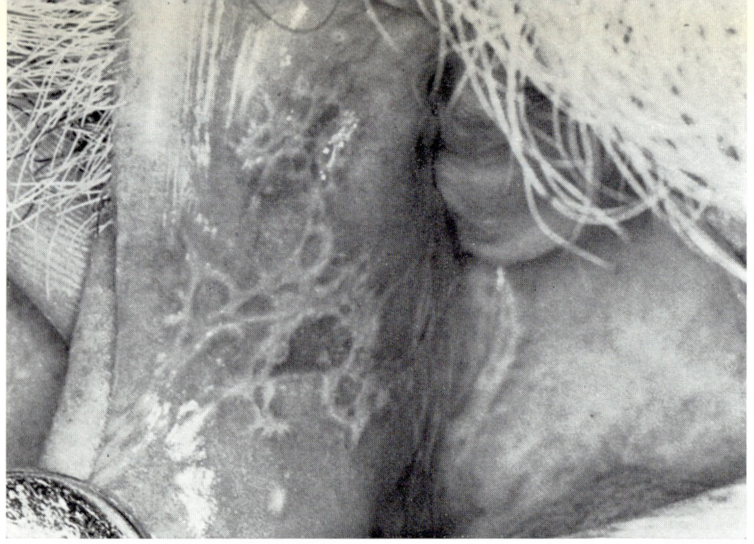

Fig. 101.—Reticular type of lichen planus on the buccal mucosa. Symmetrical appearance on the left and right.

incidence in the oral cavity. Generally two types are to be distinguished:—

First, there is the *hyperkeratotic type*, associated with a white lace-like pattern and patches on the buccal mucosa (*Fig.* 101). In some cases the picture may be fine reticulated patches (*Fig.* 102), sometimes the lesion appears as papules or plaques (*Fig.* 103), while in very rare cases white ring-like structures occur (annular type) (*Fig.* 104).

Secondly, there is the *erosive type*, which may be very troublesome for the patient (*Fig.* 105). It is characteristic that both types are of almost symmetrical appearance in the oral cavity, in contrast to leucoplakia.

Differential diagnosis may give rise to difficulties. In these cases biopsy is necessary. In the case of lichen planus there is a band-like inflammatory infiltrate just under the lesion. Treatment of the hyperkeratotic type is not required and of the erosive type only in cases of marked complaints. As the aetiology is still unknown, appropriate treatment is not easy. In former times arsenic and bismuth were administered; at present vitamins, sedatives, and corticosteroids are prescribed. Hydrocortisone lozenges or submucous injections of this hormone under the lesion are sometimes

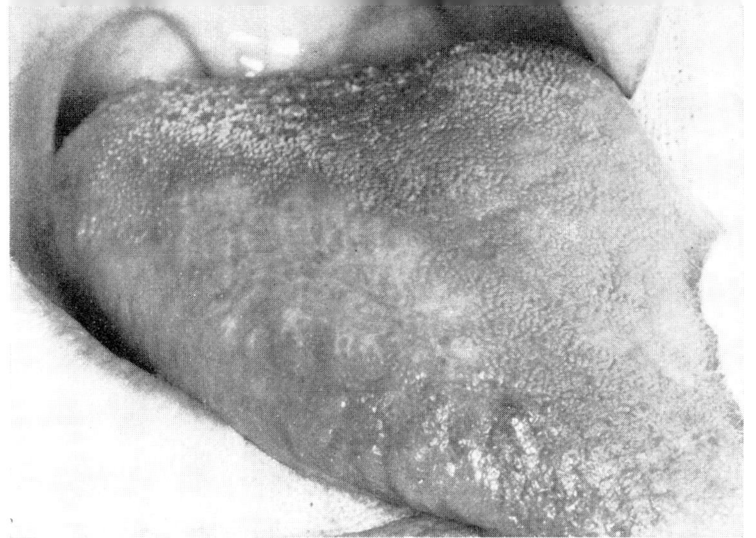

Fig. 102.—Fine-reticulated type of lichen planus on the tongue.

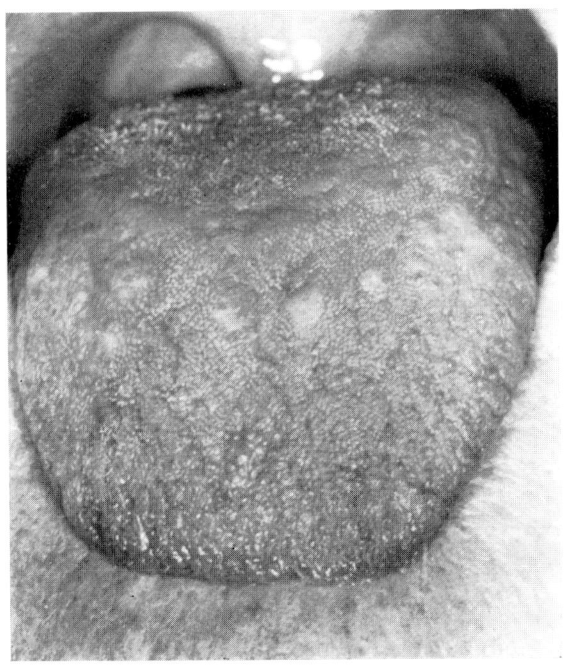

Fig. 103.—Plaque and papular type of lichen planus.

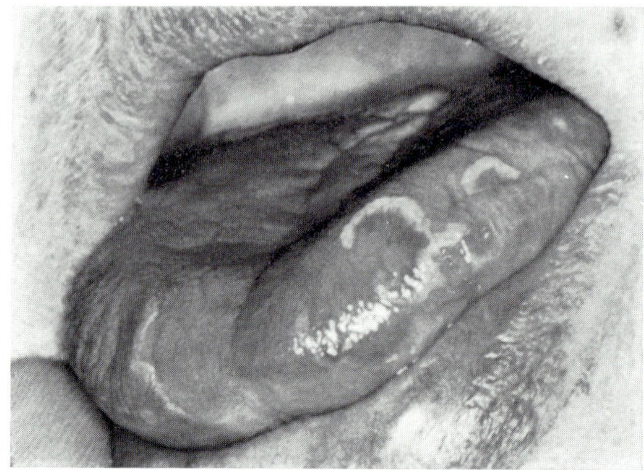

Fig. 104.—Annular type of lichen planus.

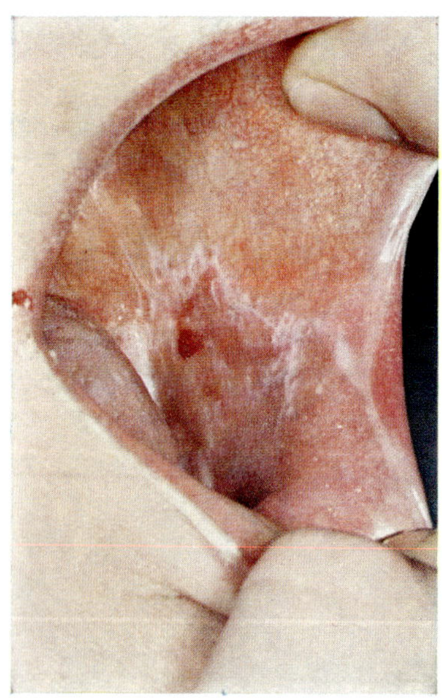

Fig. 105.—Erosive type of lichen planus. The reticular type occurs along its peripheral border.

advised. In the case of the erosive type Kenalog (triamcinolone acetonide) in Orabase may be applied.

Moniliasis (Candidiasis).—Moniliasis of the oral cavity, caused by the yeast-like fungus *Candida albicans*, is characterized by flaky white patches, mostly somewhat elevated and consisting of merged colonies of *Candida*. Around the periphery solitary colonies can be observed (*Fig.* 106). It is difficult to wipe off the white patches; they

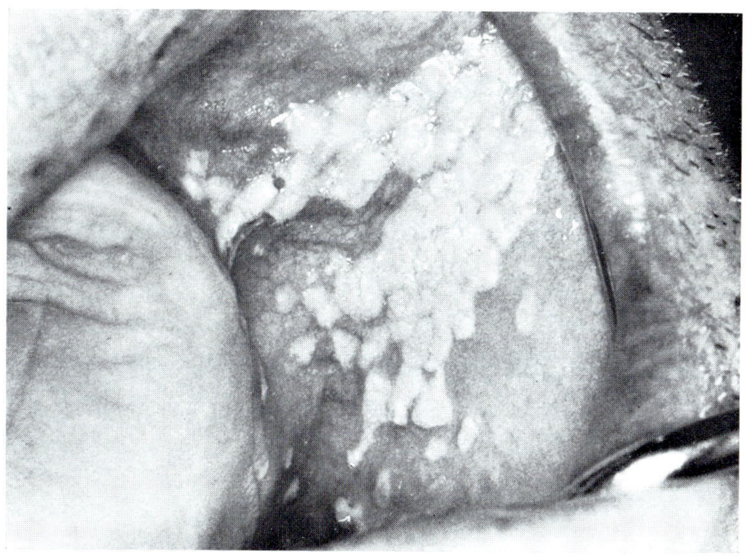

Fig. 106.—Acute *Candida albicans* infection of the buccal mucosa in a 51-year-old patient with carcinoma of the upper jaw. Healing within 5 days by painting with gentian violet.

leave a lightly bleeding erosive surface. A dense network of *Candida* organisms in the form of hyphae and spores can be demonstrated microscopically by adding a drop of a 10 per cent potassium hydro-oxide solution to a specimen on a slide and heating gently.

The lesions occur in very young children and in adults who are debilitated owing to, for instance, diabetes or treatment with cyto-statics, or when the balance of the oral flora is disturbed owing to prolonged administration of antibiotics. *Candida albicans* is resistant to antibiotics and therefore its growth is favoured when, due to use of antibiotics, the normal microbiotic balance is disturbed. The fungus *Candida albicans* is often seen under dentures and in the corners of the mouth, where rhagades occur. Common complaints are a burning or itching sensation and pain, often combined with xerostomia.

Treatment of moniliasis (thrush) may consist of painting or spraying with a 0·5 per cent solution of gentian violet in water. Recently local application of the antibiotic fungicidin (nystatin) in the form of ointment, cream, or a suspension has been recommended (rinsing with a suspension of 100,000 units per ml. four times a day until healing is complete). Good results can also be obtained with natamycin (Pimaricin, Pimafucin) 2 per cent as ointment and amphotericin-B as cream 3 per cent (Fungizone).

Aphthae.—Aphthous ulcers are usually small (3–5 mm.), sharply demarcated, practically round, with a scarlet, non-elevated margin, and covered with a yellowish-grey layer. The lesion is very painful, especially in the early stages. Generally the lesion occurs solitarily, but multiple lesions are known (aphthous stomatitis). The latter form may be very troublesome when eating, speaking, or swallowing. The form and size of the ulcers and absence of small speckles around the larger merged defects differentiate between herpetic stomatitis. The lesion is of unknown origin. Some authors are of the opinion that psychological factors, others that food allergy, play a part (nuts, chocolate, mustard, some toothpastes, and so on). A causal therapy is not yet known; the aphthae disappear spontaneously within 10–14 days without leaving scars (*Fig.* 107). Treatment of solitary, very painful lesions may consist of the application of 5 per cent phenol, with Pyralvex Berna,* or a viscous solution of lidocaine hydrochloride 2 per cent or Kenalog in Orabase.† Treatment is mainly aimed at the relief of pain. In multiple or frequently occurring very large and painful aphthae hydrocortisone-sodium-hemisuccinate lozenges can be prescribed in order to decrease

---

* The following prescription may be used: Acid. salicyclic. 900 mg.; extract aloes aq. sicc. 900 mg.; spirit dil. ad 30 ml.

† The following prescription may be used: Lidocaine hydrochloridum 600 mg.; methylcellulosum 400 centipoise 600 mg.; aqua ad 30 ml.

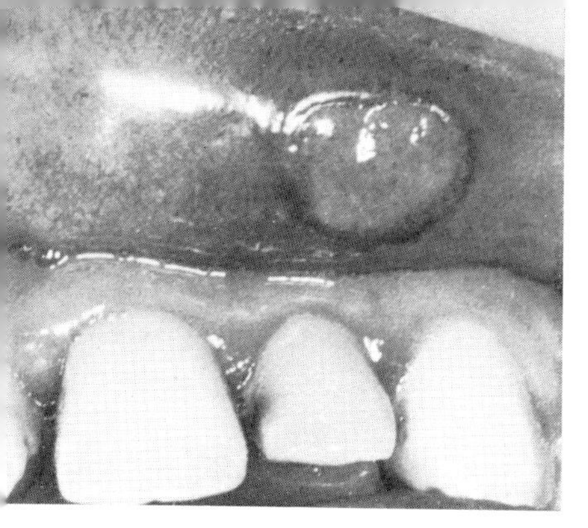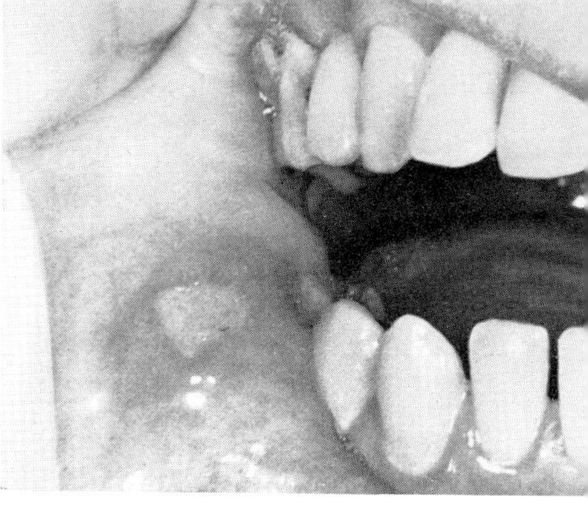

a   b

Fig. 107.—a, Big aphthous ulcer on the upper lip. b, Healing aphthous ulcer.

the inflammatory symptoms. The dose is a maximum of 10 mg. (= 4 tablets) per day, for 2–4 weeks. The lozenges should be sucked as close as possible to the lesion in the mouth. Recurrences are seen, notwithstanding the use of lozenges for months. Continuous prophylactic dosage must be kept as low as possible. Initially 2 lozenges (of 2·5 mg. each) per day can be prescribed, which number may, if necessary, be increased to 4 lozenges a day. Caution has to be observed when using this long-lasting hormonal medication. An effective therapy, excluding recurrences, is unknown. The patient may be warned of a possible connexion between the occurrence of aphthae and certain foods taken in the preceding 2 or 3 weeks, so that he can avoid those foods afterwards.

Erythema Exudativum Multiforme.—On the skin this disease has a multiform character with, as a rule, annular rash, often with centrally or peripherally a circular vesicle. Sites of predilection of the lesions are hands, back of the feet, forearms, knees, left and right sides of the neck, and the face. Sometimes the eruption of the lesions on the skin is associated with a feeling of illness.

The lesion in the oral cavity usually starts as a vesicle, usually rupturing early. Multiple and rather large and irregular superficial mucosal defects covered by a fibrinous layer, often symmetrical and mainly occurring on the lips, dominate the clinical picture (*Figs.* 108 and 109).

The Stevens-Johnson syndrome, which is definitely related to erythema exudativum multiforme and is also called ectodermosis

127

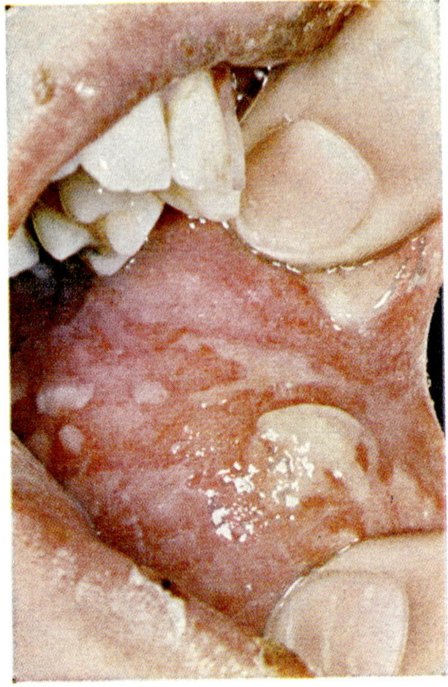

Fig. 108.—Erythema exudativum multiforme on cheeks and lips.

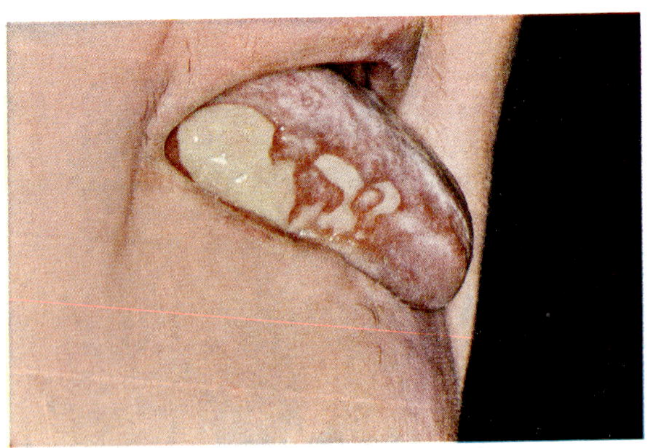

Fig. 109.—Erythema exudativum multiforme on the tongue.

erosiva pluriorificialis, shows foci on the mucosa of mouth, nose, eyes, and genitalia, with the formation of a tough, mucous secretion, which leads especially in the mouth to the formation of diphtheria-like false membranes. The origin of the disease is generally unknown; treatment is given by a dermatologist.

Herpes.—Herpes may occur as herpes labialis or as herpetic gingivostomatitis. Herpes labialis is known as 'fever blister' and may occur during periods of lowered resistance.

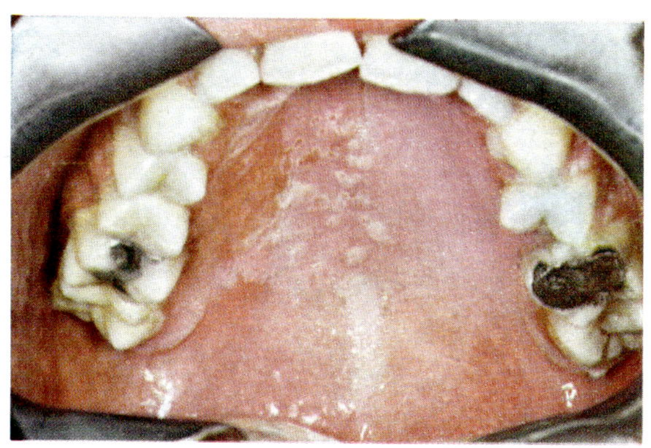

Fig. 110.—Herpetic vesicles shortly after appearance.

Herpes labialis is almost always a recurrence. Lesions of herpetic gingivostomatitis occur anywhere in the oral cavity (gingiva, tongue, palate, cheek). Vesicles are hardly ever seen, because they rupture soon after appearance (*Fig.* 110). In most cases the mucous membrane is covered with very small yellowish-grey ulcers (much smaller than aphthous ulcers) with a red margin and with a tendency to merge into irregular patterns (*Fig.* 111). Solitary lesions are seen along the periphery (*see also Fig.* 136).

The lesions are very painful. The highest incidence is seen in very young children. Usually an initial contact with the herpes virus is concerned. Herpetic gingivostomatitis in its very extensive form does not recur as such, but normally in the form of a more localized lesion or as herpes labialis. The diagnosis may be confirmed

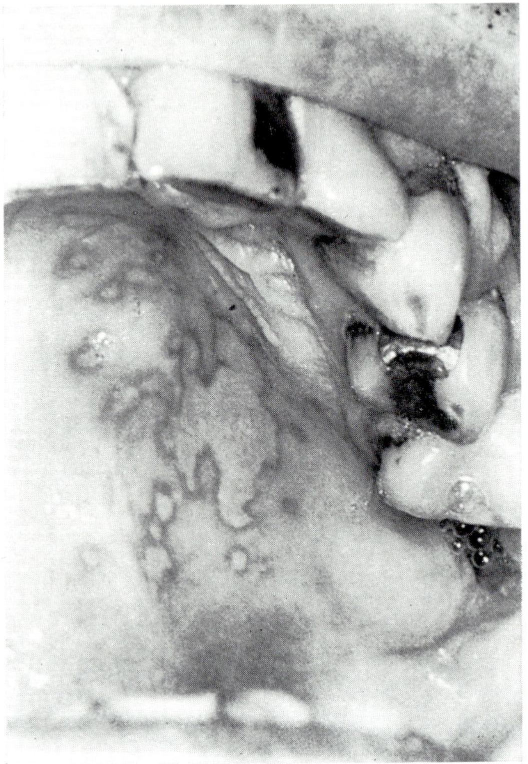

Fig. 111.—Small herpetic ulcers merged into irregular structures with peripheral solitary lesions.

by virus culture and serological investigation. Early in the initial stage the lesions cause a gross lymphadenopathy, which may remain for a very long time. The herpes virus cannot readily be influenced therapeutically. Generally, treatment can only be palliative: good oral hygiene and in very serious cases bed-rest and local application of an analgesic (viscous solution of lidocaine hydrochloride). Application of idoxuridine in ointment (0·5 per cent) is sometimes advised. Experience with this medicament in the oral cavity is limited. It is mainly used to treat viral infections in ophthalmology.

After 3 days (spontaneous) healing begins, to be complete within 7–14 days.

Inflammations following Administration of Drugs.—Patients treated for a long time (and sometimes even after a short period) with orally administered antibiotics may show stomatitis-like lesions. The mucous membrane is red and the epithelium gives an atrophic impression. The tongue is red, painful, and smooth owing to loss of filiform papillae.

The real origin is unknown. Presumably *Candida albicans* plays a part though no marked colonies are to be seen. The concurrent incidence of perlèches in the corners of the mouth (which may also be caused by *Candida albicans*) makes some authors think of vitamin-B deficiency (suppression of intestinal flora). Tetracyclines are considered to have a direct effect on epithelial cells by influencing the enzyme system, in which lactoflavin plays a part. Therapy must include the treatment of *Candida albicans*.

Treatment with cytotoxic drugs may cause serious stomatitides. *Candida albicans* plays a part in some of them. A serious stomatitis is sometimes considered a favourable sign in the treatment of malignant lesions.

Denture Sore Mouth.—By this term is understood a painful and burning mucosa under a prosthesis. It is a very troublesome lesion, mainly occurring under the upper denture. Sometimes the mucosa is fiery red and glassy transparent in appearance; sometimes, however, its aspect is papillomatous (*Figs.* 112 and 114). In some cases no lesions are visible at all. Often the oral cavity of these patients gives a dry impression. It is usually difficult to trace the cause of the lesion. An ill-fitting prosthesis with friction over the mucosa during mastication or during execution of masticatory habits at periods of psychological tension is probably the most common cause. Maceration and infection (*Candida albicans*) of the mucosa under the denture, under which normal cleansing by saliva, tongue, and food is impossible, may play a role. Fungicidin (nystatin) ointment or cream (100,000 units per g., tube à 15 g.) gives relief of complaints if infection with *Candida albicans* plays an important part. Hypersensitivity to the acrylic resin, of which the prosthesis is made, is often mentioned, but is rare (*Fig.* 113). It is also possible that this hypersensitivity may be related to the bacterial plaque occurring

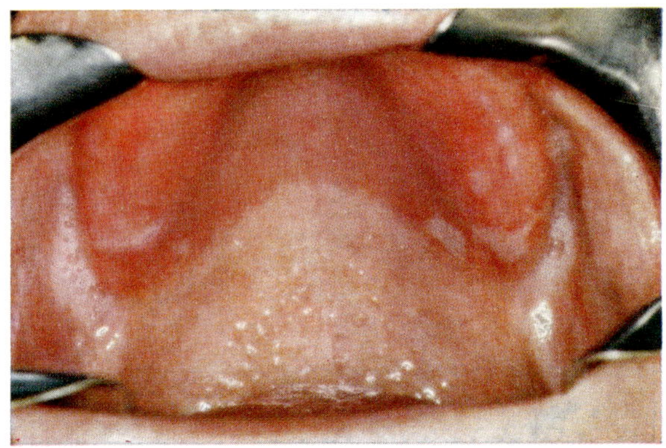

Fig. 112.—Denture sore mouth.

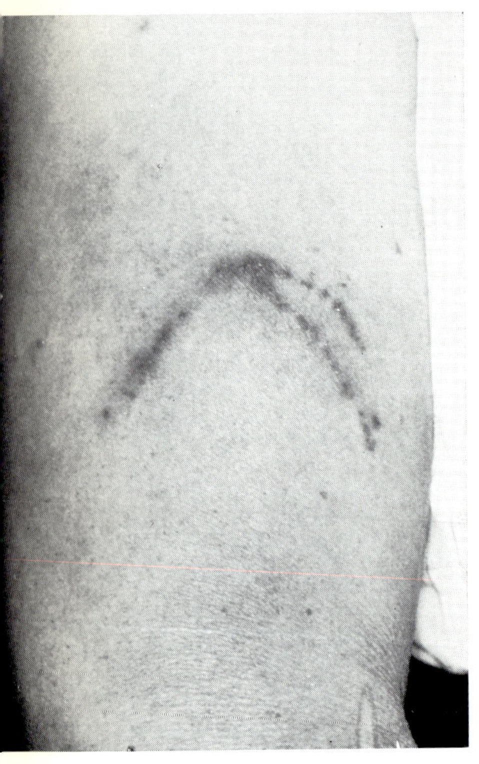

Fig. 113.—Allergic reaction of the upper arm appearing as small vesicles and hyperaemia after the patient had kept her prosthesis there for 24 hours by means of a wet bandage.

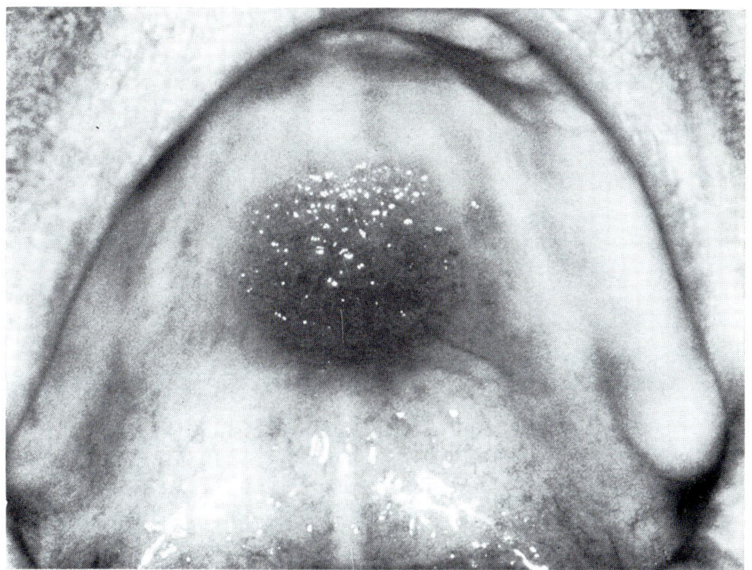

Fig. 114.—Papillary hyperplasia of the palatal mucosa, generally caused by ill-fitting dentures. Treatment consists of correcting the prosthesis and, in serious cases, of excision of the whole papillary area.

on the prosthesis. Disinfection of the prosthesis during the night, after good mechanical cleaning, should also be employed. When the effect is negative, it is advisable to make a well-fitting prosthesis of a totally different plastic, for instance of Luxene, a synthetic resin in a polyvinyl base (manufactured by Hownet) or Andoran (Bayer). Occasionally one has the impression that psychological factors play a part.

If, notwithstanding correction of the prosthesis and therapy directed to *Candida albicans*, the burning sensation remains, this may be controlled by corticosteroids in ointment or in a substance adhering to the oral mucosa (Kenalog in Orabase).

Rhagades.—Wet, inflamed corners of the mouth may be caused by either general or local factors. General factors are: vitamin-B deficiency (ariboflavinosis) and hypochromic anaemia due to an

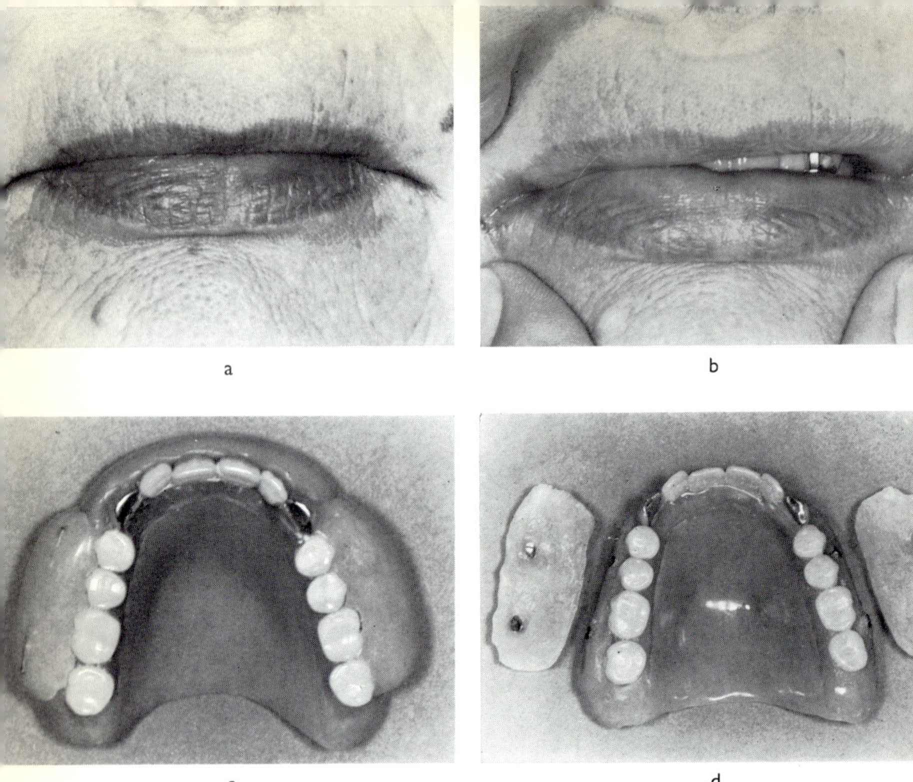

Fig. 115.—a, b, Very deep rhagades owing to wearing a prosthesis of insufficient vertical dimension and inadequate cheek and lip 'filling'. c, d, Prosthesis extended in width by means of detachable extensions, and aimed at adequate stretching of the corners of the mouth so that they remain dry and will heal (Berendsen's method). The extensions are worn during the night and at daytime as often as possible. After healing an adapted prosthesis has to be made.

iron deficiency. Amongst local factors are included: leakage of saliva from the angles of the mouth and the habit of continuous licking the corners of the mouth. In most cases, however, the lesions occur in patients wearing a prosthesis of insufficient vertical dimension with insufficient 'filling' of cheeks and lips, causing inadequate stretching of the buccinator muscle. The angles of the mouth are insufficiently stretched and remain continuously moist. Superinfection with *Candida albicans* may be present. If the rhagades are caused by an unsatisfactory prosthesis therapy consists of making

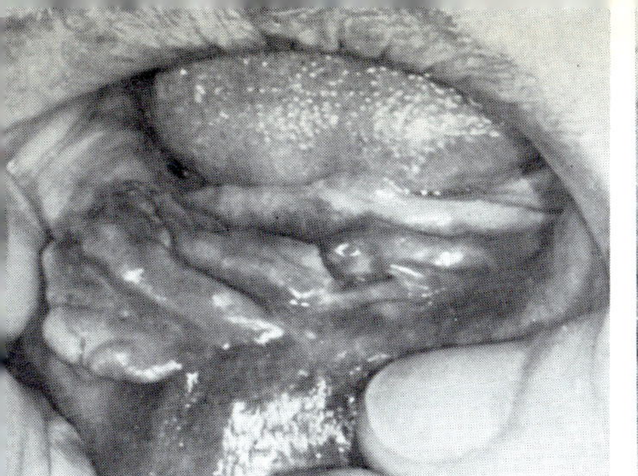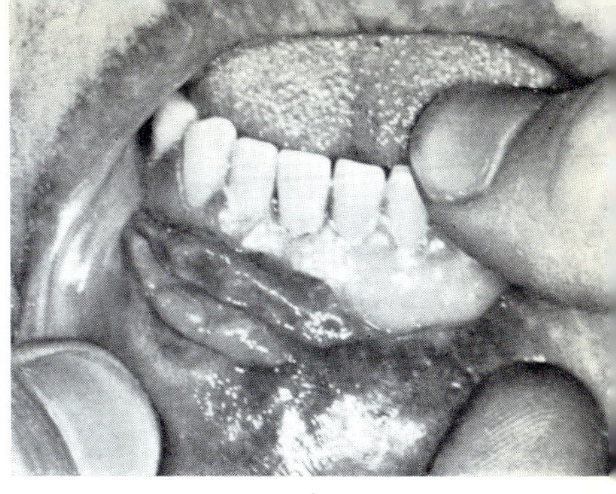

a   b

Fig. 116.—a, Irritation fibromas owing to an ill-fitting lower denture. b, The relation is shown between the border of the prosthesis and the fibromas.

another prosthesis with adequate lip- and cheek-filling (good tonus of the buccinator muscle and stretching of the folds in the corners of the mouth) with a good vertical dimension, and finally of treatment of the *Candida albicans* infection by antibiotics with a local effect in a cream or ointment base (nystatin, pimaricin, amphotericin B). The longer the rhagades exist the more difficult treatment will be. In persistent cases it may be necessary to provide the buccal side of the lower and upper denture in the premolar region with temporary and detachable extensions in order to stretch the folds of the corners of the mouth completely, so that they will remain dry (*Fig.* 115).

Decubitus Ulcer and Irritation Fibromas.—A decubitus ulcer owing to irritation by the border of a prosthesis is of common occurrence in the lower jaw. It is an oblong mucosa defect covered by a fibrinous layer, occurring in the buccal sulcus and causing pain if the prosthesis is loaded. It is formed rather rapidly and disappears within some days after correction of the prosthesis. If the irritational factors remain, elevated margins arise labially and lingually of the ulcer, which are the initial stages of irritation fibromas. The latter occur most frequently in the lower buccal sulcus in people with a strongly resorbed alveolar process and an ill-fitting denture and consist of multiple, oblong, parallel, rather firm hyperplasias on the mucous membrane. They are of pale pink colour and painless on palpation (*Fig.* 116). There is no adequate term for this lesion. Synonyms are: irritation fibromas, prosthesis fibromas, fibrosis localis, epulis fissuratum, dentive granuloma, and so on.

135

Treatment of irritation fibromas consists of excision and, of importance in preventing recurrence, correction of the dentures or making new ones. It may be necessary to deepen the buccal sulcus or the floor of the mouth surgically in order to create sufficient retention for the prosthesis.

Traumata.—Traumata of the oral mucosa occur mostly in children who may fall having an oblong object in their mouth (blow-pipe, flute, handle-bar of a scooter, and so on). Treatment is only indicated when the soft palate is perforated, when there are wounds in the dorsal free margin of the soft palate, or in a case of serious haemorrhage. In the case of deeper lesions inspection of the pharynx is necessary.

Burns.—Burns in the mouth may be caused by hot food or drinks or by drinking a caustic fluid. The most serious burns are seen in children who put the loose end of the flex of a vacuum cleaner or an electric iron into their mouth while the other end is still in the socket. Clinical observation of these patients is necessary in connexion with extensive oedema, which may occur sometimes, resulting in respiratory difficulties. It is advisable to decide upon tracheostomy at an early stage.

Chemical burns in the form of white etched spots are sometimes seen in persons suffering from a toothache who have sucked an aspirin tablet.

Tumours of the Oral Mucosa.—
Benign Tumours.—Tumours of the oral mucosa are relatively rare. The following benign tumours can be mentioned: *Papilloma,* white in appearance and having a cauliflower-like aspect (tongue, palate, cheek, and lips) (*Fig.* 117 a); *fibroma* (true fibromas with a marked capsule are rare, generally the lesion is a hyperplasia occurring after irritation), mostly pedunculated, pale in colour, and of rather firm consistency (cheek) (*Figs.* 117 b and 119); *lipoma,* yellowish in appearance and very soft on palpation (many transitional forms occur with more or less fibrous tissue) (*Fig.* 120); *haemangioma,* located in and under the oral mucosa (bluish-red in colour); and *lymphangioma* with a somewhat granular and glassy aspect. Occasionally in patients wearing dentures a very compressed tumour is seen, hanging on a very thin peduncle. Histologically the lesion may be either a small

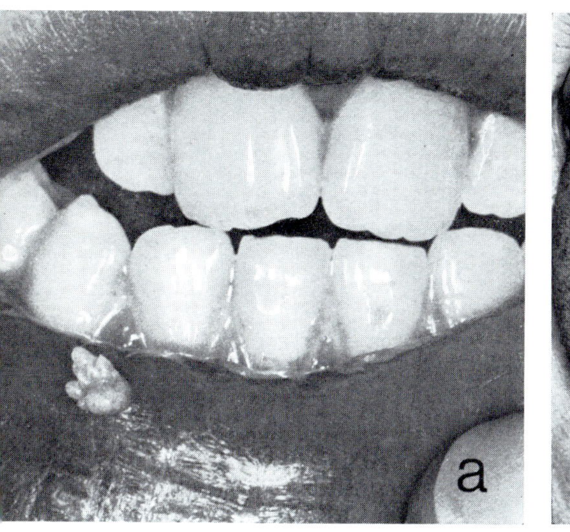
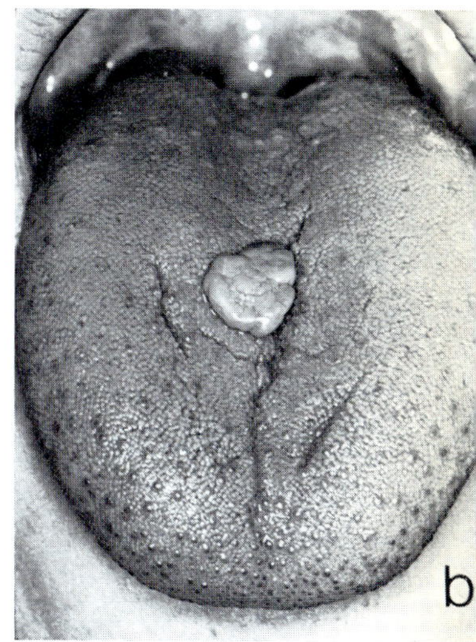

Fig. 117.—a, Papilloma on the lower lip (present for 2 years). b, Small pedunculated fibroma, clinically resembling a papilloma.

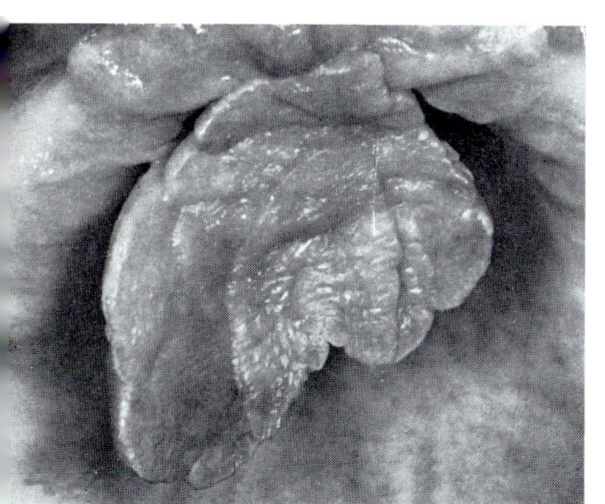
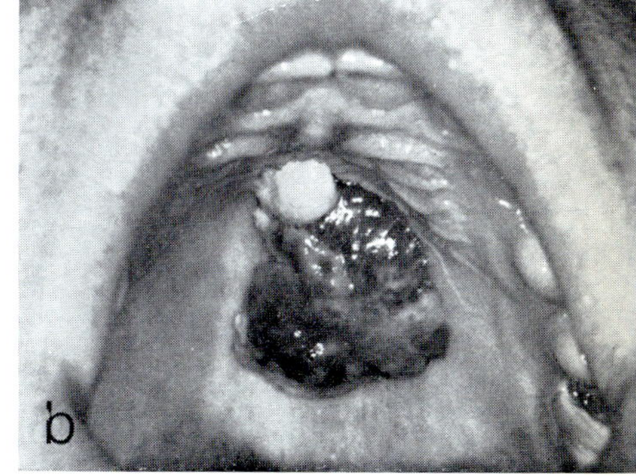

Fig. 118.—a, Small pedunculated fibroma compressed under a prosthesis. b, Granuloma telangiectaticum which has arisen in 4 weeks following injection of a local anaesthetic.

fibroma or a compressed granuloma telangiectaticum (*Fig.* 118). Dorsally on the hard palate a broadly based mixed tumour may occur, originating from a mucous gland, mostly globular in shape with a broad base (1–2 cm. in size), either of firm consistency or fluctuating (cystic) (*Fig.* 121; *see also Fig.* 122).

Treatment of these benign tumours consists of wide excision including the underlying tissue. Though a mixed tumour is a benign lesion, it is widely excised, because of its tendency to recur.

Malignant Tumours.—Carcinoma of the oral mucosa is of the planocellular type. Often the lesion is a very painful ulcer with an elevated margin and a granulomatous, speckled aspect (strawberry-like) (*Figs.* 122 b, 123, 124, and 125). This ulcer is often found on the actual gingiva.

This neoplasm occurs in middle-aged patients and is usually diagnosed late. The lesion fails to heal, even after elimination of any irritating factor. Aetiological factors may be: irritation by sharp teeth edges, sharp edges of a prosthesis, tobacco-chewing, and smoking (pipe and cigars). Initially there is only slight bone resorption; only after some time is irregular bone-resorption visible on the radiograph. *The teeth will get loose.* Extraction is *not* indicated owing to the possibility of metastases occurring. Metastases may occur in the submandibular and cervical lymph-nodes. Early diagnosis is of major importance. Treatment can best be done by an oncological team. The smaller the tumour the less mutilating the operation and the greater the chance that the operation will be successful. Very superficial tumours may be treated by radiation. The patient is advised not to smoke or chew tobacco any more in order to reduce the chance of a recurrence. Multicentric tumours are known (*Fig.* 99 b).

Cylindroma malignum (often classed as adenocarcinoma) originating from a mucous gland and occurring in the transitional area of the hard and soft palate (smooth or nodulous, firm or elastic, with a marked vascular pattern) grows slowly, but is a malignant lesion with regard to its clinical features. The tumour may sometimes be bluish in colour and of rather soft consistency (*see Fig.* 122 a, p. 140). In this case it may be difficult from a diagnostic point of view to differentiate between a benign mixed tumour and a mucous cyst. The cylindroma infiltrates the surrounding structures by means of long extensions (along the perineural lymphatics) and cannot easily be removed completely by excision; moreover, the

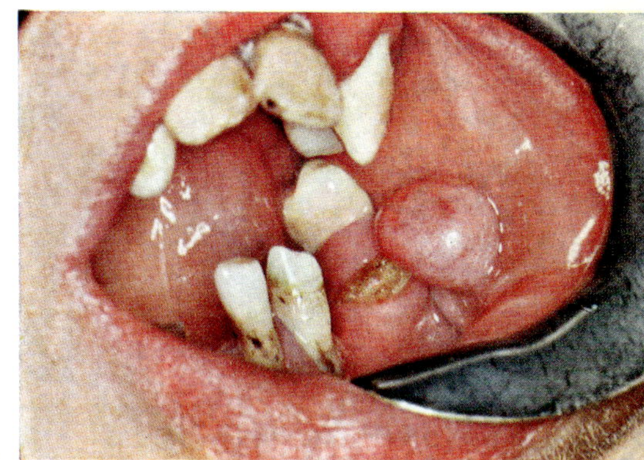

Fig. 119.—Pedunculated fibroma.

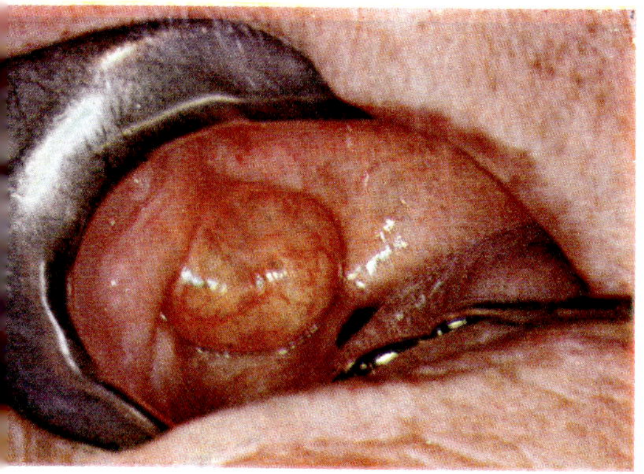

Fig. 120.—Lipoma on the
buccal mucosa.

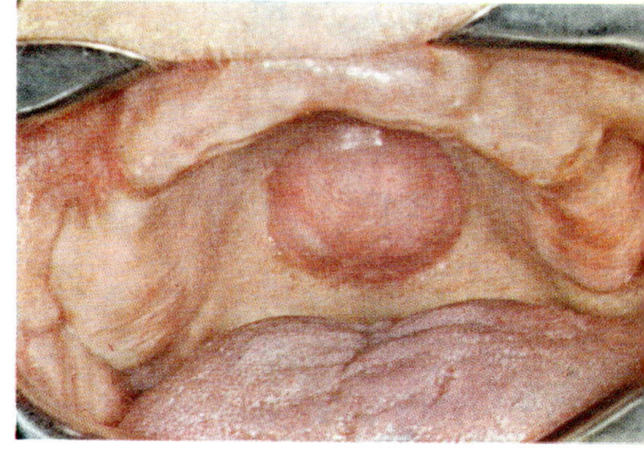

Fig. 121.—Benign mixed tumour
on the palate in a 59-year-old
woman. Soft consistency. Wide
local excision.

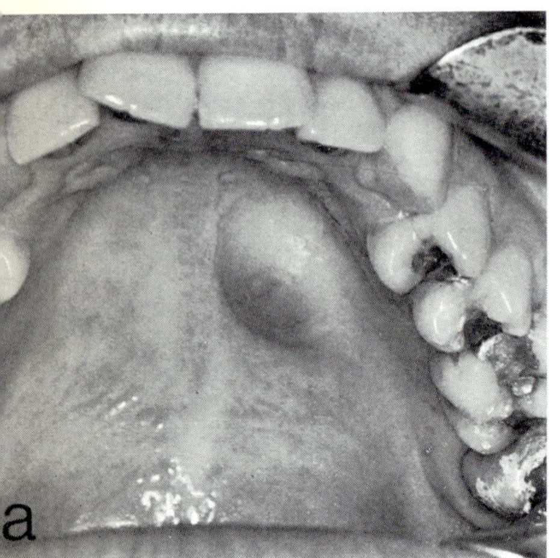
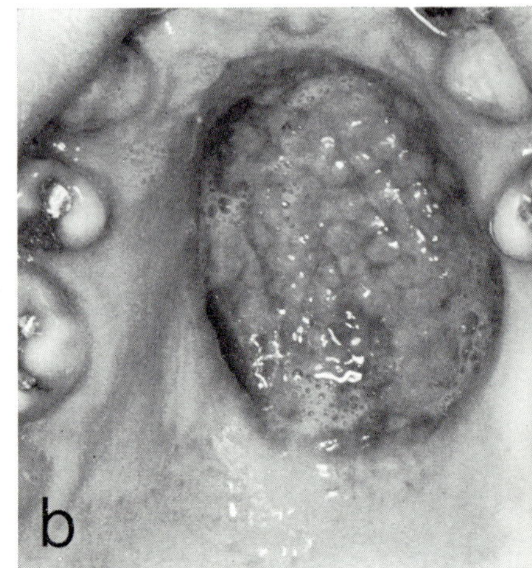

Fig. 122.—a, Cylindroma on the hard palate (22-year-old woman). Firm-elastic consistency. Radical excision. b, Carcinoma of the palate in a 22-year-old woman. Radical excision inclusive of a great part of the adjacent bony palate. Closure by prosthesis.

tumour is notorious for its late manifestation of metastases. Therefore the prognosis is generally poor (*see also* p. 240 and *Fig.* 71, p. 89).

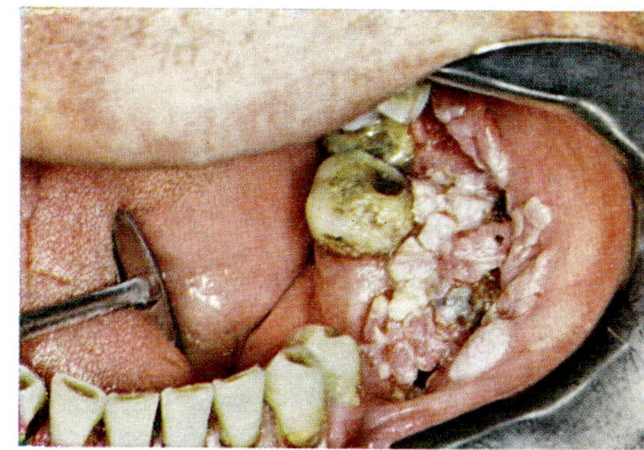

Fig. 123.—Planocellular carcinoma of the gingiva in a 54-year-old man (tobacco-chewer).

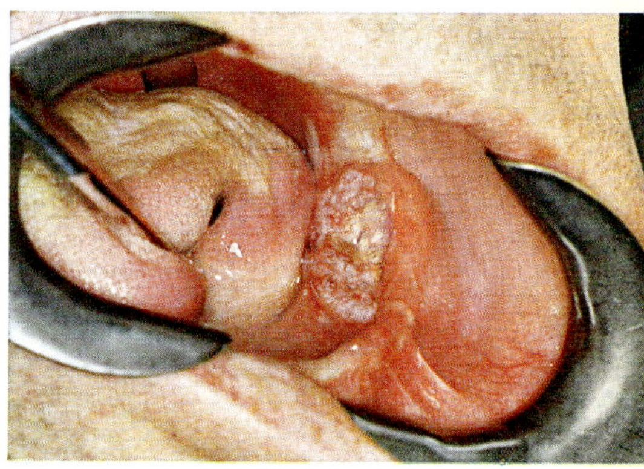

Fig. 124.—Infiltrating planocellular carcinoma of the gingiva in a 35-year-old male patient. Granulomatous aspect. Involvement of the jaw bone.

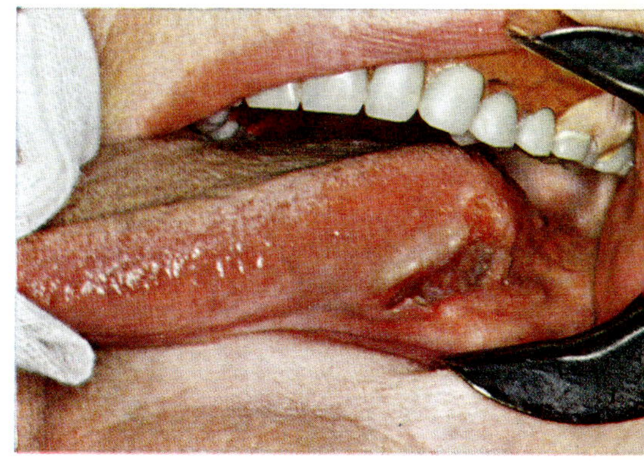

Fig. 125.—Planocellular carcinoma of the tongue in a 71-year-old woman. Painful: present for 3 months.

CHAPTER 5

THE TONGUE

Coated Tongue.—A coated tongue is less important in medical diagnosis than was formerly believed. The lesion may occur without a clearly demonstrable reason. In general, a moist coated tongue is clinically insignificant. A dry coated tongue may occur owing to infections of the respiratory tract, but especially in the case of dehydrating diseases (fever), owing to mouth-breathing, or irritation by tobacco smoke.

Fissured Tongue (Scrotal Tongue).—In some people the tongue shows deep fissures, the surface seems to be strongly folded. The fissures tend to pass in a dorsoventral direction. It is a congenital lesion, often with a large tongue. Sometimes the lesion is combined with a geographic tongue. The lesion is mostly asymptomatic; on the bottom of the deep fissures (difficult cleaning) debris may accumulate and give rise to inflammation, which may cause a burning sensation. Treatment is impossible and usually not required (*Fig.* 126).

Geographic Tongue.—Geographic tongue is characterized by loss of filiform papillae in circumscribed areas, often surrounded by a slightly elevated white margin. Such an area is hyperaemic and therefore fiery red in colour. The fungiform papillae are clearly visible. The lesion may occur both on the dorsal part of the tongue and along the borders (*Fig.* 127). The fanciful form may change rapidly and the lesion may move about the tongue (glossitis areata migrans). Clinically the lesion is insignificant and mostly asymptomatic. The lesion is of unknown origin. There is no known treatment. It is of importance to reassure the patient.

Lingua Villosa (Hairy Tongue).—Lingua villosa is characterized by very long filiform papillae, occurring on the median dorsal third part of the tongue. The colour may vary from white, via yellowish

142

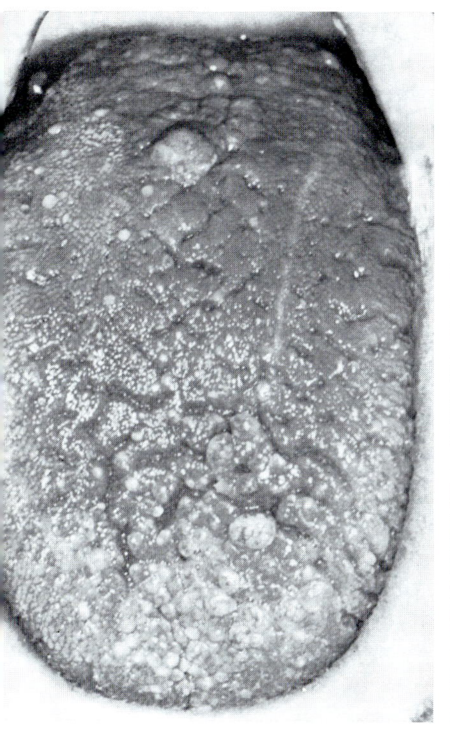

Fig. 126.—Fissured tongue.

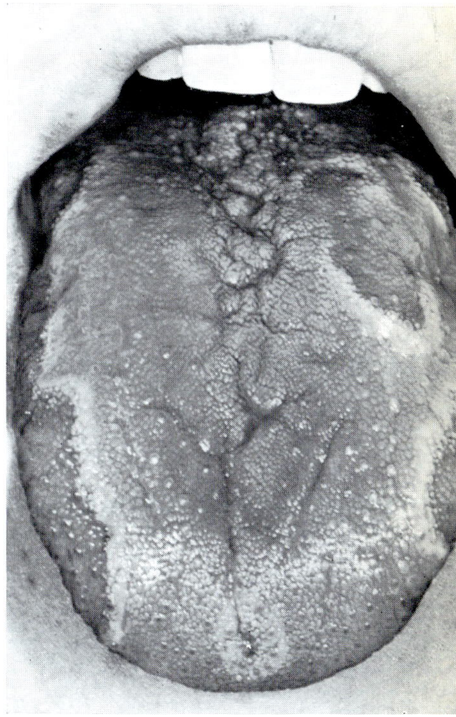

Fig. 127.—Geographic tongue.

to brown and black. The dorsal part of the tongue seems to be covered by a thick hairy coat (*Fig.* 128). The lesion is harmless and there are only aesthetic complaints. In general the cause is unknown. Long-lasting and frequent rinsing with hydrogen peroxide is conducive to a brown hairy tongue.

Lengthy treatment of inflammations elsewhere in the body with antibiotics may disturb the microbiological balance in the oral cavity and may cause black discoloration of the dorsal part of the tongue, but with only moderate elongation of the papillae, because pigment-producing cocci are dominating (*Fig.* 129). Adequate treatment of lingua villosa is not known; in case of serious aesthetic complaints an attempt may be made to remove the 'hairy coat' by mechanical means. The lesion may last for years but may

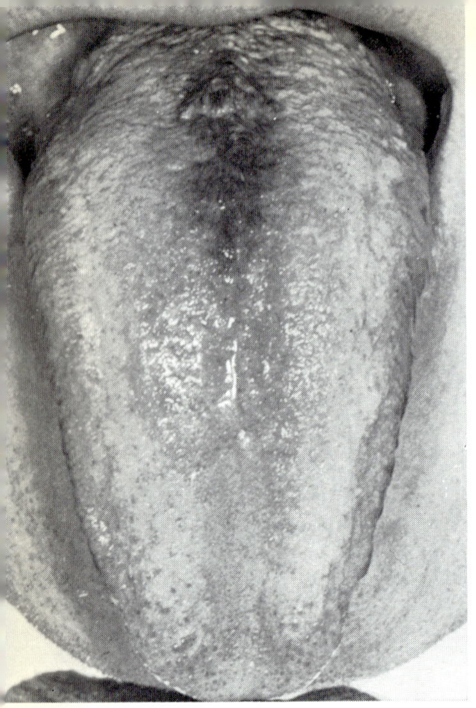

Fig. 128.—Hairy tongue (heavy smoker).

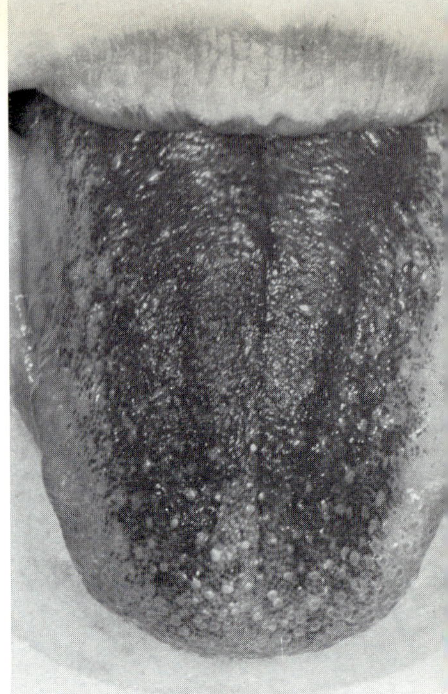

Fig. 129.—Black tongue in a 16-year-old girl after prolonged administration of penicillin.

also disappear spontaneously. It is of importance to reassure the patient.

White Tongue.—Nearly the whole surface of the tongue is of an even white colour without elongation of the papillae. The surface appears etched. The cause is unknown and adequate treatment impossible. The lesion is of rare incidence (*Fig.* 130).

Atrophic Glossitis.—Marked atrophy of the tongue mucosa, causing a smooth and thin mucosa, is very troublesome. Spontaneously or after use of sour, salt, or spicy food a burning sensation may occur. The cause is not always clear. An atrophic red tongue may, for instance, occur in Sjögren's syndrome, hyperchromic anaemia, as part of the Plummer-Vinson syndrome, and due to hypochromic anaemia (Hunter's glossitis). Also in the case of vitamin-B deficiencies, for instance in pellagra, a swollen, burning,

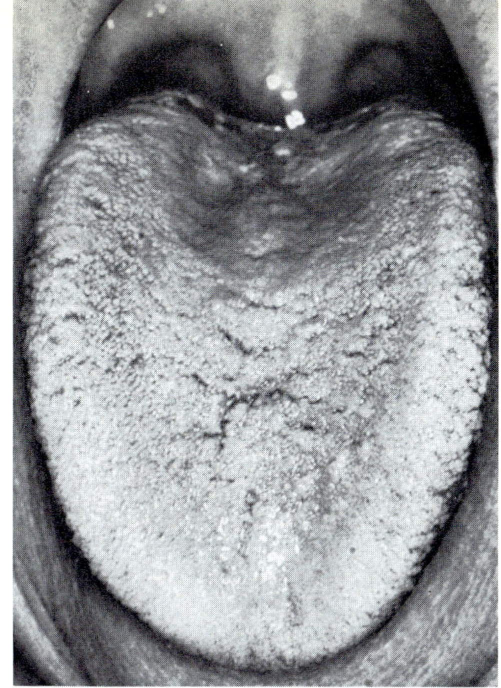

Fig. 130.—White tongue in a 55-year-old woman. Healing in 2 months after administration of vitamin B and painting with gentian violet.

and painful tongue may occur. At first, there is a white coating, and later on the tongue becomes fiery red ('Cardinal's tongue'). The first manifestation of the lesion is atrophy of filiform papillae at the borders of the tip of the tongue.

Strawberry Tongue.—This fiery red, speckled tongue occurs during scarlet fever. Also after long-lasting treatment with antibiotics such a fiery red, painful tongue may be seen (*see* p. 131).

Non-specific Ulcer of the Tongue.—This rare and peculiar lesion appears as a rather large, almost or completely painless ulcer, often very superficial, without marked hyperaemic or indurated elevated margins. The base of the ulcer is smooth and covered by a fibrinous layer (*Fig.* 134). The border of the tongue is the usual site. Perhaps traumata and irritation play a part (neurotic tongue habits, sharp edges of teeth). Elimination of these causal factors is necessary, but

145

is not always immediately followed by complete healing. Possibly there is a relation to the erosive type of lichen planus. The lesion may exist for one or two months without being very troublesome. Taking a biopsy to exclude malignancy is essential. A non-specific ulcer may occasionally occur on the mucosa of an edentulous alveolar process. After radiation of the tongue mucosa such a painless mucosal defect may exist for a long time. Moreover, it should be kept in mind that syphilis may also cause an ulcer (tip of the tongue) which heals with difficulty.

Leucoplakia of the Tongue.—In principle the lesion is identical to leucoplakia elsewhere in the oral cavity. Also on the tongue a flat, more extensive form and a localized hypertrophic form may be found (*Fig.* 131). Taking biopsy specimens from suspect areas is necessary. Small areas should be excised *in toto* (*Fig.* 132). The patient must be examined periodically.

Carcinoma of the Tongue.—Carcinoma of the tongue presents as a painful ulcer without a tendency to heal. There is an elevated, often indurated margin and a base with a granulomatous aspect. There may be gross foetor oris and many patients complain of earache. The dorsal borders of the tongue have to be inspected thoroughly (*Fig.* 125). Be careful when the following diseases are mentioned in the previous medical history: Plummer-Vinson syndrome, syphilis, alcoholism, or anaemia.

Often, metastases from tongue carcinoma are found in the cervical lymph-nodes.

Therapy of a superficially located tumour consists of radium implantation and, in the case of an infiltrative tumour, hemiglossectomy, if necessary combined with radical cervical block dissection.

Ankyloglossia (Tongue Tie).—Treatment is hardly ever required. In many cases the condition disappears spontaneously. Only when the fraenum is attached too far forward towards the tip of the tongue and interferes with either drinking or the speech of the child (disturbed articulation) is extirpation indicated (*Fig.* 133). Following the careful cutting of the fraenum along the lower surface of the tongue, a diamond-shaped defect is left. It is not necessary to cut the fraenum from the floor of the mouth and to remove it completely.

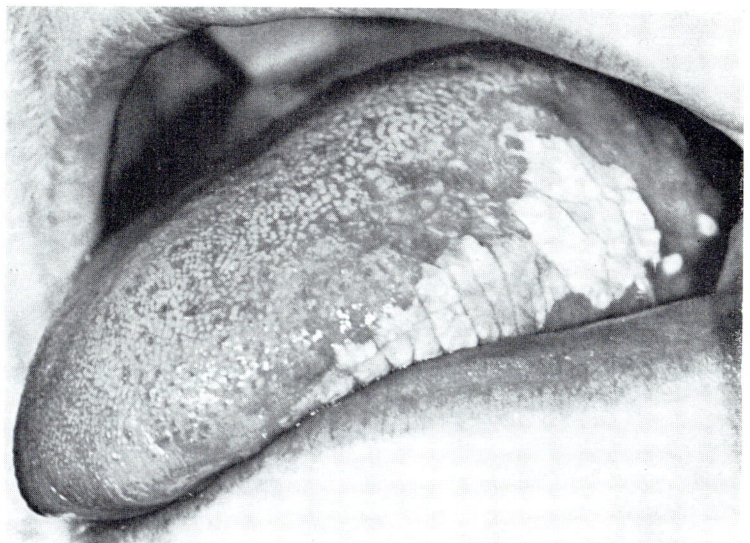

Fig. 131.—Leucoplakia of the tongue in a 51-year-old woman. Very suspect for malignancy.

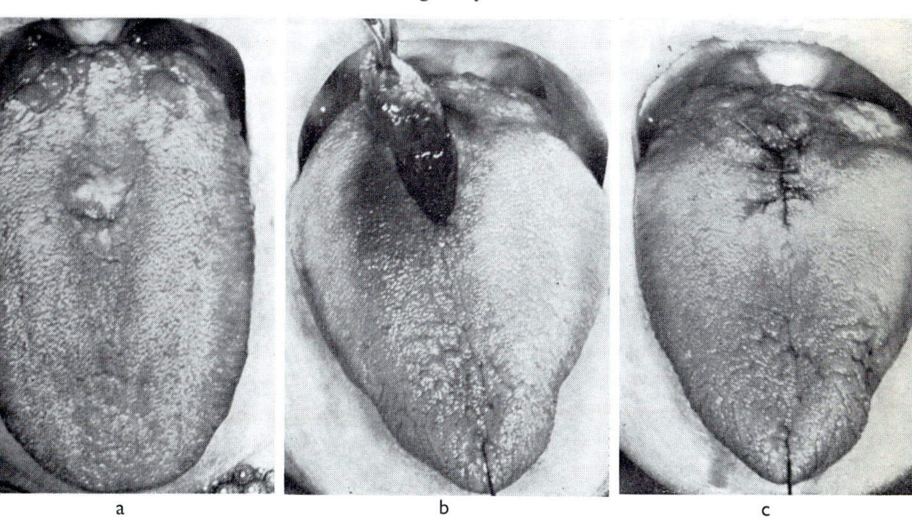

a   b   c

Fig. 132.—a, Small area of leucoplakia on the dorsal part of the tongue. b, Elliptical excision. c, Primary closure.

147

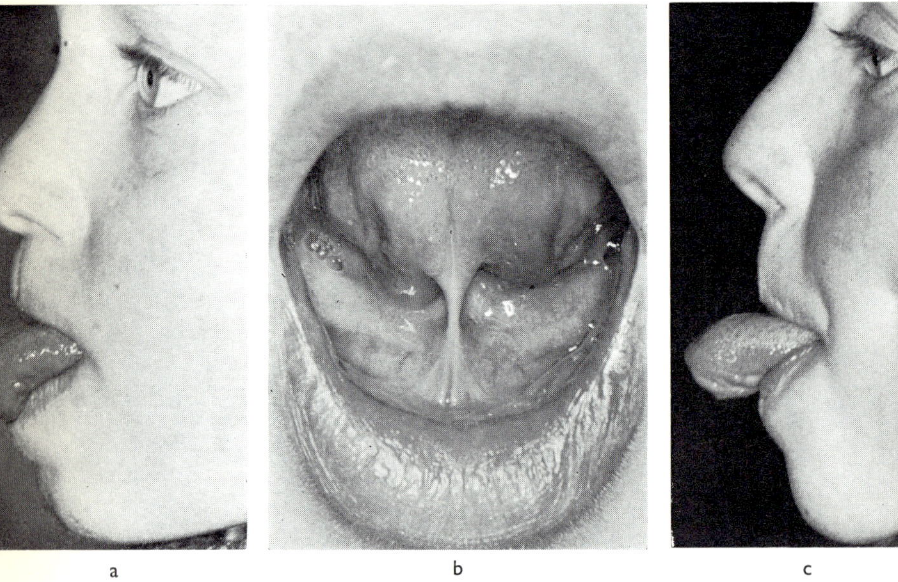

a   b   c

Fig. 133.—a, Ankyloglossia in an 8-year-old boy. The tongue cannot be put straight out. b, The hypertrophic lingual fraenum. c, Result 1 year after fraenectomy.

Cutting just above the floor of the mouth may result in scar contraction and obliteration of the submandibular duct. The rhomboid defect has to be sutured carefully, so that no scar contraction occurs, which will also cause limitation of movement. Cutting without suturing is quite a mistake. Elongation may also be obtained by means of a Z-plasty. The effect of fraenum extirpation is often disappointing, presumably because in many children the mobile part of the tongue is underdeveloped. Sometimes a combination of an enlarged fraenum and a cleft tip of the tongue is seen.

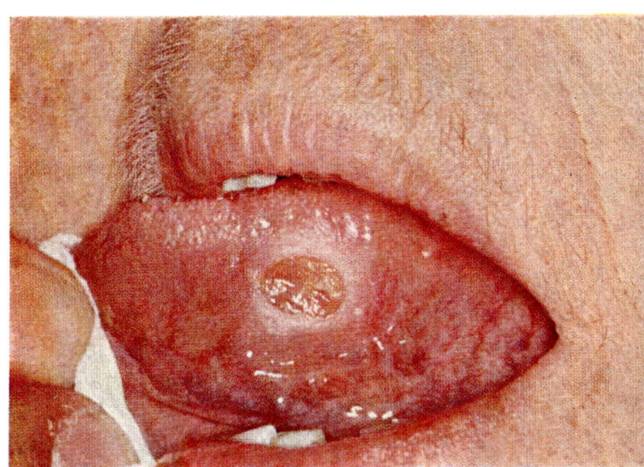

Fig. 134.—Non-specific ulcer of the tongue in a 58-year-old woman.

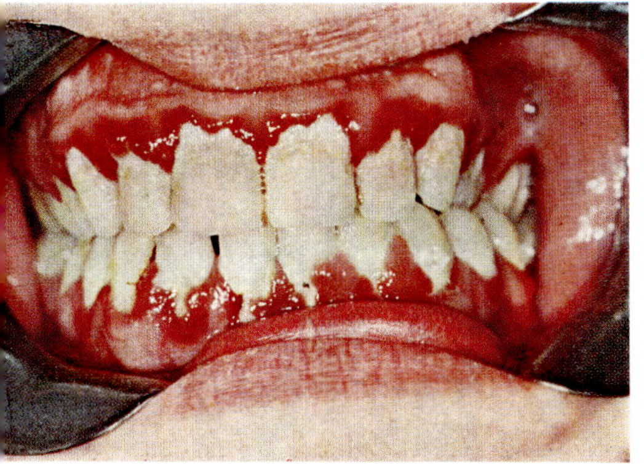

Fig. 135.—Marginal gingivitis.

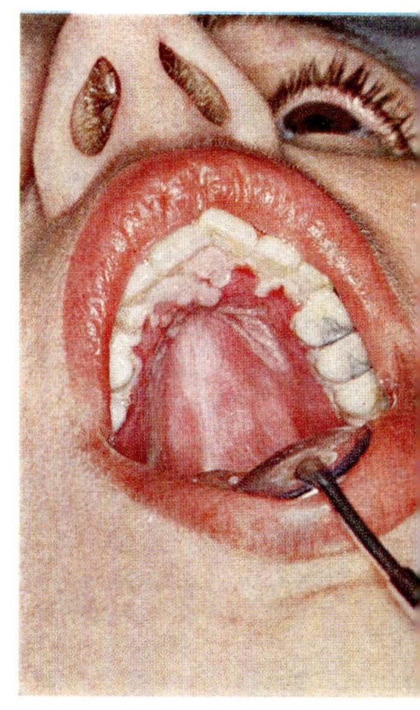

Fig. 136.—Herpetic gingivitis.

149

CHAPTER 6

THE GINGIVA

Pigmentation.—Melanin pigmentation is always present in the dark races, but may also occur on the gingiva in white people (*Fig.* 137 a). Sometimes a broad, dark-coloured band can be seen along the gingival margin (*Fig.* 137 b).

The rarely occurring Addison's disease and Peutz-Jeghers syndrome may cause gingival pigmentations.

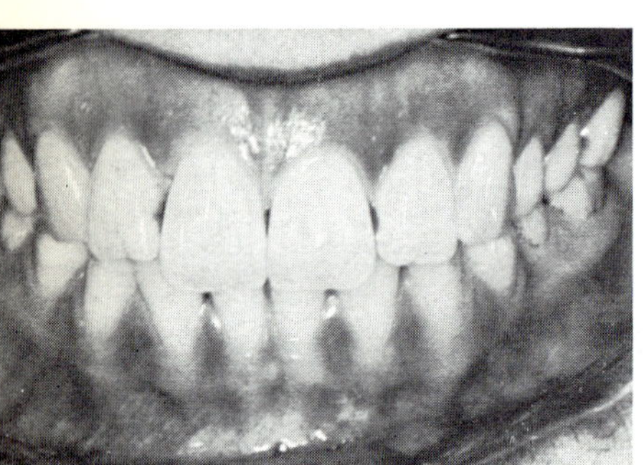
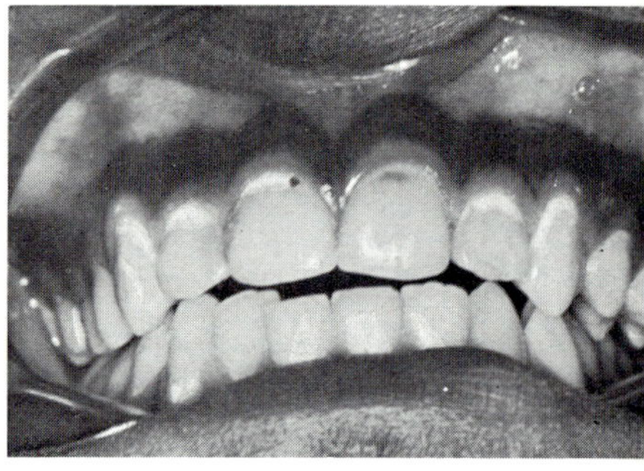

a   b

Fig. 137.—a, Gingival pigmentation in a white patient, mainly localized at the level of the interdental papillae. A narrow line along the teeth is free of pigment. b, Band-like gingival pigmentation in a Negro. The pictures of the lower and upper jaws are identical.

Exogenous pigments have been described, but are of rare incidence. A distinct lead line (found only in persons with natural dentitions) is seldom seen. From a differential diagnosis point of view the presence of dark-coloured subgingival calculus must be considered. This may easily be demonstrated by lifting up the gingiva from the tooth by means of a dental probe.

Marginal Gingivitis.—Chronically inflamed gingiva, characterized by a 1–2 mm. wide fiery red line along the marginal gingiva, which

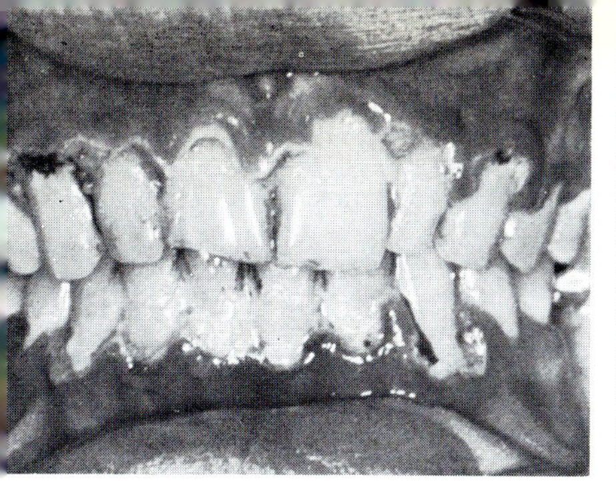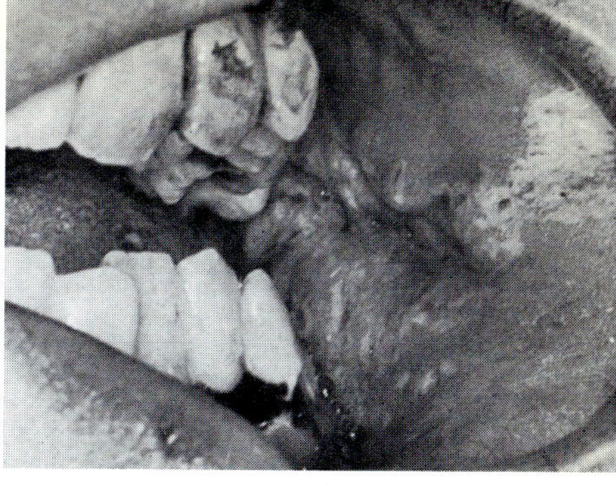

a   b

Fig. 138.—a, Serious acute necrotizing gingivitis. b, Contact ulcers in the buccal mucosa.

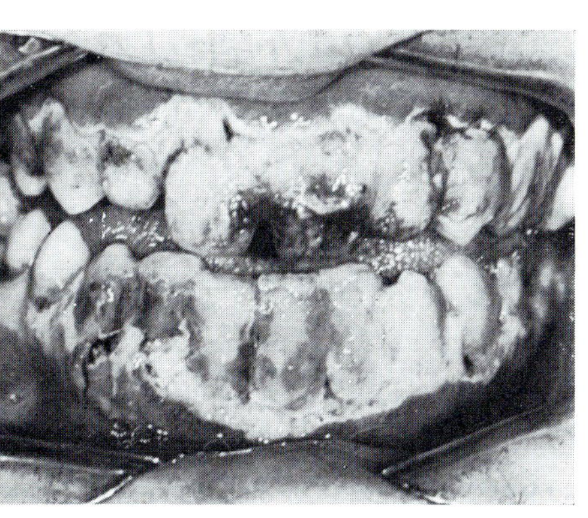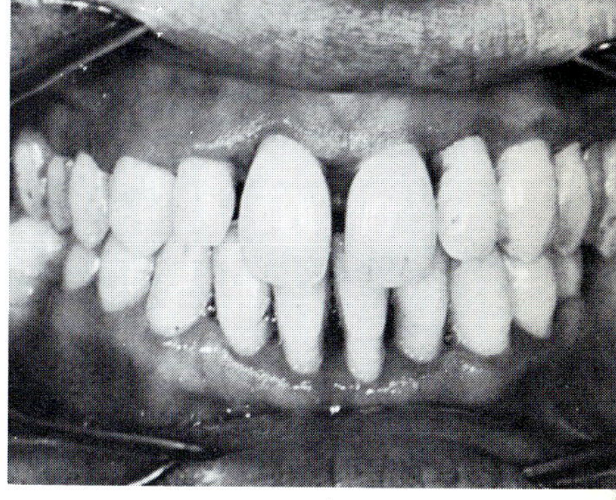

a   b

Fig. 139.—a, Very serious acute necrotizing gingivitis. b, Fifteen days after (local) treatment.

is not very painful, but which bleeds easily. There are no distinct ulcerations (*Fig.* 135). This inflammation is mainly seen in patients with a poor oral hygiene. The teeth are covered by a thick deposit of materia alba. Treatment consists of thorough cleaning of the dentition by a dentist, after which the patient has to ensure good oral hygiene.

Necrotizing (Ulcerative) Gingivitis.—Necrotizing gingivitis is of rather common occurrence. By the term is understood a more or less acute inflammation of the gingiva, presumably caused by Vincent's fuso-spirochaetal infection.

151

In the case of chronic inflammation complaints are few, there is little pain, there is a more or less distinct foetor oris, and the interdental papillae are necrotic. In acute cases the gingiva is very painful, bleeds easily, and is covered by a greyish layer (*Fig.* 138 a). The interdental papillae are usually affected first and may disappear completely within a very short period (*Fig.* 139). There is a strong foetor oris. The alveolar bone is generally not involved. In serious cases contact ulcers may occur on the tongue, cheeks, or lips (*Fig.* 138 b). The lesion may occur endemically in closed communities (crews of submarines, in monasteries, and so on), because the infection is spread by food utensils. Causative factors may also be: consumption of exclusively very soft and mushy food, which has no cleaning effect on gingiva and dentition, excessive use of tobacco, and poor oral hygiene. Treatment consists of spraying the gingiva with hydrogen peroxide (1·5 per cent) and thorough cleaning of the dentition by a dentist. In connexion with pain and swelling of the gingiva this cleaning will take several sittings. The patient himself has to apply, three times daily, packs saturated with hydrogen peroxide on the buccal and lingual side of the gingiva for 5 minutes. A prescription can be given of 500 ml. 3 per cent hydrogen peroxide.* The patient dilutes some in a glass with an equal quantity of warm water. The formation of foam of the hydrogen peroxide has a cleansing action and, moreover, it has a favourable effect on the mixed anaerobic flora owing to liberation of oxygen. The maintenance of good oral hygiene after healing is of major importance if chronic persistence of the inflammation, which may easily lead to recurrence, is to be avoided. Accumulation of debris is greatly increased by the loss of the interdental papillae. Treatment consisting only of rinsing with hydrogen peroxide is not very effective. Vitamin-C administration or prescription of citrus fruits is useless. Penicillin lozenges are quite a mistake.

Only in very serious cases with contact ulcers and general illness with a clinical picture resembling noma is intramuscular injection of penicillin indicated, in addition to local treatment. In these cases haematological examination is necessary (in order to exclude such conditions as agranulocytosis).

Noma (cancrum oris) is a rapidly spreading necrosis, mainly occurring in tropical countries. The causal agents are the same as in

---

* Solutio hydrogenii peroxidi 3 per cent.

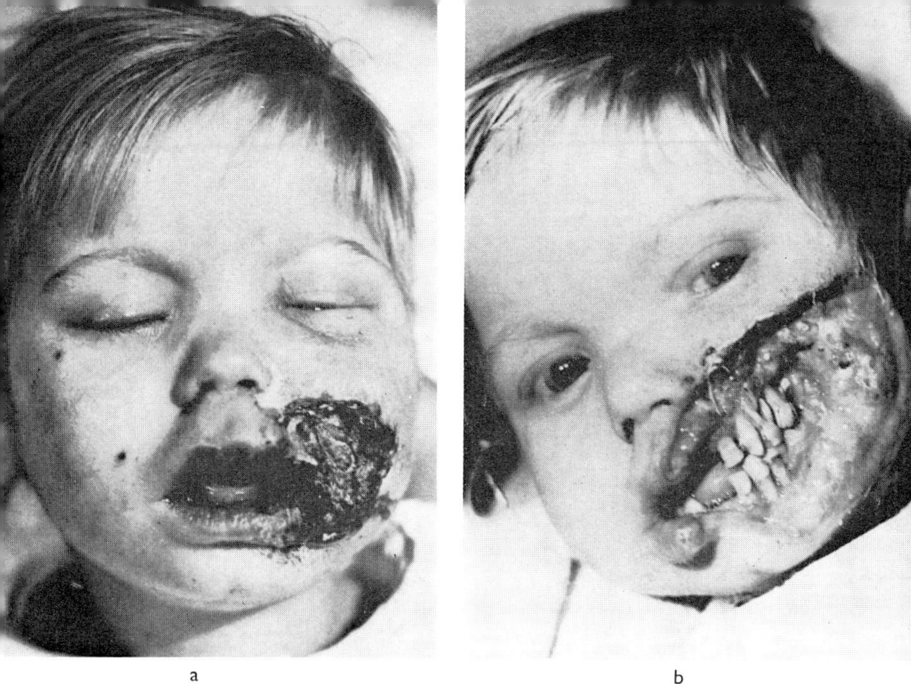

a   b

Fig. 140.—a, Noma; 4-year-old boy referred at the end of the Second World War with characteristic necrosis of left-cheek tissue. b, After detachment and removal of necrotic tissue.

gangrenous gingivitis. Within a very short period extensive defects (also of the bone) may occur, mainly arising from the corners of the mouth or cheek (*Fig.* 140).

Herpetic Gingivitis.—A painful lesion characterized by the occurrence of small circular herpetic lesions, covered by a greyish-yellow layer, which may merge. This inflammation caused by the herpes virus can be distinguished from necrotizing gingivitis by the fact that in the case of the former there is no foetor oris, the papillae are not flattened, and there is an occurrence of small solitary lesions (*see also* p. 129) (*Fig.* 136).

Hyperplastic Gingivitis.—This chronic gingival inflammation may occur owing to poor oral hygiene, calculus, or dehydration caused by mouth-breathing. Gingival pockets are a common finding (*see* p. 29). These are the most common causes of a swollen gingiva.

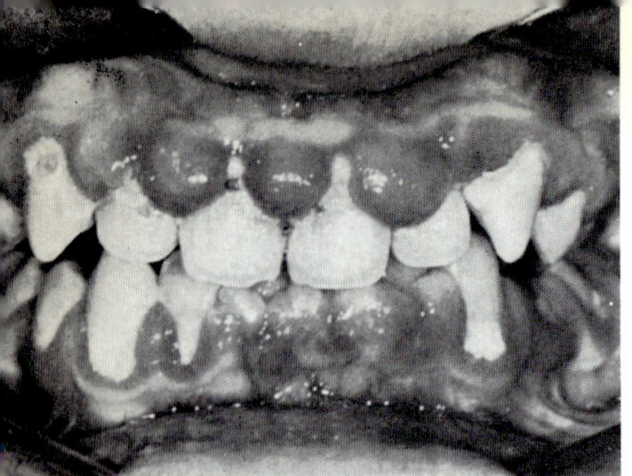
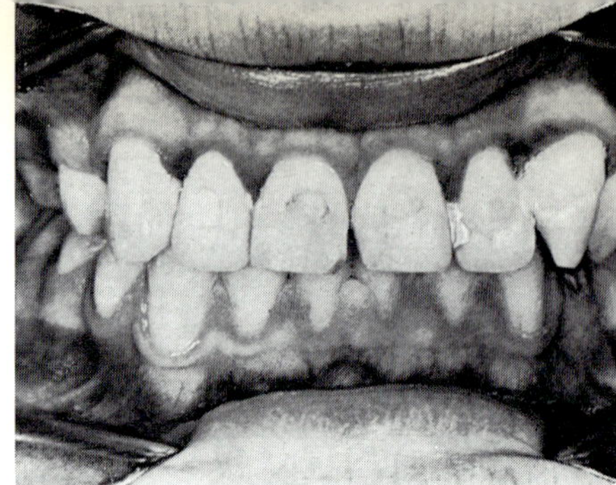

a   b

Fig. 141.—a, Hyperplastic gingivitis in a 16-year-old boy. b, Same patient after gingivectomy.

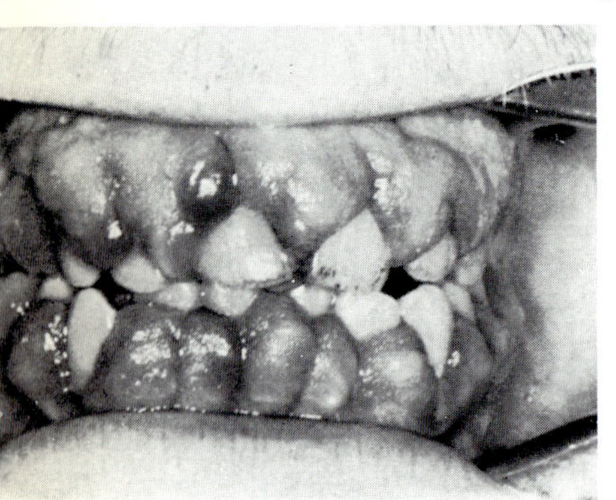
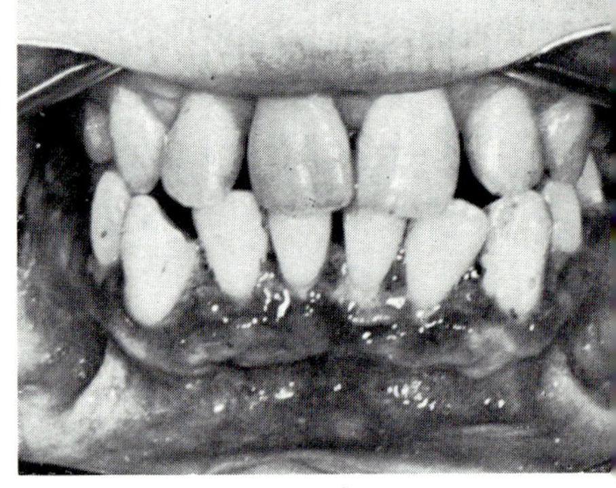

a   b

Fig. 142.—a, Gingival hyperplasia following administration of the anti-convulsant, phenytoin, in a 16-year-old boy. b, After gingivectomy in lower and upper jaw.

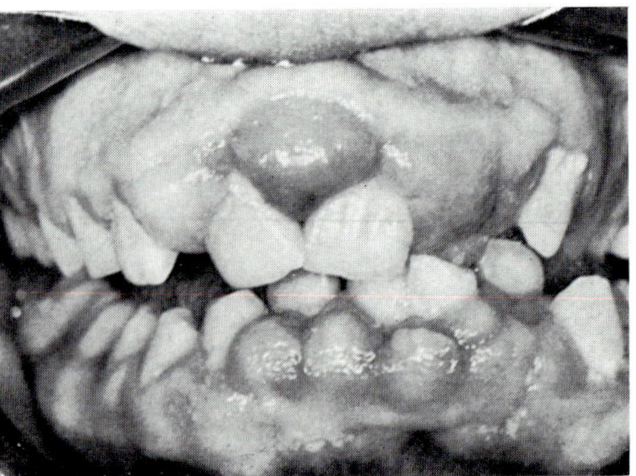

Fig. 143.—Familial gingival hyperplasia in an 18-year-old girl. Microscopic findings: dense connective tissue with chronic, non-specific, inflammatory infiltrate.

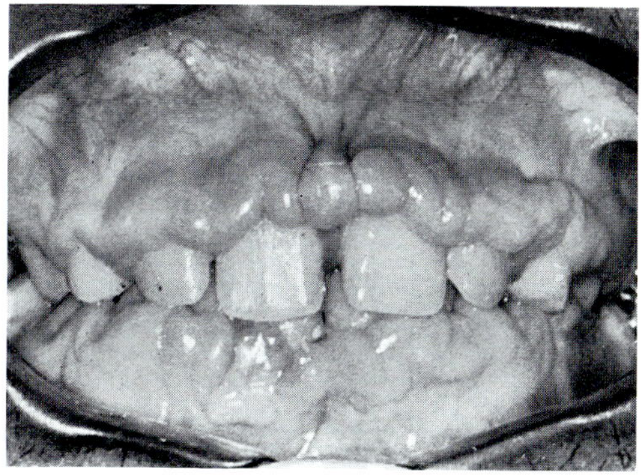

Fig. 144.—Gingival swelling in an 11-year-old patient suffering from leuk-aemia (mercaptopurine may have been a possible aetiological agent as well).

Hormonal factors (at puberty) may play a part in some cases. Pregnancy may also be associated with gingivitis, characterized by swelling and increased bleeding tendency. Generally therapy consists of periodical cleaning of the dentition by a dentist and good oral hygiene. In serious cases gingivectomy is the treatment of choice (*Fig.* 141).

For localized gingival swelling *see* p. 156.

Dilantin Hyperplasia.—Patients suffering from epilepsy, treated by Dilantin sodium, may show a very pronounced hyperplastic gingiva. Sometimes the teeth are hardly visible. The gingiva is pale pink in colour and the swelling is rather firm on palpation. The interdental papillae are generally affected first. By retention of debris between tooth and swollen gingiva chronic inflammation may increase the swelling. Many inflammatory cells are found, including many plasma-cells; possibly an allergic reaction is concerned. The occurrence of Dilantin hyperplasia is related to the presence of teeth. After extraction of the dentition the lesion disappears.

Treatment consists of removal of the excess gingiva tissue (gingivectomy) and, if possible, complete or partial change to another anti-convulsant drug in order to prevent recurrence. Good oral hygiene is very important (*Fig.* 142).

Fibromatosis Gingivae.—In some families a type of hereditary gingiva hyperplasia occurs. The clinical picture resembles Dilantin hyperplasia; a pale pink, somewhat nodular, firm gingival swelling in both lower and upper jaw. Treatment consists of gingivectomy each time the swelling becomes troublesome (*Fig.* 143).

Leukaemia.—In very rare cases a gingival swelling may be caused by leukaemia owing to the accumulation of leucocytes, especially in acute forms (*Fig.* 144). In a further stage excessive gingival bleeding is a common finding. Blood examination may confirm the diagnosis of leukaemia.

Avitaminosis C (Scurvy).—This disease may lead to marked inflammation-like, purple swelling of the gingiva with ulcerations and necroses. Finally, marked loosening or loss of teeth occurs. The lesion only occurs after prolonged complete or partial lack of vitamin C in the food. Avitaminosis C does not occur with a 'normal' diet and therefore the lesion is of extremely rare incidence in western Europe. As a rule haemorrhage and infections of the gingiva are not caused by vitamin-C deficiency (*see* pp. 29 and 51).

Amyloidosis.—Also of very rare occurrence is a gingival swelling owing to accumulation of amyloid in amyloidosis. Formerly a gingival biopsy was often used as an aid in diagnosis, but at present a rectal biopsy is usually taken.

Epulides.—These benign tumours of the gingiva may occur in both lower and upper jaws. A site of predilection is the buccal side of the alveolar process, while the base is usually an interdental papilla. Most epulides can be classed as proliferative inflammations. Their size may range from 0·5 cm. to 1 cm. The following types can be distinguished:—
Epulis Granulomatosa.—A soft swelling, fiery red in colour, easily bleeding on palpation owing to the richness in blood-vessels. Histologically the picture resembles an inflammation (*Fig.* 145).
Epulis Telangiectatica (gingival pyogenic granuloma).—A soft swelling of the gingiva, characterized by a granular aspect and a reddish-purple colour. Easy bleeding is caused by the abundance of excessively dilated capillaries. This bleeding tendency, rapid growth, resorption of bone, and recurrence after incomplete removal may clinically resemble a neoplasm. This impression is emphasized when the tumour becomes almost black due to haemorrhages or shows

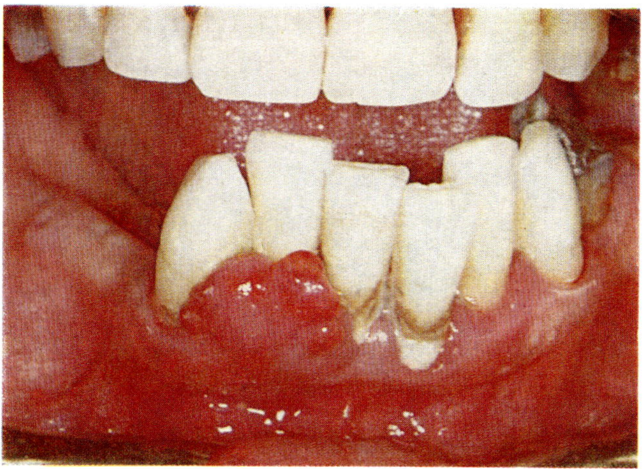

Fig. 145.—Epulis granulomatosa.

extensive ulcerations (dental trauma). The lesion is both clinically and histologically classed as inflammation (*Fig.* 146).

Pregnancy Tumour (Granuloma telangiectaticum in Graviditate).—This tumour, only occurring in combination with pregnancy, shows the histological picture of a granuloma telangiectaticum. The epulis may involve several interdental papillae and may cause loosening of teeth following resorption. Characteristic are its rapid growth and spontaneous diasppearance or regression after parturition. In a subsequent pregnancy recurrence at the same site may occur (*Figs.* 147 and 150).

Epulis Fibrosa.—This epulis has the characteristics of a fibroma. The swelling is firm on palpation and is covered by a pale pink, normally speckled gingiva. It is a slowly growing lesion. On histological examination a primary proliferation of connective-tissue-like cells is found, whereas a marked inflammatory component is lacking. Bony tissue and a cementum-like substance may occur in this lesion. Presumably the lesion is a hamartoma (*Fig.* 148).

Epulis Gigantocellularis (Giant-cell Epulis).—An elastic, soft tumour of bluish-purple colour, with a milky bloom. The lesion may be of considerable size (1–3 cm.). Bone resorption is a common finding. The tendency to recur in case of incomplete excision is

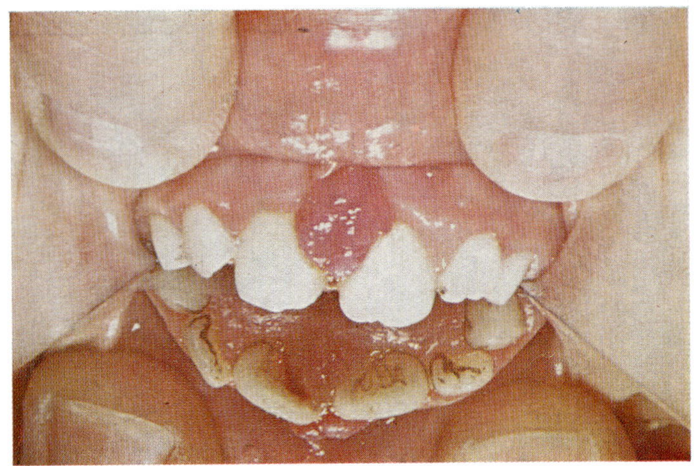

Fig. 146.—Epulis telangiectatica (gingival pyogenic granuloma).

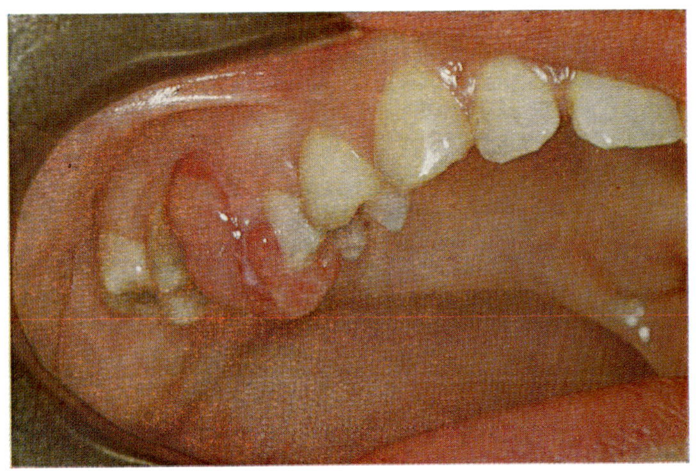

Fig. 147.—Epulis gravidarum (pregnancy tumour).

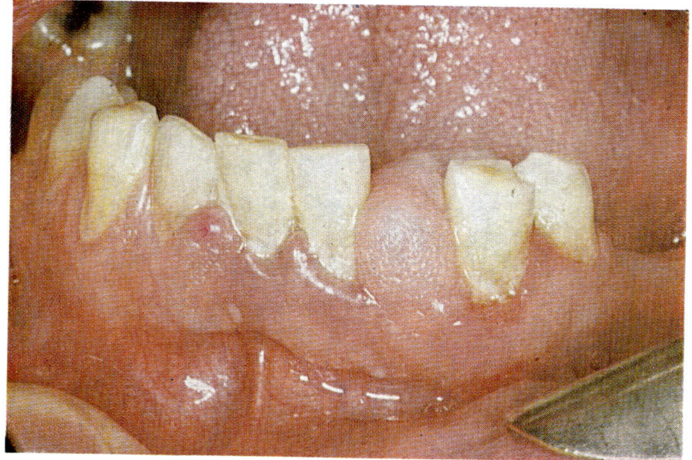

Fig. 148.—Epulis fibrosa.

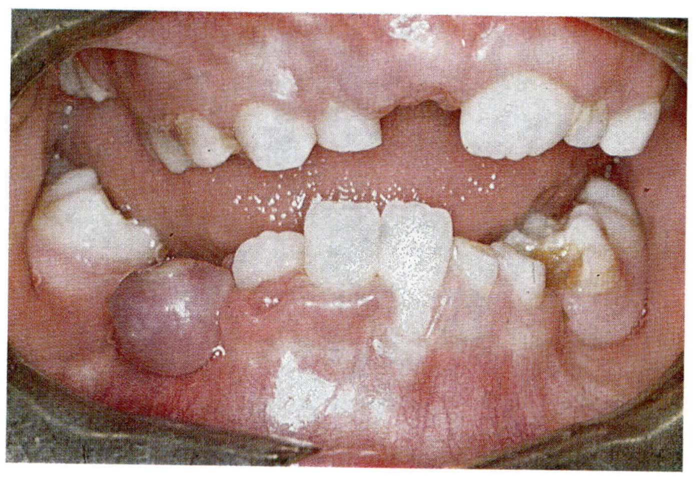

Fig. 149.—Epulis gigantocellularis (giant-cell epulis).

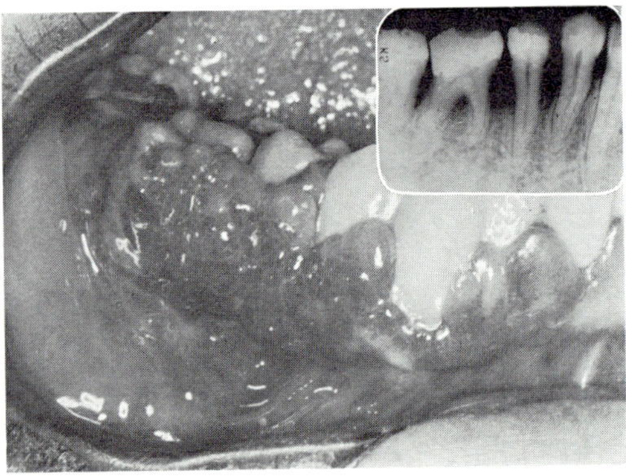

Fig. 150.—Extensive pregnancy tumour. The dental radiograph shows marked resorption of the alveolar margin.

generally greater than in other types. It is not clear whether these giant-cell lesions are true tumours or reactive neoplasms. Histological examination reveals a stroma of connective-tissue-like cells with numerous capillaries. In this stroma big multinucleated giant cells are found, mostly located in the walls of the capillaries (*see also* p. 96, *Fig.* 149, and *Fig.* 79, p. 100).

Symmetric Fibromas.—These strongly fibrous gingival swellings occur on either side palatally of the upper molars and in rare cases lingually of the lower molars. They are pale pink in colour and of firm elastic to very firm consistency (*Fig.* 151). Mostly they are asymptomatic. Sometimes they grow so large that they meet in the midline. Excision is only indicated when they are troublesome to the patient. If full dentures are made, it is better to remove the fibromas in advance.

Leucoplakia and Gingival Carcinoma.—In essence the clinical picture is not different from that described on pp. 118 and 138 (*see Figs.* 123 and 124).

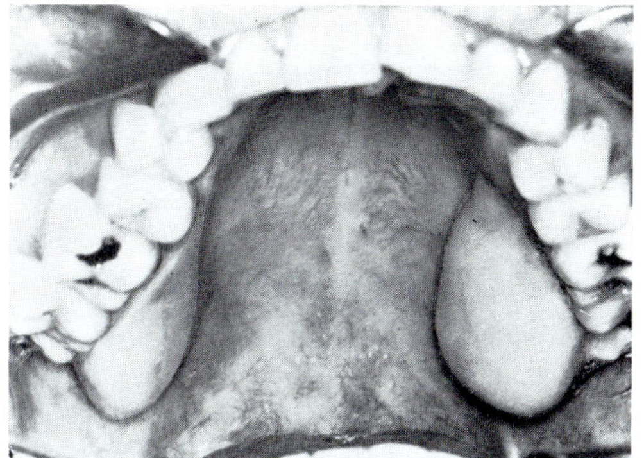

Fig. 151.—Symmetrical fibromas.

CHAPTER 7

INFECTIONS IN THE MANDIBULAR AND MAXILLOFACIAL REGION

ODONTOGENIC INFECTIONS

BY odontogenic infections are meant infections in which the dentition plays a part. In most cases the nature of the bacteria is of secondary importance. Mostly a mixed infection is composed of non-specific, mostly Gram-positive cocci (indifferent streptococci, haemolytic streptococci, *Streptococcus viridans*, *Staphylococcus aureus* and *Staph. albus*) or a mixed anaerobic flora. Fortunately most of them are sensitive to penicillin and other frequently used antibiotics.

Elimination of the *odontogenic cause* is of major importance in all infections, either as a therapeutic measure or to prevent recurrence. Therefore odontogenic infections can be divided according to their odontogenic 'origins'. The following infections can be distinguished: *periapical* infections (starting as a root-tip infection), pericoronal infections (starting as an infection of the follicle of a partly erupted tooth), and finally *periodontal* infections (starting at the bottom of a deep gingival pocket). These infections may extend chronically into bone or soft tissues, but it is also possible that extension takes place by means of subacute or serious acute inflammation. Reactions of the soft tissues may be either absent, slight, or very extensive, resulting in a wide range of clinical pictures. Extension into the bone is fortunately rare (*see also* pp. 47–54).

Acute Odontogenic Inflammation.—
Acute Odontogenic Inflammation without Marked Reaction of the Soft Tissues.—Toothache may be caused by:—

a. Total acute pulpitis: There is a violent, radiating pain, which cannot easily be located, and which increases when drinking hot or cold liquids (prolonged pain) and at night when the patient goes to sleep. The affected tooth contains either a big cavity or a big restoration, or has recently been treated by a dentist (buccal amalgam filling). Sometimes the tooth feels overerupted and is usually painful on percussion. At an earlier stage of pulp hyperaemia this is usually not seen (pain is not long-lasting after thermal vitality tests). Cold gives relief of pain in partial purulent pulpitis. Pulpitis does not heal. Treatment may consist of extraction or endodontic (root-canal) treatment.

b. Acute exacerbation of periapical granuloma (acute periapical or alveolar abscess): Initially there is a gnawing pain, increasing rapidly and becoming throbbing in nature. In general the pain can easily be located; the tooth responsible is somewhat loose, feels overerupted, and is painful when bitten upon (hyperaemia of the periodontium). There is pain on palpation and redness at the level of the root-tip, but no increase of pain when eating hot or cold food. There is, however, as in pulpitis, percussion pain. The associated tooth is often dark (blue or grey in colour) and less transparent, because the pulp is necrotic. Usually the tooth contains either a big cavity, large filling, or a crown. The dental radiograph reveals a periapical radiolucency (periapical granuloma).

Treatment consists of:—

Extraction (drainage of pus through the socket);

Opening of the pulpal chamber and cleaning of the root canal (draining of pus through the root canal);

Trepanation (via a small incision the buccal bone lamella at the level of the apex is perforated so that drainage of pus is effected).

The method of choice depends upon whether or not the tooth is to be retained and, in the first method, whether the root canal is open or not (dowel crown). Extraction is impeded because it is very difficult to achieve good local anaesthesia in the case of acute inflammation (an extra injection in the periodontal space may make the pain bearable). Short-acting general anaesthesia facilitates treatment considerably. When the acute symptoms subside adequate root-canal treatment or apicectomy has to be carried out in order to prevent recurrence.

c. Pericoronitis: By this term is meant acute infection around the crown of an erupting tooth. This type of infection is predominantly seen around the lower third molar, which usually cannot easily erupt owing to lack of space or abnormal position. The mucosa, still partly covering the tooth (operculum), is painful, red, and swollen. On pressure pus is discharged from the space between the crown and follicle (pseudopocket). Sometimes the operculum is bitten, namely

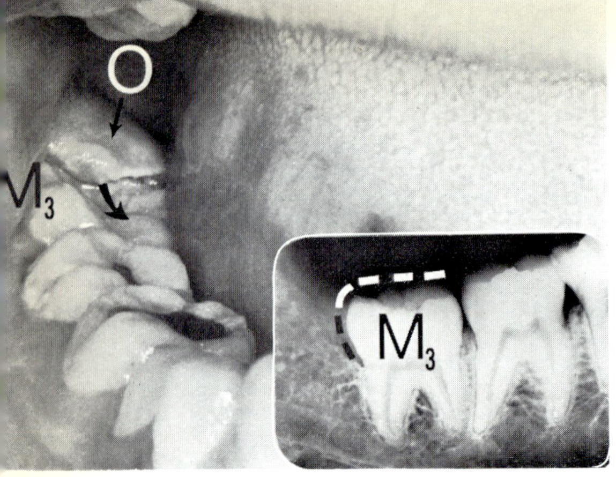

Fig. 152.—Pericoronitis of the lower right third molar. The crown is partly covered by the operculum (O). On pressure pus exudes out of the pseudopocket (*see* arrow), which can be probed as far as the cemento-enamel junction (*see* dotted line inset).

when the upper third molar is also erupting or has already erupted. Complaints are of dull or sometimes severe pain in the third molar region, pain on swallowing, on occluding (sometimes), and on excessive opening. There is often slight trismus. There is no swelling of the soft tissues of the face (*Fig.* 152).

Therapy consists of rinsing the pseudopocket with 3 per cent hydrogen peroxide, diluted with an equal quantity of warm water. A record syringe is used with rather a thick, bent, blunt needle, which can easily be brought into the pericoronal fissure. If necessary, infra-red radiation may be prescribed. When the acute symptoms have

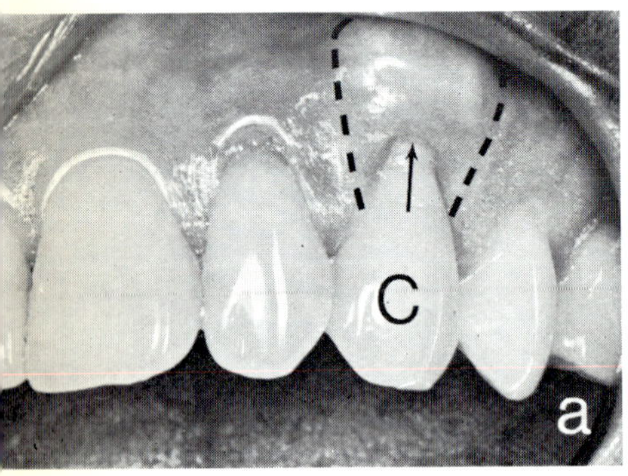

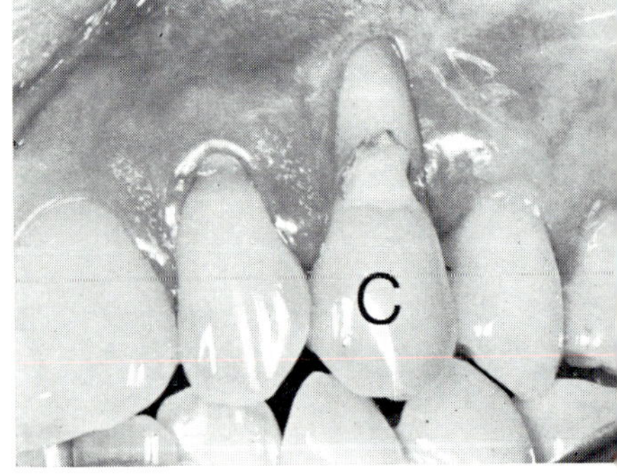

Fig. 153.—*a*, Periodontal abscess, upper left cuspid. A deep pocket can be demonstrated at the level of the arrow. Local gingivectomy along dotted line. *b*, Healing after elimination of the pocket. Part of the root remains uncovered.

subsided the tooth responsible can best be extracted. If the position of the tooth is good and an antagonist is present, it may be retained; removal of the operculum is indicated to prevent recurrences.

d. Periodontal abscess: In advanced periodontal disease with deep gingival pockets the ever-present chronic inflammation at the bottom of the pocket may become acute, when for instance the normal drainage along the neck of the tooth is obstructed. At first there is a dull pain which later becomes pulsating; palpation produces pain on the alveolar process at the level of the tooth responsible. Sometimes the tooth can be moved and is painful on percussion, but may respond normally to vitality tests (vital pulp). Finally a submucosal abscess develops about 0·5–1·0 cm. in size, mostly buccally, about half the height of crown and root tip (*Fig.* 153 a).

Therapy usually consists of cleaning the root and providing pus drainage along the marginal gingiva. If the acute symptoms are subsiding curettage of the pocket or local gingivectomy may be carried out (*Fig.* 153 b). Of course, extraction of the tooth also removes the unfavourable anatomical relationship.

e. Periodontitis: By this term is meant inflammation of the periodontal membrane and the immediate surroundings, and is clinically characterized by percussion pain and a feeling that the tooth is overerupted. It may be caused by overloading (too high filling), by trauma, or be the result of an infection (total pulpitis, acute periapical abscess, periodontal abscess). Treatment should be aimed at the causative factors. Corrective grinding of the tooth may give relief of symptoms.

Acute Odontogenic Inflammations with Marked Reactions of the Soft Tissues.—In almost all cases of the so-called *swollen face* owing to an infected tooth an *acute exacerbation of a chronic odontogenic inflammation* is concerned. This may be a periapical granuloma at a tooth with a non-vital pulp or a root fragment, or a chronic inflammation around the crown of an erupting tooth (third molar).

a. Periostitis: The inflammation often begins with pain. After 1 or 2 days a swelling develops (periostitis with soft-tissue oedema) (*Fig.* 154). The swelling increases and indurates (infiltrate), the pain increases and becomes pulsating when after 3 or 4 days an abscess develops (subperiosteal abscess). This abscess may become a submucosal abscess when the periosteum is breached, or it may extend into the soft tissues of the cheek and floor of the mouth. Which of the two possibilities is to occur is largely dependent upon the location of the primary inflammation in relation to the buccal sulcus (*Fig.* 155). After the periosteum is breached the pain subsides rapidly because of the decrease of pressure. The swelling increases considerably especially in the case of extension into the soft tissues of the cheek. Treatment of periostitis depends on the seriousness of the symptoms; infra-red radiation or wet compresses, combined with opening of the pulpal chamber and root canals, is occasionally sufficient to restrain the process or to let it localize. In other cases administration of penicillin will be the treatment of choice. A course of penicillin has to consist minimally of administration for 5 days, for example: five times 900,000 units of procaine penicillin and 300,000 units of penicillin. Administration for more than 7–10 days is generally

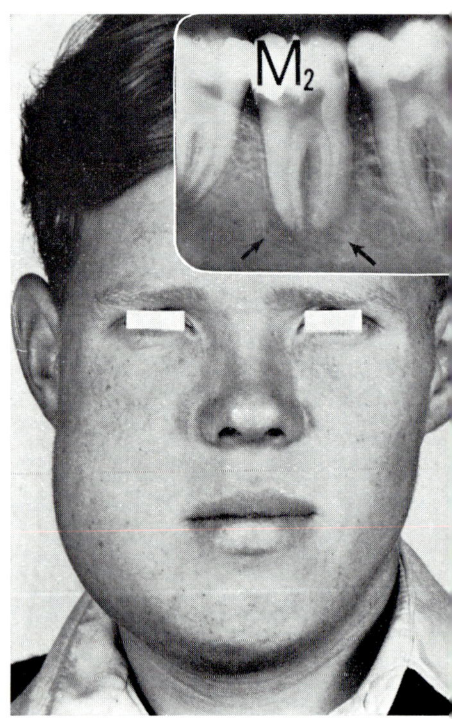

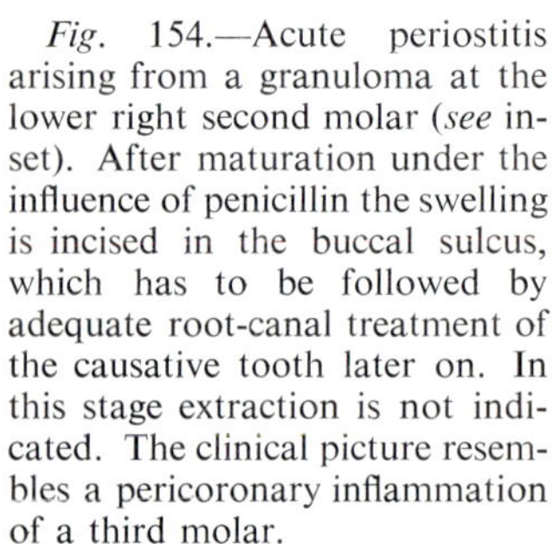

Fig. 154.—Acute periostitis arising from a granuloma at the lower right second molar (*see* inset). After maturation under the influence of penicillin the swelling is incised in the buccal sulcus, which has to be followed by adequate root-canal treatment of the causative tooth later on. In this stage extraction is not indicated. The clinical picture resembles a pericoronary inflammation of a third molar.

rather useless. If no favourable reaction takes place after about 3 days another antibiotic should be used. As soon as pus can be demonstrated or is presumed (after 3 or 4 days) incision is necessary. It is better not to extract at this stage.

b. Submucosal abscess (vestibular space abscess): This type of abscess is usually visible and palpable adjacent to the associated tooth in the buccal sulcus (*Fig.* 156).

A palatal abscess originates as a rule from an upper lateral incisor (*Fig.* 157) or from the palatal root of an upper molar.

A submucosal abscess (sublingual abscess) of the floor of the mouth is rather rare. It originates from the teeth of which the apices are situated above the mylohyoidean line (attachment of the mylohyoid muscle) (lower central incisor–lower first molar). The swelling often has a glassy aspect.

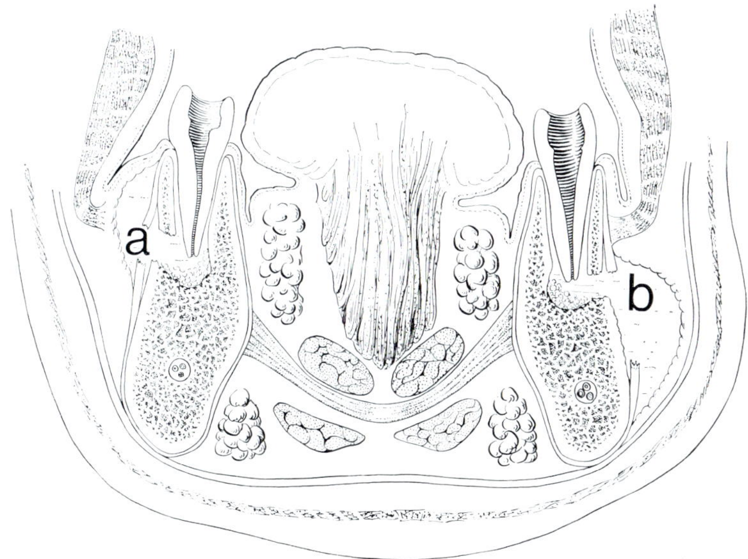

Fig. 155.—Extensions of a periapical inflammation: a, To the buccal sulcus (submucosal abscess). b, To the soft tissues of the cheek (subcutaneous abscess). Of less frequent occurrence are lingual extensions; these may lead to a sublingual abscess (above the mylohyoid muscle) or a submandibular (dorsally) respectively submental abscess (ventrally) (beneath the mylohyoid muscle according to Axhausen).

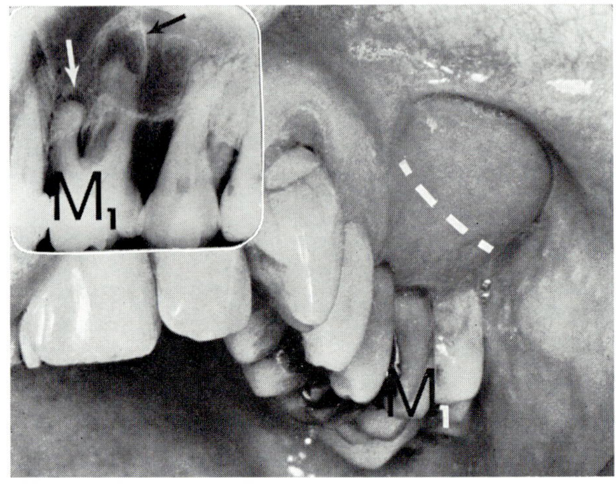

Fig. 156.—Submucosal abscess originating from a granuloma at the upper left first molar (*see* inset). Treatment: incision along dotted line and root-canal treatment of upper left first molar or extraction.

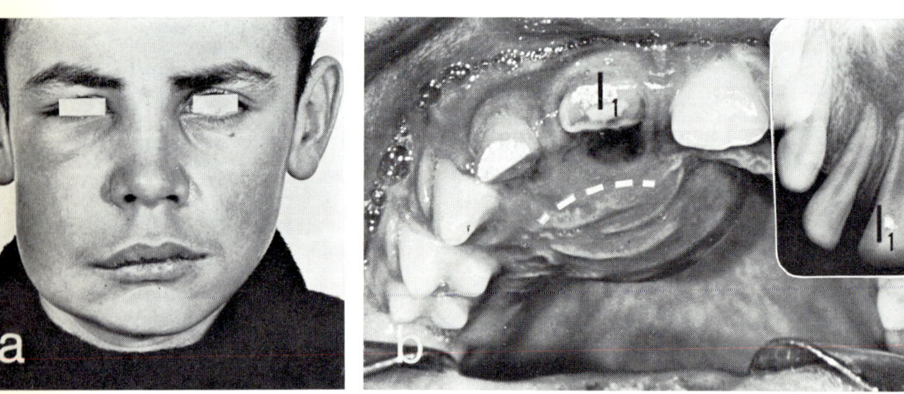

Fig. 157.—a, Collateral oedema. b, Palatal abscess, arising from granulomas at the upper right central and lateral incisor. The pulps are necrotic owing to trauma. Treatment: incision along dotted line and drainage. After the acute symptoms have subsided apicectomy of both central and lateral incisor is indicated.

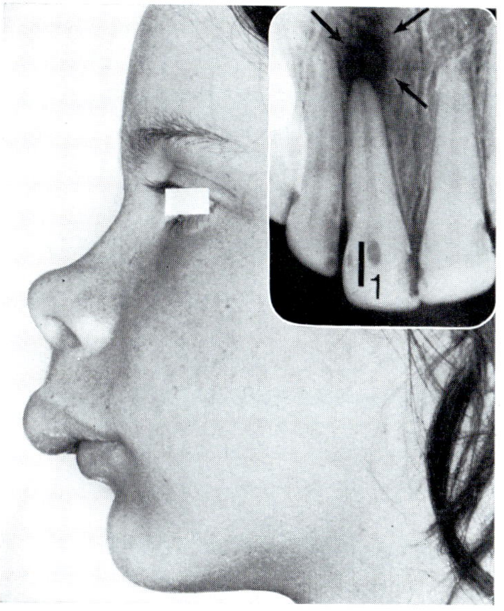

Fig. 158.—Submucosal abscess with marked oedema of the upper lip, arising from the upper right central incisor (gangrenous pulp and periapical granuloma, *see* inset). Therapy: incision in the labial sulcus and drainage. When the acute symptoms have subsided, incision must be followed by root-canal treatment or apicectomy.

Submucosal abscesses, localized in the buccal sulcus, are as a ruie associated with oedema of the facial soft tissues (*Figs.* 158 and 159). Extra-orally marked infiltration cannot usually be palpated.

In the case of a palatal or sublingual abscess extra-oral reaction is mostly slight (*Fig.* 157 a).

Treatment consists of incision and drainage. An incision in the buccal sulcus is usually placed adjacent to the tooth responsible. If this tooth is a lower premolar regard must be paid to the mental nerve, which leaves the mandibular canal in this area. In the case of a palatal abscess attention must be paid to the course of the greater palatine artery (parallel to the midline in a postero-anterior direction, in the region where the vertical alveolar process passes into the horizontal palatal roof). If the associated tooth need not be retained, extraction will sometimes give sufficient drainage and make incision unnecessary (*Fig.* 156). In order to prevent the wound from too

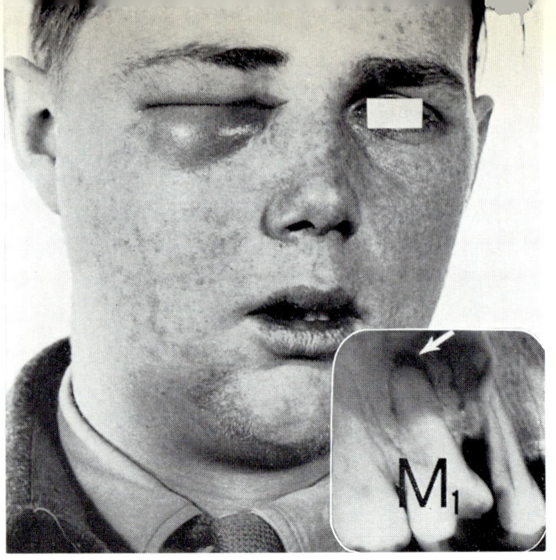

Fig. 159.—Massive oedema due to an abscess in the canine fossa originating from the upper right first molar (*see* inset). Developed in 5 days. Treatment: intra-oral incision in the buccal sulcus. Extraction of the molar when acute symptoms are over.

early closure a drain can be inserted (iodoform gauze in petroleum jelly) or, when a palatal abscess is concerned, an elliptical piece of mucosa can be excised. The latter method cannot be applied when the cause is an infected cyst for it will interfere with treatment and especially the healing of the cyst. Administration of antibiotics is usually not necessary.

c. Subcutaneous abscess: The initial stage of this abscess starts as a periostitis, also with slight oedema of the soft tissues. Afterwards the very painful (pulsating pain) subperiosteal abscess arises. When breaking through the periosteum after 2–4 days the violent pain subsides, but is followed by a very extensive oedema of the soft tissues (phlegmonous stage). In about 3–6 days an induration (infiltration) develops centrally in this oedema. After 4–6 days there is a centre which is painful on palpation and this is a sign of early abscess formation. Finally, after about 4–7 days, it will be possible to elicit fluctuation (subcutaneous abscess). The skin, originally not involved in the process, will redden later (*Fig.* 160), changing colour to reddish-blue and finally the top of the swelling becomes yellowish, because of the presence of pus close to the surface. Hereafter the swelling may burst. The abscesses may be distinguished according to their localization, for example: cheek abscess (*Fig.* 160), chin

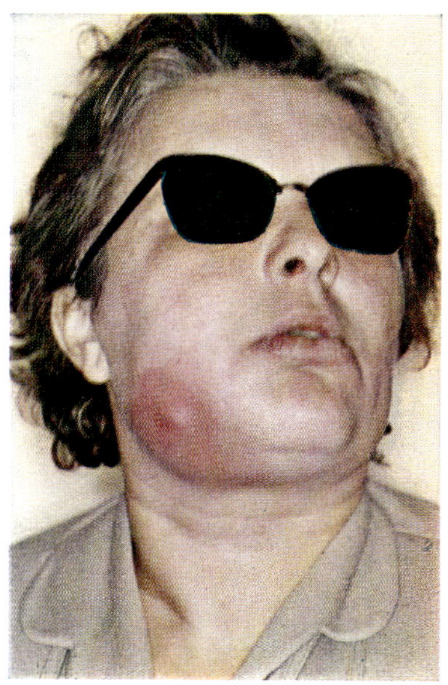

Fig. 160.—Extensive inflammation of the soft tissues (infiltrate). Tendency to abscess formation (central swelling). Treatment: extra-oral incision, drainage, wet bandage. Removal of causative tooth or root-canal treatment when acute symptoms are over.

abscess (*Fig.* 162), etc. After drainage of pus acute symptoms subside and finally only a fistula remains.

The phlegmonous stage of acute inflammation of soft tissue is sometimes called *cellulitis* (*Fig.* 160).

Not every subcutaneous abscess arises in this way, sometimes there are no violent reactions of the surrounding soft tissues. Then the inflammation is subacute or chronic. There is only slight oedema, which is very well localized. Via the infiltrative stage a subcutaneous abscess is formed (chronically) (*Figs.* 161 and 162) (*see also* p. 180 and *Figs.* 166 and 167).

Treatment of a subcutaneous abscess consists of incision and drainage (rubber drain or iodoform gauze in petroleum jelly) as soon as pus can be demonstrated (by fluctuation) or is expected (after 4–5 days, when there is a centre which is painful on palpation). The site of incision is chosen so that the scar will be almost invisible (for instance along the lower mandibular border or submentally) (*Figs.* 161 and 162)).

The course of the facial artery must be kept in mind when making an incision in this region; this artery crosses the lower mandibular

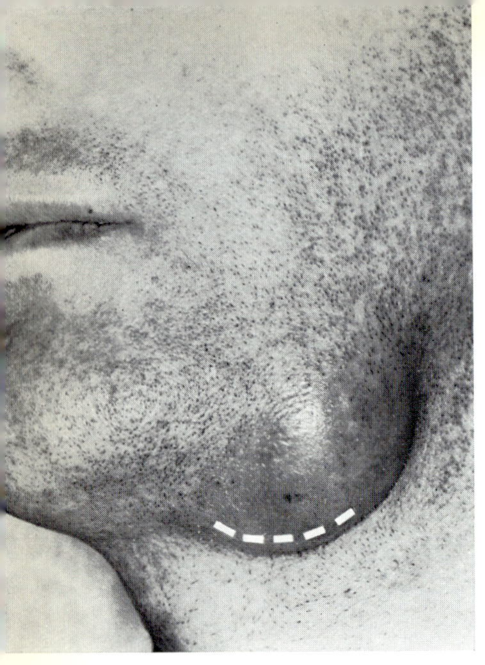

Fig. 161.—Subacute subcutaneous abscess, originating from granulomas at lower left first and second molar. Treatment: incision along dotted line, drainage, and wet bandage. Extraction of the two molars when the inflammation has decreased.

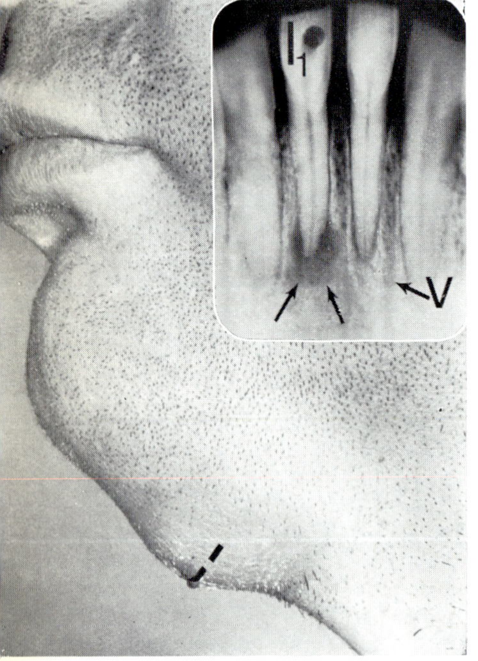

Fig. 162.—Submental abscess, recurred four or five times in the previous 1½ years, arising from the lower right central incisor. Treatment: incision along dotted line, followed by apicectomy of the tooth (v = vascular channel).

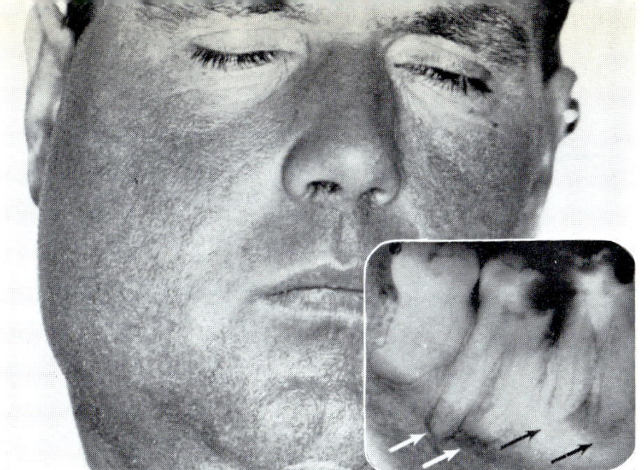

Fig. 163.—Phlegmonous stage of a severe acute inflammation originating from the lower right first and second molars (*see* inset). Developed in 1 week. Tendency to abscess formation in the deeper spaces. Treatment: hospitalization, antibiotics; afterwards extra-oral incision beneath the mandibular angle and drainage. Extraction of the two molars.

border in the region of the anterior border of the insertion of the masseter muscle. Antibiotics may be administered in the case of very severe inflammation, as long as the infiltrative stage is not yet over and there is no formation of an abscess (for instance: 900,000 units of procaine penicillin and 300,000 units of penicillin intramuscularly daily for at least 5 days). Infra-red radiation and wet compresses may be helpful in accelerating the process.

d. Exceptional extensions: Acute odontogenic inflammations may spread into the different spaces into which the face is divided by fasciae and muscles. Generally, however, in the case of these often severe inflammations it is very difficult to determine where exactly the abscess is situated (*Fig*. 163).

General anaesthesia is indicated to enable exploration and incision of these abscesses. Hospitalization is necessary.

Acute inflammations following tooth extraction are discussed on p. 196.

Ludwig's angina is a rapidly spreading, very acute infection of the floor of the mouth, which may develop in 4–6 hours and which is probably due to haemolytic streptococci. The tongue is greatly swollen and protruding and the patient often extends his neck in order to be able to breathe. Large doses of antibiotics, adequate drainage, and tracheostomy, in the case of respiratory difficulties, are indicated. Fortunately this kind of inflammation is very rare.

Odontogenic maxillary sinusitis may originate from a granuloma at an upper molar or premolar or from a deep gingival pocket. In most cases of odontogenic sinusitis the inflammation is caused by a *perforation of the floor of the sinus*, following tooth extraction. In general, odontogenic sinusitides are very putrid, in contrast with rhinogenous sinusitides. Treatment of *acute odontogenic sinusitis* may consist of puncture and irrigation via the inferior nasal meatus (every other day, four or five times in total), oral administration of antibiotics (for instance ampicillin, 250–500 mg. 6-hourly, for 5 days, or tetracycline hydrochloride, 250 mg. at 6-hourly intervals, for 5–7 days). It is obvious that the odontogenic cause must be eliminated as soon as possible.

In the case of *chronic sinusitis* treatment consists of irrigating the maxillary sinus every other day, either via the inferior nasal meatus or via the perforation in the sinal floor, with physiological salt solution, until the fluid remains clear. Treatment may be supported by inhalations and nasal decongestants (for instance, xylometazoline 0·1 per cent solution (Otrivine)).

When there are many polyps in the maxillary sinus removal is indicated by means of a Caldwell-Luc operation. The odontogenic cause must be eliminated also and any possible perforation in the antral floor must be closed.

e. Remarks: Teeth in the upper jaw generally tend to the formation of a submucosal abscess. Cellulitis and subcutaneous abscesses usually originate from teeth in the mandible.

A swelling at the mandibular angle combined with marked trismus in a patient between 17 and 21 years of age is, in the majority of cases, due to an inflammation originating from a third molar erupting with difficulty.

Except for clinical investigation, *radiographic examination* is of major importance in finding the odontogenic cause and should never be omitted. Deeply situated root remnants, impacted teeth, residual infected cysts, and so on can be demonstrated radiographically. Periapical lateral-oblique radiographs are the most useful.

The question whether the *tooth responsible can be extracted during the stage of acute inflammation* should be considered in each individual case. If the patient is anxious to retain the tooth and the tooth can be treated endodontically or by apicectomy and its crown is of such quality that restoration is possible, the tooth need not be extracted. Neither is extraction necessary to make acute inflammatory symptoms subside faster. Only in early periostitis may progression be stopped by extraction of the causative tooth.

It is often stated that during acute inflammation extraction is in principle incorrect. In our opinion this is not true. If it is expected that *extraction will be easy* and that drainage will be promoted, there is no objection at all (submucosal abscess). The clinical pictures of *Figs*. 156, 158, and possibly *Fig*. 157 show examples. In the case of subcutaneous spread extraction will have no favourable effect; the inflammation of the soft tissues has become a distinct entity and has to be treated accordingly. Examples hereof are shown in *Figs*. 160, 161, 162, and 163. It should be kept in mind, however, that it may be difficult to achieve good local anaesthesia for extraction. In general it is advisable to treat the acute inflammation as a distinct entity and to extract or treat the causative tooth shortly after the acute symptoms have subsided, in order to prevent recurrence.

Local anaesthesia for abscess incision can best be achieved by very superficial submucosal or subcutaneous injection of 0·5–1 ml. 2 per cent lidocaine hydrochloride with adrenaline 1 : 80,000 at the point where the incision will be made. Though not completely painless, incision and exploration of an abscess can be endured in this way, at least by adults. Short-lasting general anaesthesia is indicated for nervous children, or when the abscess is located very deep and it is expected that exploration will be difficult.

Anaesthesia by freezing (ethyl chloride spray) is usually followed by a very severe, deep, dull pain and is therefore, and also because of its short duration, not a method of choice.

f. For differential diagnosis in the case of a swelling in the region of the mandibular angle an inflammation of the parotid gland (mumps, acute exacerbation of a non-specific chronic parotitis) must be considered. The localization of these inflammations is more cranially, anterior and posterior to the ear, pushing the ear lobe outward; pus may be massaged from the parotid duct and trismus is slight or absent. In the case of a submandibular swelling a swollen lymphnode has to be considered (acute non-specific lymphadenitis in children) or an inflammation of the submandibular gland (salivary calculus, epidemic sialo-adenitis).

When there is a swelling dorsally in the mouth, except for an inflammation originating from a third molar, a peritonsillar abscess must be kept in mind.

Sometimes acute osteomyelitis (mandible), carcinoma of the maxillary sinus, and cervicofacial actinomycosis are mentioned in the differential diagnosis.

Chronic Forms.—These may be in principle just like acute inflammations—apical, pericoronal, or periodontal in nature. The apical inflammations are of major importance.

a. Periapical Granuloma.—The bone around the root tip of a tooth with a necrotic pulp is replaced by granulation tissue. Such a granuloma can be considered to be a reaction to chronic irritation caused by the discharge of bacteria and their products and of debris of pulp tissue via the apical foramen of the tooth. Generally a granuloma is asymptomatic and the patient is unaware of its presence. Sometimes there is a slight, gnawing pain every now and then; there may also be a slight swelling at the apex. Sometimes a small 'pustule' is visible. The fact that the pulp of a tooth is necrotic (bluish-grey discoloration of the crown, no reaction to ethyl chloride or electric vitality tests) may excite the suspicion that there is a granuloma at the apex. A dental radiograph may confirm this suspicion, for on the dental radiograph a sharply or ill-demarcated radiolucent area 0·5–1·0 cm. in diameter may be seen, the periodontal space and especially the lamina dura of the alveolus being disrupted (*Fig.* 164).

Though a granuloma is asymptomatic it is advisable to have it treated as soon as it is discovered in order to prevent acute exacerbation (often at a most inconvenient moment) causing many symptoms. Treatment may consist of either extraction, root-canal treatment, or apicectomy (incisors, canines, and premolars). Broadly speaking there are two principles of root-canal treatment: first, the necrotic contents of the canal may be disinfected and completely removed up to the apex and afterwards the root canal can be eliminated by filling it completely by an inert material (gutta-percha). This method is only practicable if the root canal is accessible and can be reamed.

The other principle is based on removal of the contents of the pulpal chamber and of the entrances of the root canals. Following this, occasionally a disinfectant is included in the pulpal chamber (often with a formaldehyde base) to disinfect and to mummify remnants of the pulp in the root canal. After that a disinfectant with sustained action is sealed into the pulpal chamber and root entrances (Trio-paste). This method may be applied to teeth of which the root canals are not accessible.

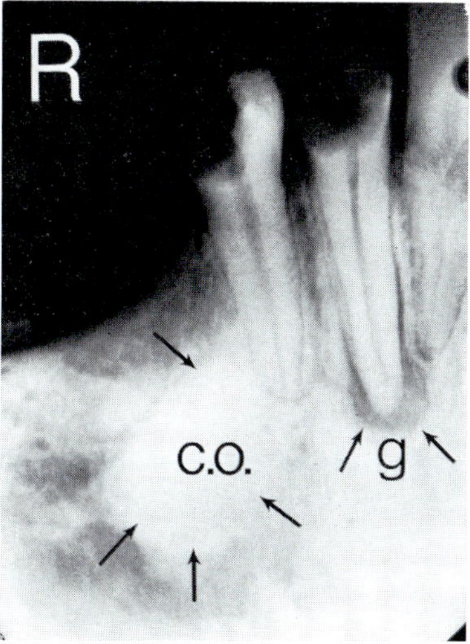

Fig. 164.—Dental radiograph showing both root-tip granuloma (g) and condensing osteitis (c.o.).

In both methods of endodontic treatment many variants are known which may all produce, provided they are carefully performed, good results.

In the case of apicectomy the root tip is exposed via an intra-oral incision and the granuloma is curetted. The root tip is resected and the root canal is filled with an inert material. Resection of the root tip is necessary because this part of the root canal has many ramifications which (with their contents) cannot easily be eliminated by other means.

b. Condensing or Sclerosing Osteitis.—When the inflammatory irritation, originating from a gangrenous pulp, is only slight, or the resistance high, an ill defined radio-opacity of gradually increasing density may develop. The lesion is usually painless and there are no clinical symptoms. Here a very slow endosteal bone formation is seen related to a primarily chronic infection. The lesion is usually found accidentally and occurs mainly periapically to a lower first molar. Sporadically such a bone sclerosis occurs in relation to a tooth with chronic pulpitis or in an overloaded tooth.

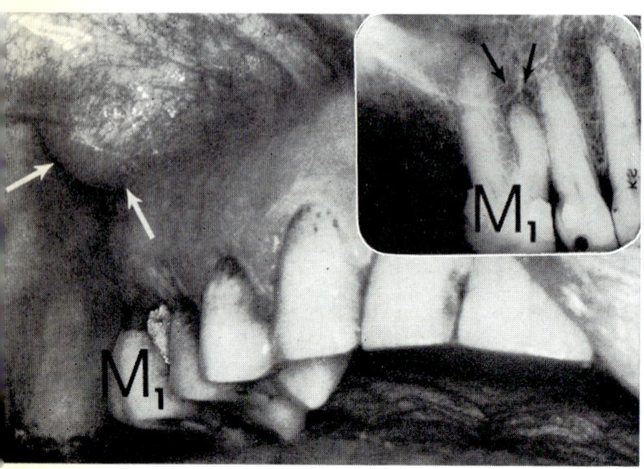

Fig. 165.—Granulating periostitis originating from the upper right first molar. Painless. (*See also Fig.* 156.)

In the lower jaw, however, in extremely rare cases similar osteo-sclerotic areas may occur, but without any apparent odontogenic origin. The cause is unknown (*see also* p. 50).

Treatment of condensing osteitis may consist either of extraction (usually not necessary) or adequate endodontic treatment of the involved tooth.

c. Chronic Granulating Periostitis.—When the apical inflammation extends to the periosteum, granulating periostitis may develop. A localized soft swelling (0·5–1·5 cm.) develops intra-orally on the jaw, which may show (pseudo) fluctuation and sometimes resembles a small submucosal abscess (*Fig.* 165). After a time the swelling may become firmer and increase slowly in size. Complaints are few or absent. Treatment consists of extraction of the tooth responsible or of endodontic therapy. When the cause is removed granulating periostitis will heal without any further treatment.

d. Periostitis Ossificans.—Very slight irritation of the periosteum may lead to bone apposition. The inflammation here is even more chronic in nature than the preceding one. A bony-hard symptom-less swelling (0·5–1·5 cm.) develops on the jaw adjacent to a tooth with a necrotic pulp, whereas there are no symptoms. From a differential diagnostic point of view a radicular cyst must be considered. A dental radiograph is decisive: if the lesion is a periostitis ossificans there are either no signs at all or the bone may be slightly more

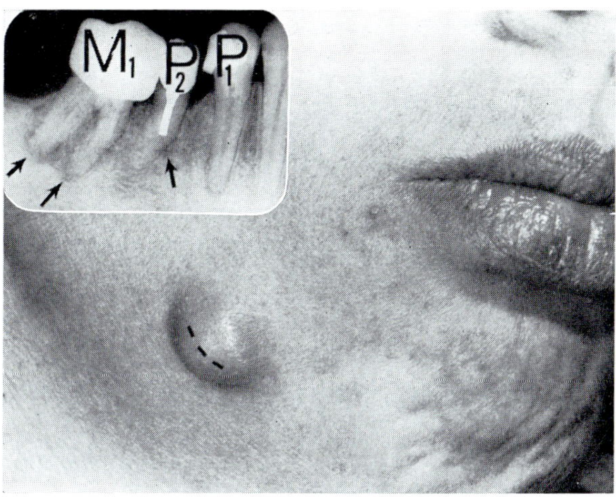

Fig. 166.—Small chronic subcutaneous abscess originating from the lower right second premolar. After breaking down, a fistula may remain. There are also periapical lesions of the lower right first premolar and molar (*see* inset).

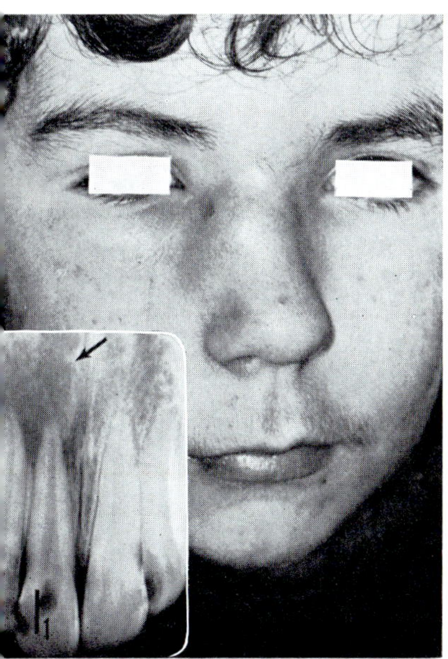

Fig. 167.—Small odontogenic abscess adjacent to the nose originating from a granuloma at the upper right central incisor. After rupturing, a fistula may remain.

dense, whereas a cyst shows a circumscribed radiolucency. Treatment consists of either extraction or root-canal treatment. The new bone need not be removed.

e. Intra-oral Dental Fistula.—If the apical inflammatory process perforates periosteum and mucosa (usually after development of a small abscess) a fistula may develop in the mucosa, mostly in the region of the apex. In general the lesion is asymptomatic. Treatment consists of removal of the dental cause.

f. Odontogenic Skin Fistula.—When the chronic inflammatory process extends apically of the buccal sulcus into the soft tissues, firstly an induration develops, for instance in the cheek ('disk', 'lump'). Initially the skin can still be moved over the induration, but later on this becomes impossible. A circumscribed discoloration develops, initially red, afterwards reddish-blue, and finally in the centre a small 'pustule' is formed. When it bursts a small quantity of sanguineous pus is discharged (*Figs*. 166 and 167). A skin fistula is then formed. This entirely chronic development does not cause many symptoms; this is, of course, not applicable to those cases in which the fistula has remained after eruption of an acute inflammation to the skin.

Usually the patient is not referred until the fistula has existed for some time. There is a troublesome 'dimple' on the cheek or the chin with a 'pustule' at its base, which fails to heal and from which every now and then some secretion is discharged. Washing and shaving give rise to difficulties at that spot. The skin cannot be moved and elevated (*Fig.* 168). Via the 'pustule' a thin probe can be inserted to the apex of the causative tooth. A strand can be felt intra-orally in the buccal sulcus, leading from the skin to the tooth; the latter shows all the characteristics, mentioned previously (p. 176), of a tooth with a necrotic pulp. A radiograph of the tooth shows the picture of a periapical granuloma or a cyst (infected). Sometimes the fistula is caused by an impacted tooth or a root remnant.

The localization of odontogenic skin fistulae is dependent on the position of the causative granuloma and of the easiest way to the skin surface. Blocking their path are, for instance: cortex, fasciae, and especially the facial musculature. Places of predilection for these fistulae are (*Fig.* 169):—

Laterally or caudally of the lower mandibular border, immediately anterior to the insertion of the masseter muscle (lower molars and premolars);

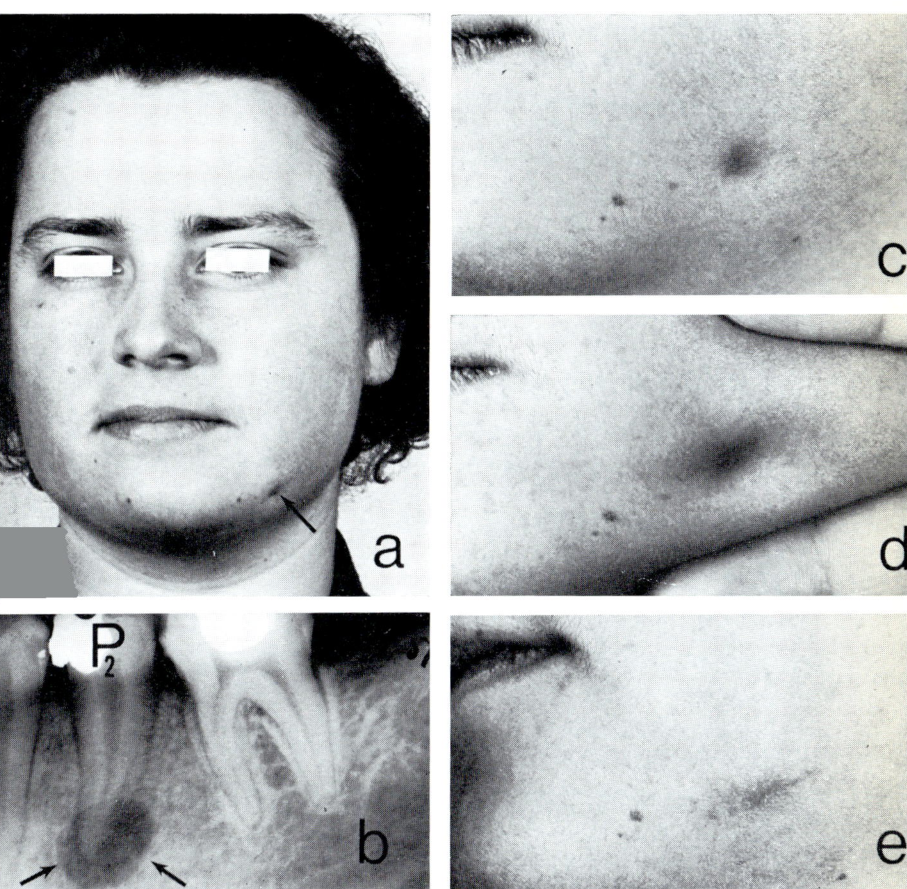

Fig. 168.—a, Characteristic picture of an odontogenic skin fistula. b, The fistula is caused by a granuloma at the lower left second premolar. c, The skin shows the characteristic dimple. d, The skin cannot be elevated. e, After treatment of the causative molar and healing of the fistula the scar was corrected.

Submentally (lower incisors);

In the mentolabial sulcus (lower incisors);

In the prominence of the cheek, immediately caudally of the most prominent part of the zygomatic bone (upper premolars);

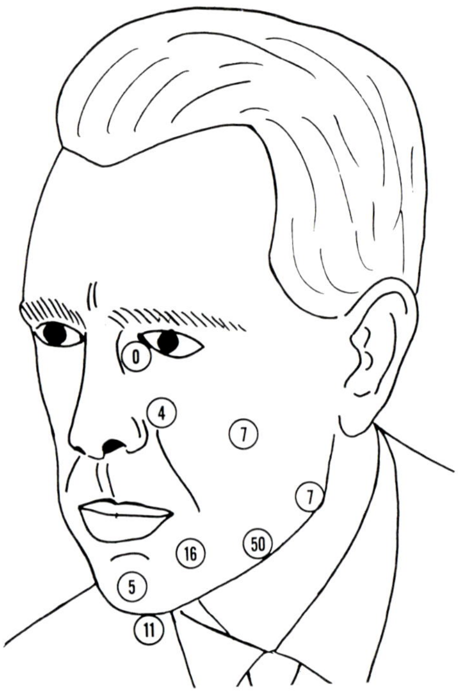

Fig. 169.—Places of predilection for odontogenic fistulae in the face. The numerals indicate the relative frequency of incidence.

In rare cases an odontogenic fistula may occur in the medial corner of the eye or behind the mandibular angle.

The clinical picture, just before the skin breaks down, may sometimes resemble a furuncle or an infected sebaceous cyst (*Figs.* 166 and 167). Also an early actinomycosis must be kept in mind (pus culture and histological examination of granulations).

Repeated surgical treatment may lead to ugly scars (*Fig.* 170).

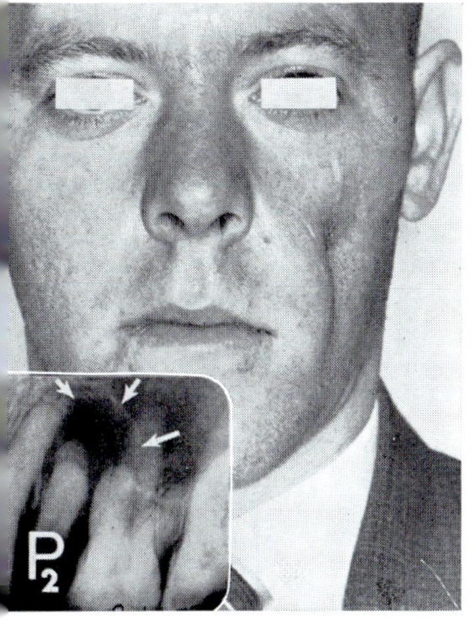

Fig. 170.—Erroneously repeated surgical treatment may leave ugly scars. The odonto-genic cause, namely a granuloma of the upper right second premolar, was overlooked (*see* inset).

Treatment of these fistulae consists of removal of the odontogenic cause (*see* inset, *Fig.* 170). Subsequently the fistula will heal spontaneously. In the course of time a simple plastic operation may remove the disfiguring scar, if desired (*Fig.* 168). Usually, however, this will be unnecessary.

Focal Infections.—Formerly much significance was attached to chronic foci of inflammation of odontogenic origin in the jaws in the aetiology of rheumatic diseases. Furthermore, they were said to play a part in eye infections (iridocyclitis) and skin diseases. Especially in Andrews's disease, with recurrent purulent foci on the palms of the hands and sometimes on the soles of the feet too, much significance is still placed on focal infection.

It is also generally accepted that thrombophlebitis migrans is maintained by a focus.

Furthermore, periapical granulomata may be responsible for a slightly raised temperature or a high E.S.R.

Periapical inflammations, chronic osteitides, root remnants, impacted teeth, and deep gingival pockets may act as foci of infection. We have an impression that the importance of elimination of these foci is only small at present, at least as far as rheumatism is concerned. It is, however, advisable to remove these foci of infection also for reasons of general health. Investigation of the dentition has to consist of vitality tests of all teeth and examination of a complete set of dental films. Prophylactic administration of antibiotics to these patients in the case of extraction is advisable.

NON-ODONTOGENIC INFECTIONS

Non-specific Acute Lymphadenitis.—Especially in children, but also in adults, a severe infection of unknown origin of a submandibular lymph-node may occur (*Fig.* 171). Inspection of the dentition and appropriate radiography must not be omitted. Treatment is seldom necessary; infra-red radiation or wet towels may speed the healing of the infection. In most cases it takes some weeks before the infection has fully subsided. Abscess formation is of rare occurrence and therefore incision is seldom necessary.

From a differential diagnostic point of view a swollen submandibular salivary gland, a lateral cervical cyst, and a tuberculous lymph-node must be considered (*see* p. 187).

Actinomycosis.—An infection by this ray fungus in the maxillo-facial area is of rare incidence. The site of entry may be a carious tooth with a necrotic pulp, a partly erupted lower third molar (many patients are between 19 and 25 years of age), or an extraction wound. The infection is caused by a mixed flora in which non-specific cocci are preceding or coexistent with *Actinomyces israeli*, which is almost always the cause of actinomycosis in man. This fungus, occurring as a saprophyte in the mouth, is anaerobic and is hardly seen outside the human body. Formerly the fungi, sometimes found in grasses or hay, were thought to be the producers of the disease, but as these fungi are aerobic they cannot possibly be the cause. In cattle, actinomycotic processes are mostly caused by the aerobic actino-bacillus and only in rare cases by *Actinomyces israeli*. The consistency of the chronic inflammation of the soft tissue is board-like, but curiously enough not painful. The skin shows a bluish-red discoloration and is immobile. There is a tendency to formation of multiple small abscesses, from which thin pus is discharged after incision, which contains yellowish-green granules (flakes), consisting of *Actinomyces* colonies. The infection is generally localized cervicofacially, i.e., in the cervicofacial tissues in the region of the mandibular angle and sometimes in the parotid gland area (*Fig.* 172).

The diagnosis depends on the characteristic clinical picture, microscopical examination of the pus, and histopathological

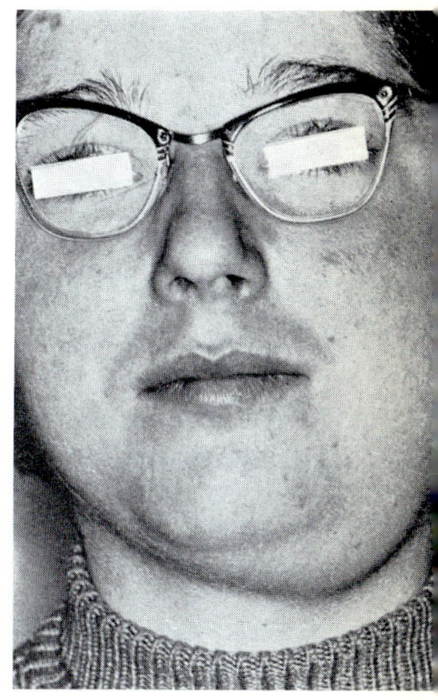

Fig. 171.—Subacute inflammation of a submandibular lymph-node in a 15-year-old girl. No odontogenic cause could be found.

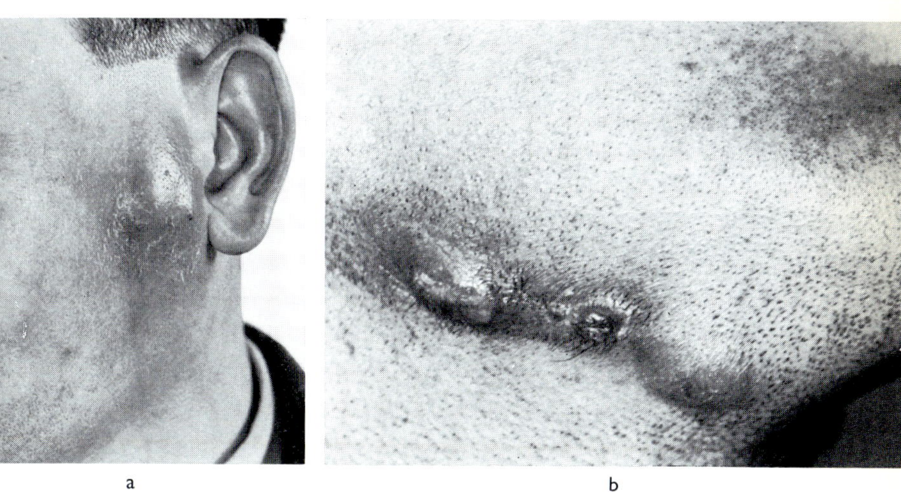

a   b

Fig. 172.—a, Persistent actinomycosis in the left parotid area. b, Characteristic cervicofacial actinomycosis. Board-like, painless infiltrate, reddish-blue discoloration, multiple abscesses. Site of entry was presumably a deep carious third molar.

investigation of the granulation tissue. Culture can only confirm the diagnosis, because it may be some time before the results are known. The radiograph may show the tooth, which has possibly been the site of entry, or an empty socket. The bone is usually unchanged. Actinomycosis of the mandibular bone is extremely rare.

Therapy consists of extraction of the involved tooth and administration of high doses (for instance 2,000,000–3,000,000 units per day) of penicillin, continued for a long period. In the majority of cases this therapy will prove to be successful. Sometimes it is advisable to change to another antibiotic (tetracycline, erythromycin, or chloramphenicol). When small abscesses are formed, they must be incised and curetted. Sometimes packs saturated with Lugol's solution are advised. Hospitalization and improvement of general resistance are necessary, especially in the initial stage. Prolonged control is indicated; the prognosis is favourable in the case of adequate treatment.

Syphilis.—Syphilis may occur in the mouth as a primary lesion on the lips, tip of the tongue, and in the tonsillar region. It appears as an ulcer with an elevated margin and a fiery red base. Secondary, highly infective lesions are mainly seen on the soft palate, deep red, patchy exanthemata, which may change into red papules. Owing to epithelial swellings, very conspicuous mucous plaques, surrounded by fiery red areolae, may arise.

Sometimes a gumma is visible on the palate; in the long run the palate may be perforated (which must not be confused with the round perforation due to a sucker on the inside of a prosthesis).

Interstitial glossitis with atrophy of the dorsal tongue mucosa is also described; it is said that the lesion can easily change into leucoplakia. Tertiary syphilis sometimes manifests itself by a gummatous swelling of the tongue. It may break through to the dorsum of the tongue, leaving a star-shaped contraction.

In some cases the picture may resemble carcinoma.

Barrel-shaped Hutchinson's incisors are hardly seen today.

All the above-described lesions are of rare occurrence in the Western countries nowadays, but they must always be kept in mind.

Tuberculosis.—This specific infection is also of very rare incidence in the oral cavity. This is especially applicable to the tuberculous ulcer, which may occur in a patient suffering from an advanced stage of open tuberculous of the lungs.

Occasionally an indurated submandibular lymph-node is found of unknown origin and which fails to heal. Sometimes there may be a skin fistula with no tendency to heal, beneath which the more deeply located gland can be palpated.

The diagnosis of tuberculosis is often only confirmed after histo-pathological examination of the extirpated gland. The lesion is usually seen in children.

In the differential diagnosis an odontogenic skin fistula, an infection originating from the dentition (dental radiograph), or from the submandibular salivary gland (sialogram) have to be considered (*see also* p. 184).

CHAPTER 8

MAXILLOFACIAL PAIN

Trigeminal Neuralgia (Tic Douloureux).—This clinically very characteristic facial pain is marked by paroxysmal violent attacks, which may occur spontaneously, but may also be elicited by, for instance, soft touching of a certain skin area ('trigger point' or 'trigger zone'), which need not be the point of exit of the nerve. The lesion is of unknown origin. Histologically the nerve is undisturbed. Often the cause is erroneously thought to be located in the dentition and several teeth may be extracted unnecessarily. Examination of teeth and jaws, however, must not be omitted.

For further information reference may be made to the neurological and neurosurgical literature. This is also applicable to other rarely occurring neuralgias in this area and to neuritis.

Neuralgia-like Pain.—

a. Pulpitis may cause severe pain, which is sometimes difficult to localize. It is not always possible to identify the causative tooth and sometimes it may not even be possible to know whether the cause of the pain is located in the upper or in the lower jaw. Although pain on percussion and an enhanced reaction to thermal tests (tooth with a big restoration) may be absent, this examination must not be omitted. Especially when the patient states that the pain increases when he has just gone to bed, pulpitis must be kept in mind. Radiographic examination of the involved side of the jaws may be helpful in finding the cause (hidden cavity). Sometimes a diagnostic injection of a local anaesthetic solution will aid greatly in the localization of the pain. For treatment of pulpitis *see* p. 162.

b. Acute Infected Granuloma (periapical abscess) may cause severe, pulsating pain, especially when the granuloma is completely surrounded by a thick layer of bone. Usually the relation to a tooth can easily be demonstrated. Vitality tests (negative reaction to cold or heat application) and a dental radiograph (apical radiolucency) may confirm the diagnosis. Treatment consists of drainage of the abscess (*see* p. 163).

c. Alveolitis may cause very severe pain, which is of a continuous nature and localized to an empty socket. The related tooth was extracted some days earlier. The contents of the socket are strongly putrid (*see also* p. 195).

d. A Deep Gingival Pocket may lead to a gnawing pain, not too severe, but very troublesome owing to its persistence. Often food is impacted between two teeth, causing periodontitis by continuous irritation. Treatment consists of cleaning the adjacent teeth, spraying the pocket with hydrogen peroxide, and restoration of the contact point.

e. Impacted Teeth (third molar, cuspid), *root remnants,* chronic foci of osteitis. In fact, all kinds of lesions which may occur in the jaws, even denticles in the pulp, have been associated with neuralgia-like pain. Clinically, however, this relation is in many cases far from being evident. Extraction of a tooth or root may indeed bring relief of pain or disappearance, but not in every case.

f. In patients wearing dentures resorption of the lower alveolar process may occur to such an extent that *dehiscence of the mandibular canal* is caused. Biting upon the prosthesis may cause a deep, dull pain, which may be long lasting. An oblique lateral radiograph of the mandible shows clearly the course of the mandibular canal.

The mental nerve may be compressed, for instance by an ill-fitting prosthesis, at the mental foramen. Pain and paraesthesiae may be the result.

g. Lesions of the Maxillary Sinus may cause vague complaints of pain in the maxillary area.

On a suspicion of such a lesion a radiograph of the sinus and examination by an ear, nose, and throat specialist must not be omitted. A dental cause must be excluded by examination of the dentition and dental radiographs.

h. Disturbances of the Temporomandibular Joint owing to Arthrosis may sometimes be responsible for difficulty in diagnosing complaints of pain in the lateral part of the face. The pain may be felt in the temporoparietal region, over the eyes, in the ear, in the zygomatic area, or in the neck (*see Fig.* 82, p. 103). Usually there has been a preceding period with clicking and/or locking or the joint is painful when the mouth is opened maximally or on pressure in the external auditory canal in a ventral direction (*see* p. 103).

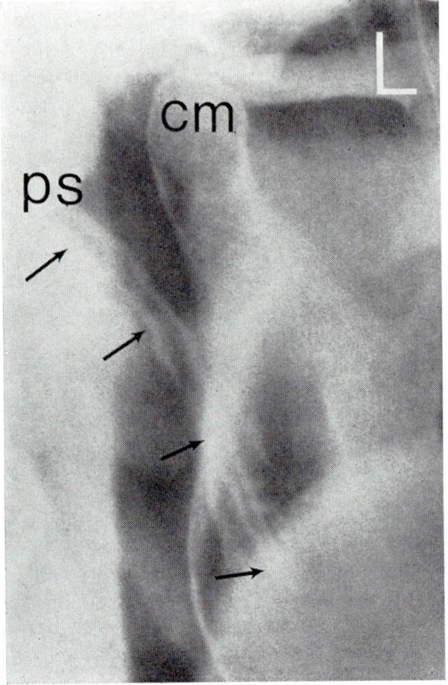

Fig. 173.—Long styloid process (ps) and calcification or ossification of the stylohyoid ligament (cm=head of mandibule) (Parma's infracranial projection).

Often there is a correlation in localization between pain, chewing side, and side of the greatest chewing ability, as far as the dentition is concerned. *Injection* of a local anaesthetic into the joint causes the pain to disappear temporarily. Radiographic examination (Parma's infracranial projection or oblique lateral transcranial projection of both joints) may sometimes give a decisive answer, but in many cases clearly visible deformities only occur in the course of years (for treatment *see* p. 103).

Spasm and pain of the masticatory muscles as accompanying phenomena of arthrosis or occurring in people with bad masticatory habits (clamping or grinding) are also mentioned in the aetiology of facial pain.

i. A Lengthened Styloid Process may be responsible for pain laterally in the neck. Sometimes pain increases when chewing or when the mouth is opened widely. Often the patient may complain of a sensation of swelling in the throat; he swallows very frequently in order to make the sensation disappear. There is pain on palpation in the tonsillar fossa area, where the long styloid process can be palpated as a hard, sometimes pointed, and immobile object. Especially on Parma's infracranial projection the deformity is clearly visible. There is often not only a lengthened styloid process, but also calcification of the stylohyoid ligament (*Fig.* 173). Treatment consists of resection.

CHAPTER 9

COMPLICATIONS FOLLOWING MINOR ORAL SURGERY

LOCAL COMPLICATIONS

Haemorrhage after Extraction.—Abnormally persistent copious bleeding following tooth extraction should be treated by the dentist who extracted the tooth. Some patients, however, ask their physician for treatment.

Haemorrhage after extraction may be caused by local or general factors.

Local Causes.—Bleeding usually occurs 2–3 hours after extraction when adrenaline in the local anaesthetic is no longer effective or when the contracting elements in the vascular walls become fatigued. Injured or torn gingival margins, multiple extractions in the same half of the jaw, and hyperaemia of the gingiva (gingivitis, periodontal disease) are conducive to haemorrhage after extraction. Bleeding is usually profuse and only in rare cases arterial (lower front teeth). In 85 per cent of the cases the bleeding is localized to the molar region.

General Causes.—These can seldom be diagnosed when the patient presents himself; the medical history is important: Is bleeding of common occurrence after tooth extraction? Is there a familial tendency to haemorrhage? Do nasal bleedings often occur? Are haematomata of common incidence after blunt traumata? Does the patient take drugs, for instance anticoagulants, or did he take abnormal high doses of salicylates or other analgesics for toothache?

In a number of cases a disturbance of the blood coagulation mechanism may be revealed by excessive haemorrhage after tooth extraction. Thorough investigation of the coagulation factors and of the platelet function is of major importance in every patient with haemorrhage after extraction or with a history of haemorrhages.

Patients suffering from haemophilia or patients taking anti-coagulants are usually aware of their bleeding tendency and do not have teeth extracted without precautionary measures.

Treatment.—Whatever may be the cause, the patient must be treated at the moment when he presents himself. The most effective method of treatment is suturing the gingival wound. After localization of the bleeding socket and local injection of a small quantity of a local anaesthetic the margins of the gingiva wound are approximated with a suture, causing local ischaemia, which makes the bleeding cease. It is not necessary and also not always possible that the margins of the wound contact each other. The number of sutures per socket depends on the size of the wound; usually two or three will be sufficient. Suture material to be used may be nylon (size 00) or catgut (00). The coagulum which is formed is thus held in the socket and is protected because the wound surface is reduced.

In case of excessive haemorrhage the socket can be filled firmly by gelfoam (Spongostan, Gelastypt, Surgicel), followed by suturing the gingival margins (the inserted sponge must not protrude from the socket); if desired, this sponge can be dipped in a concentrated thrombin solution for local application. These measures are seldom necessary.

When the wound cannot be sutured, a firmly rolled gauze which must exceed the height of the crown of the neighbouring teeth can initially be put *on* the bleeding socket. The patient is requested to bite on this pack firmly (20–30 minutes), in order to exert pressure on the margins of the wound and to protect the coagulum. Also in this case the socket can be filled with gelfoam, which must not protrude from the socket in order to prevent infection owing to absorption of saliva (dry socket).

In a case of emergency the socket can be plugged, for instance with iodoform gauze in paraffin jelly 1 cm. in width. The socket is filled firmly with this plug. Removal of this pack after 4 or 5 days, however, may cause renewed bleeding. Beware of putting cotton-wool into a socket, it may be followed by severe alveolitis!

Administration of the commonly used drugs influencing the clotting mechanism is rather useless, unless it is proved that the bleeding is due to a general cause. Many drugs recommended in the past for the treatment of haemorrhage after extraction have appeared to be ineffective (carbazochrome salicylate, calcium chloride, or calcium gluconate, vitamin K_1, or vitamin K_3).

Tooth extraction in patients treated with anticoagulants can best be done in consultation with a general physician. Extraction within a period of 6 months after the latest cardiac infarct is usually not permitted. In most patients there will be no objection to a temporary reduction in the anticoagulant therapy after this period. After consultation with the doctor who initiated the anticoagulant therapy, half the normal dose is usually given for 2 days before the extraction, on the day of extraction, and for 2 days after the extraction. The chance of haemorrhage is extremely small in patients whose thrombotest is maintained at 30–40 per cent and in whom no more than four single-rooted or two multi-rooted teeth are extracted, after which the extraction wounds are carefully sutured with nylon 00. Spongostan, Gelastypt, and similar haemostyptic agents, applied without suturing the wound, are insufficient.

Total extraction of the dentition is to be performed in several sittings with intervals of at least 10 days. It is important that in these patients the clotting mechanism is regulated after the extraction. Simple extraction of a single-rooted tooth or a root remnant can usually be done without changing the anticoagulant therapy. Also in these cases careful suturing is very important. In patients treated with Sinthrome or Marcoumar, administration of salicylic acid or phenylbutazone derivatives must be avoided. An analgesic, such as glafenine (Glifanan), may be administered.

Haemophilia.—The bleeding tendency in haemophiliac patients is so great that extraction can be performed *only in hospital.* Maximal general precautionary measures have to be taken. In the case of haemophilia A this consists of administration of fresh blood plasma or cryoprecipitate and in the case of haemophilia B of plasma or prothrombin-proconvertin-Stuart and haemophilic factor B. Sedation of the patient before and after extraction is of major importance. Local precautionary measures consist of careful suturing (nylon) and covering the wounds by an immobile plastic cover fixed by cementum, which remains in situ for 10 days (*Fig.* 174). It is advisable to extract only a small number of teeth at one time and to inject the local anaesthetic as superficially as possible in order to prevent haematomata.

Good oral hygiene and dental care from childhood are of major importance in haemophiliac patients. Many of these often young patients have already neglected dentitions with gingivitis and, partly owing to this gingivitis, have continual gingival bleeding. From the earliest possible time the dentition must be brushed carefully with a not too soft toothbrush after every meal and the dentition should be examined by a dentist at least twice a year. Local application of fluorides must be kept in mind. If the dentist is informed beforehand, there is only a slight chance of injuries during dental treatment, so

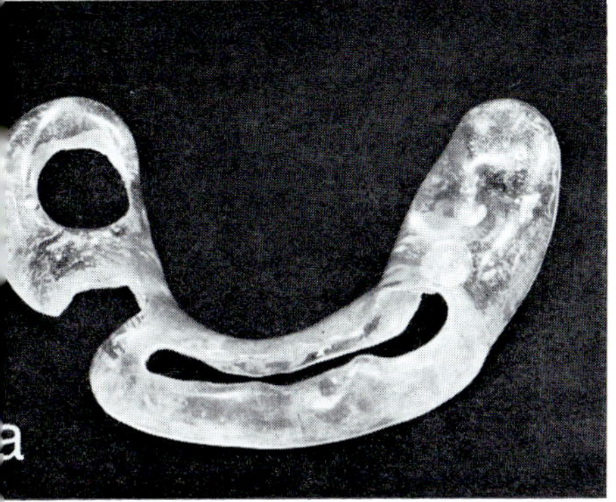

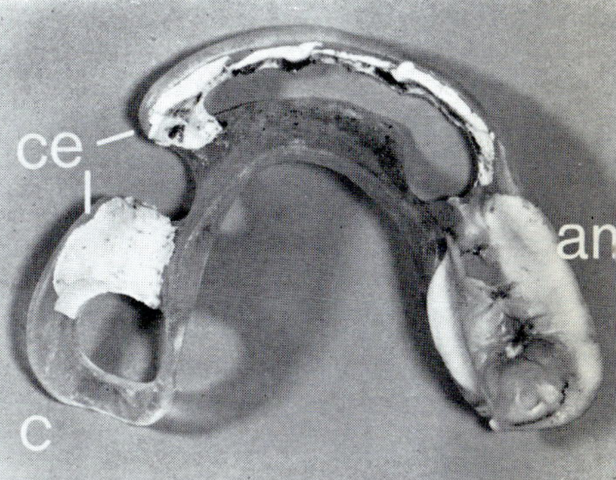

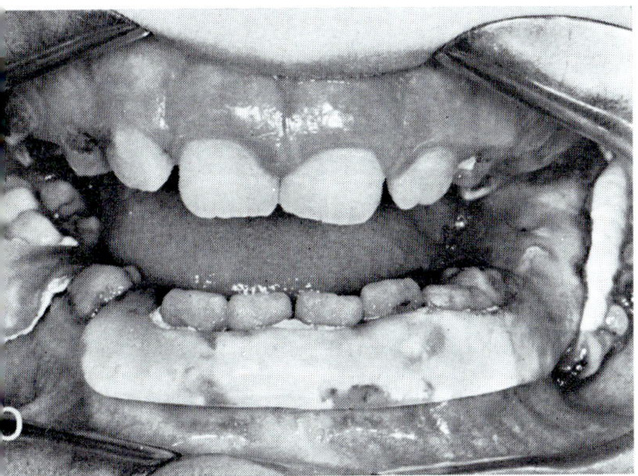

Fig. 174.—a, Plastic cover, made after a plaster-of-Paris model of the dentition of a haemophiliac patient. The right part covers the wound. b, The plate in the mouth of the patient. A lower left molar was extracted (right side in the picture). c, In order to achieve a water-tight enclosure, the part of the plate covering the wound is lined with a dressing of an elastic impression compound (am) (for instance Sta-seal); fixation of the plate to the dentition may be done by zinc phosphate cementum (ce). The cleanliness of the dressing in the wound after 10 days is striking.

that this cannot be regarded as a reason to withhold dental treatment from these patients.

Inflammations.—

Alveolitis.—From 2 to 4 days after tooth extraction a very severe radiating pain may occur. The socket is not filled by a clot, but its walls are covered by a greyish, very infected layer (alveolitis). The cause is probably a contamination with blood and saliva of the bony alveolar walls during the period that filling of the socket with blood was prevented by excessive vascular spasm, being the reaction to the vasoconstrictor in the local anaesthetic. In the case of alveolitis a very superficial osteitis of the alveolar bone is concerned.

Treatment consists of careful cleaning of the socket, daily irrigation by hydrogen peroxide (3 per cent, diluted with an equal quantity of warm water), and insertion of a pack (iodoform gauze in petroleum jelly) to prevent inflow of saliva, bacteria, and food debris. In case of very severe pain iodoform gauze in petroleum jelly can be dusted with benzocaine powder or smeared with benzocaine ointment 5 per cent. Usually it will be necessary to administer commonly used analgesics, as the inflammation takes some time to subside. After some days the pain will diminish. After separation of the superficial bone (micro-sequestra) the socket will heal by granulation.

Acute Inflammation.—Acute inflammations with swellings of the soft tissues following tooth extraction occur, but are relatively rare. It is difficult to explain these inflammations afterwards. It is possible that the 'toothache', which was the reason for extraction, was really the initial stage of an inflammation, which continued notwithstanding extraction. Obstruction of the blood circulation by the vasoconstrictor in the local anaesthetic may possibly have contributed to the acute exacerbation. It is also possible that bacteria are squeezed into the bone or soft tissues during extraction movements.

Osteomyelitis or infection following injection must also be kept in mind. Due to infections following injections large abscesses may develop in the retromaxillary area and in the pterygomandibular space, associated with swellings, which may extend into the temporal region. There is asymmetry of the soft palate and displacement of the pharyngeal arches to the uninvolved side. Sometimes the picture may resemble arthritis. The lower jaw shows a deviation towards the affected side owing to accumulation of fluid in the joint and spasm of the lateral pterygoid muscle. Hospitalization, administration of high doses of antibiotics, and timely incision are necessary.

The therapy, discussed on p. 162, is also applicable to other inflammations.

N.B.—After surgical interference in the mouth, for instance after *removal of a lower third molar*, a very extensive oedema may occur, often accompanied by a sore throat. In these cases there is hardly ever a question of infection. The temperature is often only slightly raised, and at any rate bears no relation to the extensiveness of the swelling. Cold, wet compresses or an ice pack and antiphlogistics (e.g., oxyphenbutazone (Tanderil)—first and second days 2 tablets of

100 mg. three times daily, third and fourth days 1 tablet of 100 mg. three times daily, and the fifth day 1 tablet twice) together with sedatives may lessen these postoperative symptoms. Generally they do not last longer than 5 days. Administration of antibiotics is hardly ever indicated (only in cases of considerably raised temperature).

Chronic Inflammations.—Bone fragments of the alveolus, fractured during extraction, may become necrotic and cause chronic inflammation. Usually these fragments appear spontaneously at the surface as 'sharp fragments'. Sometimes removal (curettage) is necessary.

Perforation of the Antral Floor.—Extraction of a maxillary premolar or molar may cause a perforation of the antral floor. By requesting the patient to blow with a pinched nose and opened mouth, the air escapes from the perforation as bubbles. Such a perforation has to be closed as soon as possible by suturing the gingiva (small defects) or by means of a trapezium-shaped buccal flap, aimed at the prevention of infection of the maxillary sinus. Odontogenic sinusitis is very putrid.

A root remnant pushed into the maxillary sinus must be removed on the same day. Plugging a perforation is *never* indicated. The defect is kept patent, will increase in size eventually, and is almost always followed by chronic sinusitis.

Trauma of a Nerve or Trismus of the Masticatory Muscles.—During a mandibular block injection the lingual nerve may be injured by the needle, causing unilateral numbness of the tongue. It is a very unpleasant complication which is difficult to avoid. The numbness may last for months. If the lower alveolar nerve is injured, unilateral anaesthesia of the lower lip lasting for many months may be the result. Insertion of the needle into a nerve causes the patient a 'painful shock', and the needle must immediately be withdrawn before injection. Therapeutically nothing can be done. It is of importance to reassure the patient by telling him that in most cases the numbness will disappear after some months after a period of paraesthesia.

Sometimes mandibular anaesthesia may be followed by marked trismus of the medial pterygoid muscle which may last for weeks. In most cases the trismus is of unknown origin. Therapy consists of heat application and the exercising of opening movements by the patient.

GENERAL COMPLICATIONS

Lung Complications (pneumonia).—In about 1 in 20,000 tooth extractions lung complications may arise. These may be due to a blocked air passage or aspiration of blood and saliva running into the throat under the influence of gravity. The latter occurs mainly in the case of anaesthesia of the palate and with the patient lying on his back.

In the case of aspiration of foreign bodies or when a foreign body is suspected, immediate examination by an ear, nose, and throat specialist and the removal of the object as soon as possible are indicated. One must not wait for the object to be coughed up spontaneously. It is also wrong to be tempted to omit such measures by accepting that, when the first coughing attacks are over, the object will have left the bronchus. The patient, after aspiration, should be transported to hospital in a recumbent posture in order to prevent displacement of the foreign body.

Complications in Patients suffering from Cardiovascular Diseases.—Adrenaline in a concentration contained in the local anaesthetic solutions normally used by a dentist is not contra-indicated in patients suffering from cardiovascular diseases, provided injection is given slowly and care is taken that it is not injected into a blood-vessel (aspiration). There is no objection to the administration of 2–4 ml. of a local anaesthetic with an adrenaline concentration of 1 in 50,000 or of noradrenaline 1 in 80,000 or 1 in 100,000. When adrenaline is added to the local anaesthetic solution a deeper and longer lasting anaesthesia is obtained, thus preventing the adrenals of the patient from secreting larger quantities of adrenaline into the bloodstream as a reaction against pain in the case of a less efficient anaesthesia. It is advisable not to use this vasoconstrictor in patients who know from experience that they cannot tolerate adrenaline. The patient will have to have a less efficient anaesthetic or general anaesthesia will have to be employed. Such patients are few. Often it appears that unpleasant sensations can be avoided by injecting slowly and treating the patient in a recumbent posture.

Angina Pectoris.—A patient taking nitroglycerin (or a similar drug) must always have a number of fresh tablets available when he sees his dentist. His physician must inform the patient beforehand how to use these tablets should an attack of angina pectoris occur during dental treatment.

Bacteriaemia.—Bacteriaemia occurs in the case of extractions, curettage of gingival pockets, and other kinds of surgical interference in the oral cavity. The degree of dissemination depends upon the extent of trauma and the condition of the gingiva (gingivitis). Prophylactic administration of antibiotics is indicated in patients in whom bacteriaemia must be controlled, e.g., in all patients suffering from congenital or acquired valve defects of the heart in order to prevent bacterial endocarditis, in patients who have suffered from acute glomerulonephritis, and in patients suffering from rheumatoid arthritis in order to prevent acute exacerbation.

Several schemes of treatment and several antibiotics have been advised. The advantages and/or disadvantages have yet to be determined scientifically. An example of such a scheme is: 1 or 2 hours before treatment 600,000 units of procaine penicillin together with 600,000 units of pure penicillin (both intramuscularly); for 2–4 days after treatment 600,000 units of procaine penicillin and 200,000 units of pure penicillin intramuscularly. In children a depot preparation may be given, consisting of 600,000 units of benzathine penicillin plus 300,000 units of potassium penicillin G in an aqueous suspension (Penidural D/F). Deep intramuscular administration provides a sustained action for about 1 week. Patients who are allergic to penicillin have to be treated with a different antibiotic (i.e., tetracycline or erythromycin).

Complications in Patients using Drugs.—

Antihypertensives.—These drugs give an enhanced reaction to vasoconstricting elements. Local anaesthetics containing a vasoconstrictor have to be administered with caution. Intravascular injection may produce great changes in the blood-pressure, which can be very dangerous. Also in the case of general anaesthesia these drugs are dangerous. Fainting is a more common occurrence in patients who take these drugs than in other patients.

Corticosteroids.—In patients who are regularly treated with corticosteroids (e.g., for asthma, etc.) it is advisable to increase the normal doses temporarily in the case of oral surgical interference (stress!).

Anaphylactic Shock.—Administration of penicillin may cause allergic reactions (anaphylactic shock). This is also applicable to procaine and procaine penicillin. Procaine is a derivative of para-aminobenzoic acid; these derivatives readily cause sensitivity

reactions. The injection of a local anaesthetic solution containing lidocaine gives less chance of allergic reactions (lidocaine is not a derivative of para-aminobenzoic acid).

Treatment of anaphylactic shock should consist of immediate intra-muscular administration of 0·5–1 ml. of adrenaline 1 in 1000, combined with an antihistamine (i.e., 2 ml. (50 mg.) of thiazinaminium (Multergan) intramuscularly and a corticosteroid (i.e., Oradexon 5 mg. intravenously or Di-adreson-F aquosum two or three intra-venous injections 25 mg.).

CHAPTER 10

TOOTH EXTRACTION UNDER GENERAL ANAESTHESIA

EXTRACTION under general anaesthesia is indicated in psychologically disturbed patients, also in patients who are extremely fearful and nervous or who have unpleasant experiences from previous treatments under local anaesthesia. Finally, general anaesthesia may be indicated in patients with abnormally firmly attached teeth or with impacted teeth which cannot easily be removed. Frightened little children can usually be treated satisfactorily under local anaesthesia after a talk or administration of sedatives.

For the remainder the indications differ from country to country and are partly governed by the availability of an anaesthetist to administer the anaesthetic and of postoperative hospitalization. An increasing need for treatment under general anaesthesia is to be expected.

Before indicating extraction under general anaesthesia consultation with the patient's physician is necessary. He can provide data regarding the general health of the patient and the use of drugs which may be of interest to the anaesthetist. If possible, a quiet talk with the patient is advisable with regard to the advantages and disadvantages of treatment under general anaesthesia. Most people have a wrong conception of general anaesthesia ('just be put to sleep').

By taking a complete set of dental radiographs beforehand impacted teeth or remaining root remnants are not overlooked.

Extraction of a complete dentition under general anaesthesia is often an extensive operation, so that hospitalization is usually necessary (for instance from half a day before the operation to 1 or 2 days afterwards). Extraction must always be performed in co-operation with a qualified anaesthetist. The extraction wounds are sutured in order to prevent haemorrhage after extraction and aspiration of blood.

Disadvantages of extraction under general anaesthesia are: more risks, loss of time, and higher expense.

Though there is an increasing tendency to give dental treatment to psychologically disturbed and spastic patients under general anaesthesia (not only extractions) the demand cannot yet be satisfied because of lack of manpower and hospital space.

CHAPTER 11

IMMEDIATE DENTURES

By this term is understood dentures which are fitted immediately after extraction of the natural dentition. This is made possible by making plaster casts of the dentition and jaws beforehand and removing the remaining teeth and as much of the gingiva as is expected to shrink after extraction from them. The resulting models of the lower and upper jaws are used as casts for the dentures.

After extraction, the sockets are sutured to prevent haemorrhage; after which the denture is inserted. It must not be taken out for the first few days, because a postoperative oedema can make reinsertion impossible. After 2 or 3 days the denture can be taken out to be cleaned. When extraction is performed under general anaesthesia, it is necessary to see that the patient is well awake after the operation in order to prevent any respiratory difficulties due to the prosthesis.

Immediate dentures are designed in deference to the desire of the patient not to walk about without teeth; furthermore, the dentures are very effective as a wound protection and they limit 'sinking' of the face, as well as 'sagging' and broadening of the tongue, so that it is easier to get accustomed to the dentures. Moreover, it is seldom necessary at present to be without dentures for 3 months as was formerly the case. The aim was to wait until the accelerated resorption of the alveolar process resulting from the extraction was no longer effective, before making the dentures. When making immediate dentures it is necessary, partly due to this resorption, to readapt the dentures after 3–6 months, for instance by means of rebasing.

CHAPTER 12

FOETOR ORIS

AN evil-smelling breath may be caused by disease of mouth, nose, or throat, by disturbances of the digestive tract, of the lower part of the respiratory tract, or may be due to the exhaling of scented substances. Lesions *in the mouth* which may cause a foetor are:—

Periodontal disease, especially in the case of deep gingival pockets (*see* p. 29);

Acute or chronic ulcerative gingivitis (*see* p. 151), which is often localized interdentally;

Poor hygienic condition of the dentition with many carious teeth (also in children);

Alveolitis (*see* p. 195);

Oro-antral fistula with maxillary sinusitis (*see* p. 197).

Finally metabolic diseases may cause a foeter oris: liver disease (foeter hepaticus), diabetes (acetone odour), uraemia (uriniferous odour), as well as an insufficient intake of liquids and xerostomia.

In general thorough cleaning of the dentition and treatment of cavities and teeth with gangrenous pulps by a dentist may eliminate the foetor. Good oral hygiene which includes cleaning of the interdental spaces by the patient is of major importance (electric toothbrush, toothpicks). Limited use of tobacco and sugars between meals may also produce a favourable effect.

THE SALIVARY GLANDS

CHAPTER 13

FUNCTIONAL DISORDERS

Xerostomia (Aptyalism.)—In healthy adults the total quantity of saliva produced in 24 hours is about 1–2 litres. A decreased production causes zerostomia, an extremely troublesome condition with atrophy of the mucous membrane, which may be chronically inflamed owing to the lack of self-cleansing of the mouth (burning sensation, foetor). Another result is a very rapid decay of the dentition. The saliva which is present in the mouth looks 'foamy'.

Xerostomia may occur: due to chronic inflammation of the salivary glands, Sjögren's syndrome (hypofunction of salivary, lacrimal, sweat, and sebaceous glands, causing dryness of nose, mouth, and throat, and keratoconjunctivitis sicca; furthermore affections of the joints resembling rheumatoid arthritis occur; *see* p. 229), treatment by irradiation, dehydration (vomiting, diarrhoea, fever, diabetes), psychological factors, use of drugs with anticholinergic (atropine-like) effects (neuroleptics from the phenothiazine series, the sedative glutethimide (Doriden) and the ataractic benactyzine (Suavitil, Phobex), antihistaminics, atropine, etc.).

Generally the cause of the hypofunction is unknown. Most patients are middle-aged or older women.

Treatment of xerostomia of known origin has to be directed to the cause. In most cases, however, treatment can only be palliative. This may consist of mouth-washing, chewing-gum, sparkling drinks, acid sweets (only in edentulous patients and not in diabetics), pilocarpine (pilocarpini hydrochlor. 0·25; aqua dest. 10·0; S. : 1st day 5 drops in a small quantity of water and then every day 1 drop more to a maximum of 10 drops). Advised also are: Pilocarpini nitras, powders of 5 mg. each, maximally one powder four times a day (max. 20 mg. p.d.). Side-effects which may occur are: sweat secretion, vomiting, diarrhoea, cardiac weakness, and convulsions; the antidote being atropine sulphate. No preparation is known for permanent stimulation of salivary secretion. They all have a temporary effect only. Dryness of the mouth resulting from treatment by irradiation may disappear spontaneously after 2 or 3 years.

Hypersalivation (Ptyalism, Sialorrhea).—Hypersalivation is in most cases of unknown origin. Patients who wear artificial dentures sometimes complain of hypersalivation for the first few weeks. Some of them have the neurotic habit of sucking the prosthesis continuously. All kinds of lesions causing pain in the oral cavity may cause hypersalivation (herpetic stomatitis, aphthous stomatitis, or ulcerative gingivitis). Sometimes ptyalism occurs in association with neurological disorders (e.g., Parkinson's disease), when using drugs, for instance the rauwolfia derivative reserpine, and in combination with diseases of the gastro-intestinal tract.

Treatment is the removal of the cause; often this is unknown and in that case a palliative therapy has to be instituted (e.g., atropine sulphate, three times a day 0·25–0·5 mg.; beware of tachycardia!). In serious cases it may be decided to ligate one parotid duct in order to make the gland atrophy.

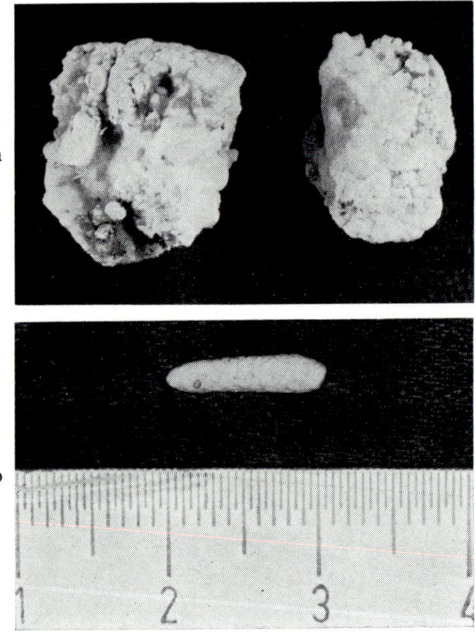

Fig. 175.—a, Salivary calculus from the hilus of the submandibular gland. b, Elongated stone from the submandibular duct. These so-called 'date stones' are mainly seen in the parotid duct (*see Fig.* 180).

CHAPTER 14

SIALOLITHIASIS (SALIVARY CALCULI)

SALIVARY calculi occur predominantly in the submandibular gland
or duct (80 per cent of cases). The occurrence of calculi in the
parotid duct and gland is relatively rare. Calculi in the submandibular duct are round or elongated, those located in the gland are
mostly irregular in shape. In the parotid duct elongated stones are
usually found (*Fig.* 175).

The cause of stone formation is not known; it is not clear whether
the often associated chronic inflammation is either primary or
secondary. There is no connexion with the incidence of stone
formation elsewhere in the body. The lesion is of more common
incidence in men than in women. Most patients are middle-aged.
Salivary calculi are hardly ever seen in children.

The lesion is characterized by attacks of pain and swelling of the
gland at or shortly before meal times, especially when the stone is
located in the duct and forms an obstruction (salivary colic). Such a
swelling may last for 1 or 2 hours. Sometimes acute inflammations
occur with long-lasting indurations of the gland. In the long term
they have a tendency not to disappear (*Fig.* 176 a).

By bimanual palpation of the cheek or floor of the mouth a stone
in the duct can often easily be felt; care must be taken that the stone
is not displaced in the direction of the gland (*Fig.* 176 b).

The radiograph often shows the stone clearly. Calculi in the submandibular duct or gland can be shown in an occlusal film of the
floor of the mouth (*Fig.* 177) and a lateral radiograph of the jaw
(*Fig.* 178 a). If a stone is suspected in the parotid duct or gland a
dental radiograph can be taken of the soft tissues of the cheek
(*Fig.* 180), an infracranial projection according to Parma or an
anteroposterior projection of the parotid area. Sialography (radiographic examination of the gland after injection of a contrast
medium, for instance, Lipiodol) is in general not indicated when the
stone is located in the duct. It might cause displacement of the stone;
if the stone is located in the hilus there is no such objection (*Fig.* 178 b).

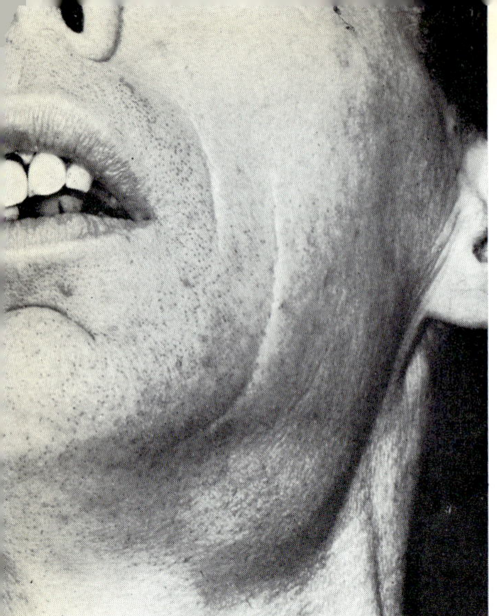

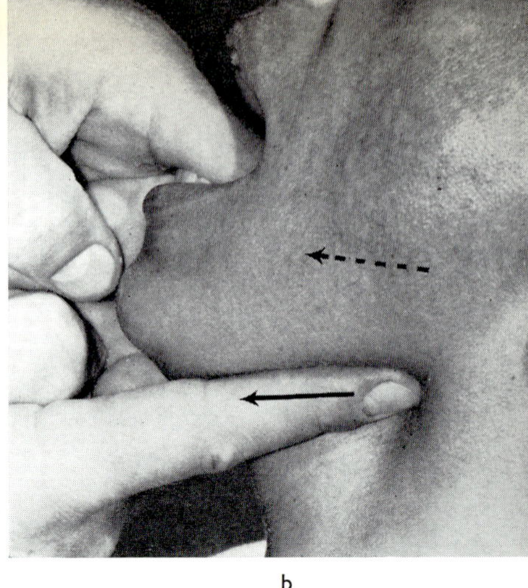

b

a

Fig. 176.—a, Acute exacerbation of chronic inflammation of the left submandibular gland, originating from a salivary calculus in a 51-year-old man. b, Bimanual palpation of the floor of the mouth.

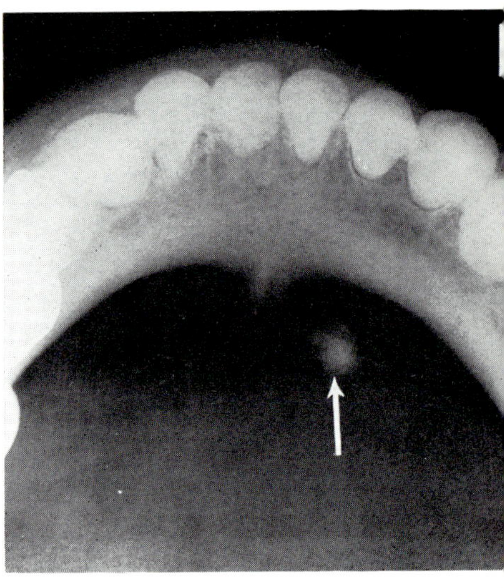

Fig. 177.—Occlusal radiograph of the floor of the mouth, showing a small, round stone, just anterior to the orifice of the submandibular duct.

Fig. 178.—a, Lateral jaw radiograph showing a big salivary calculus, probably located in the hilus of the submandibular gland. b, Sialogram of the submandibular gland of the same patient. The stone is to be seen as a recess in the contrast medium in the hilus of the gland. The duct is dilated and the glandular parenchyma has become atrophic due to the chronic inflammation. Extirpation of the gland is indicated if the complaints remain after removal of the stone.

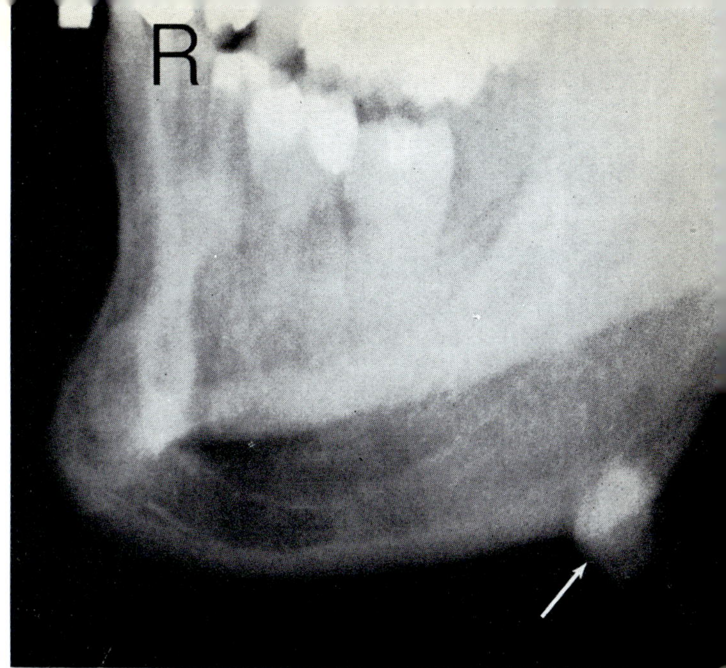

(*Fig.* 178 a)

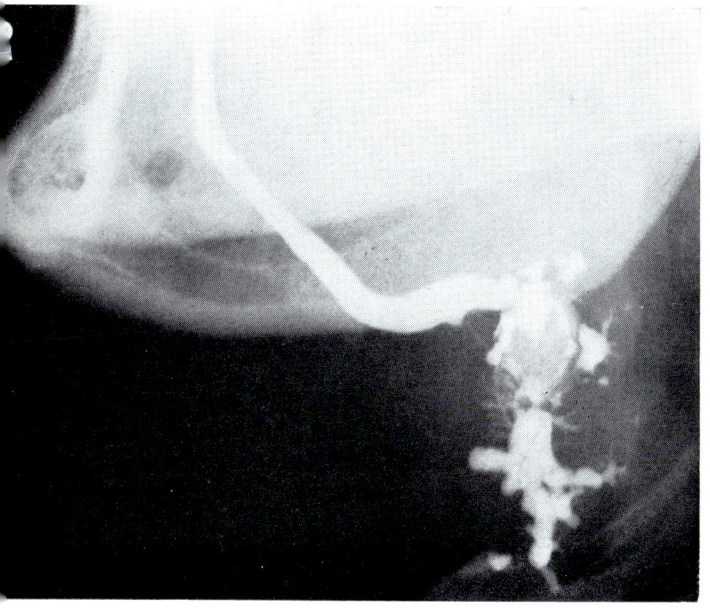

(*Fig.* 178 b)

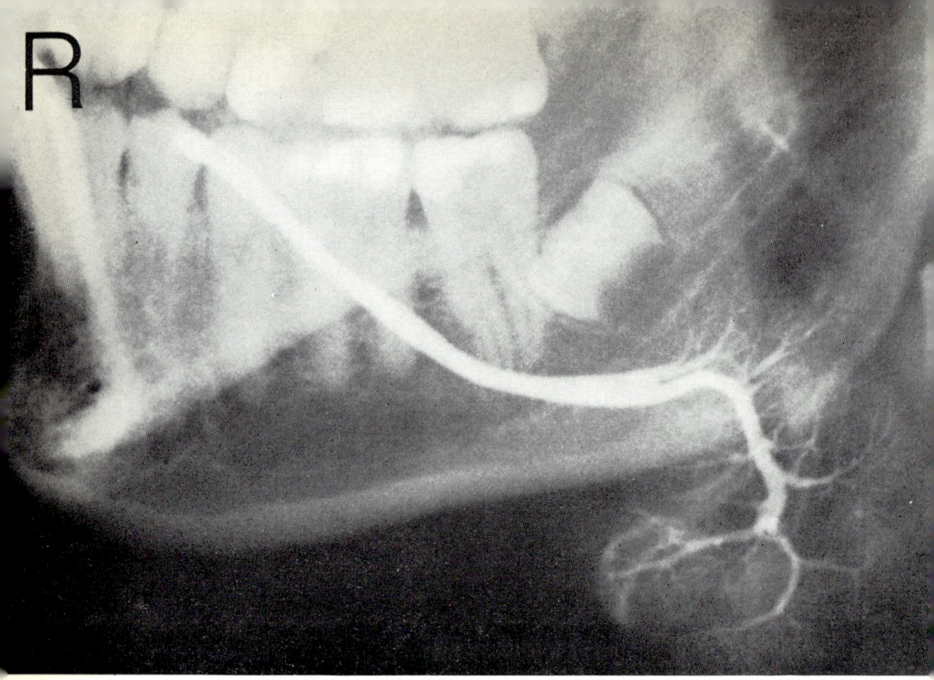

Fig. 179.—Sialogram of a normal right submandibular gland in an 18-year-
old woman.

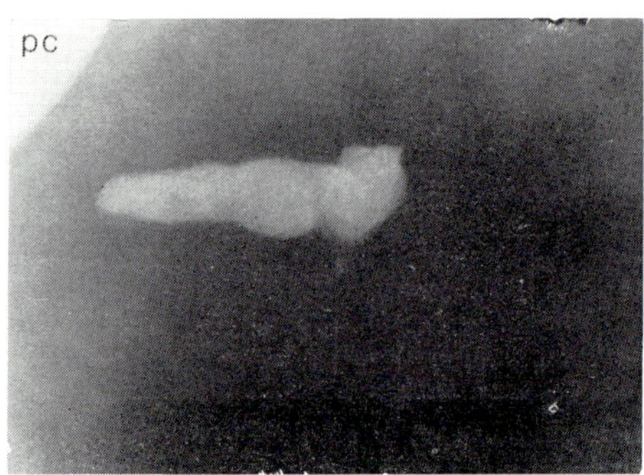

Fig. 180.—Dental radiograph of the parotid duct with an elongated salivary
calculus. (pc=Coronoid process of the mandible.)

An example of a sialogram of a normal submandibular gland is
shown in *Fig.* 179.

Treatment consists of removal of the stone. Stones in the parotid
duct can generally be removed easily. If, however, they are situated

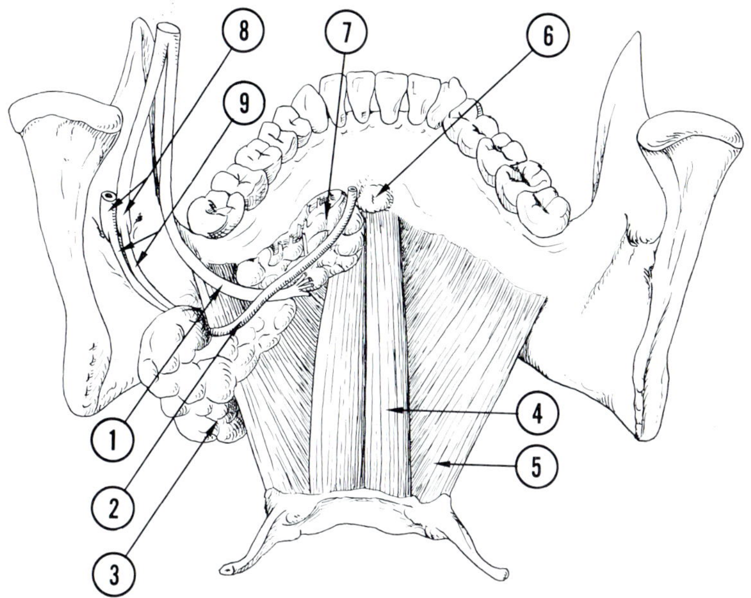

Fig. 181.—View of the floor of the mouth. Note the crossing of the submandibular duct and the lingual nerve. 1, Lingual nerve; 2, Submandibular duct; 3, Submandibular gland; 4, Geniohyoid muscle; 5, Mylohyoid muscle; 6, Mental nerve; 7, Sublingual gland; 8, Inferior alveolar artery and nerve; 9, Mylohyoid artery and nerve.

within the parotid gland (rare), partial or total parotidectomy may be necessary.

In the case of removal of stones from the submandibular duct or gland (intra-orally) the lingual nerve, which crosses the duct caudally, must be exposed and spared (*Fig.* 181). Removal of stones located dorsally in the duct or gland demands a lot of experience. General postoperative symptoms are few. Sometimes marked oedema of the floor of the mouth occurs. We have the impression that this oedema is caused by discharge of saliva into the soft tissues of the floor of the mouth if the operation wound is closed too carefully. Temperature is only slightly raised (for treatment *see* p. 196). After removal of the calculus recurrences may occur, probably due to degenerative changes in the duct or gland (*see* p. 232).

CHAPTER 15

INFLAMMATIONS OF THE PAROTID GLAND

ACUTE INFLAMMATIONS

BECAUSE most of these patients present with a common picture of acute parotitis, care must be taken when making a diagnosis.

Acute parotitis is characterized by a painful, smooth, tight elastic swelling anterior to and caudally of the ear, pushing the ear-lobe outward, which is plainly visible when the patient is viewed from behind. In serious cases the skin is shiny, tight, and hyperaemic and the orifice of the duct (papilla salivalis) is red.

Sometimes pus can be massaged from the duct; usually this cannot be done and then the gland gives a 'dry' impression in the acute stage.

In the case of acute parotitis the following diseases must be considered:

Mumps (epidemic parotitis) (in children, sometimes adults; mostly bilateral; other affected children in the neighbourhood; submandibular salivary glands may be involved; no recurrence; positive virus culture and serology) (*see below*);

Acute exacerbation of chronic, recurrent parotitis (in babies, children, young adults, seldom older people; mostly unilateral symptoms; recurrent; characteristic sialogram) (*see* p. 218);

Acute exacerbation of chronic parotitis with changes of the duct (30 years and older; recurrent; unilateral; colon-like dilated duct) (*see* p. 226);

Exacerbation of chronic parotitis due to stone formation (salivary colics; a filling defect in the sialogram) (*see* p. 226);

Primary acute bacterial parotitis (rare) (*see* p. 215).

Acute postoperative parotitis (rare) (*see* p. 218).

Epidemic Parotitis (Mumps).—This disease of the salivary glands is of very common occurrence and is usually seen by physicians. It is part of a general infectious disease caused by the mumps virus. Besides the parotid gland the other salivary glands may be involved.

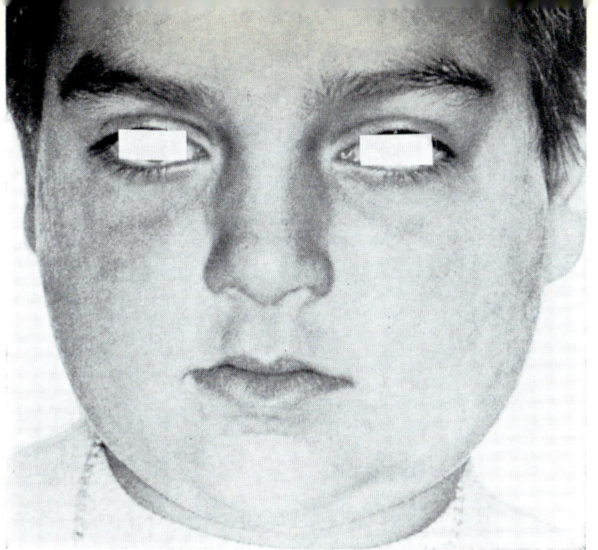

Fig. 182.—Epidemic parotitis (mumps) (left).

The infection occurs mainly in children between 5 and 15 years of age. The incubation period is 2 or 3 weeks.

Generally the picture is characterized by:—

a. Swelling of the salivary glands (both parotid glands in two-thirds of cases). Usually the disease starts unilaterally (*Fig.* 182) and after 3–6 days swelling of the other gland occurs. In about one-third of cases only one parotid gland is involved and in one-tenth of cases the submandibular gland only. In less than one-quarter of cases all major salivary glands are swollen. The swelling reaches its maximum after about 48 hours and remains 7–10 days; the fever may last for 1 week.

b. The production of saliva is greatly reduced; a marked dry mouth is not seen as a rule, because the minor glands generally maintain their function.

c. The blood-picture is not very characteristic. The complement-fixation reaction becomes positive after 1 or 2 weeks. In the initial stage of the disease the virus can be cultivated from the saliva.

Usually the patient becomes immune for the rest of his life. Treatment is unnecessary; it can only be palliative. Complications of the central nervous system and of the sexual glands are rare.

Primary Acute Bacterial Parotitis.—Primary acute parotitis caused by common organisms is rare and mainly seen as an ascending

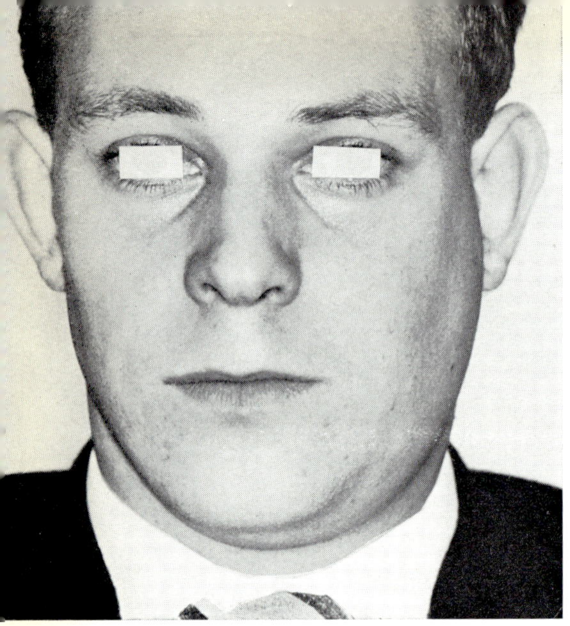

(*Fig.* 183 a)

(*Fig.* 183 b)

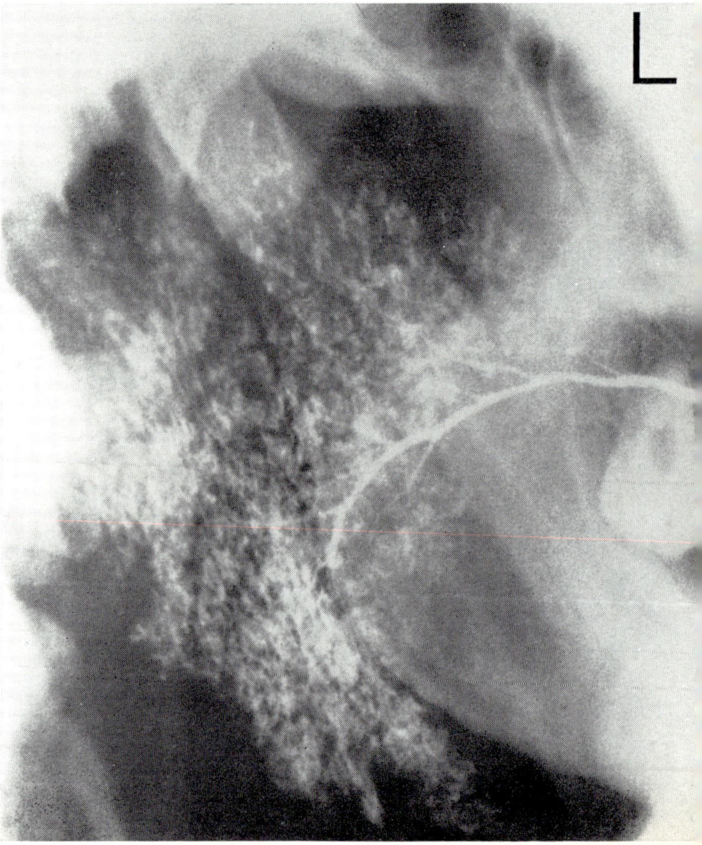

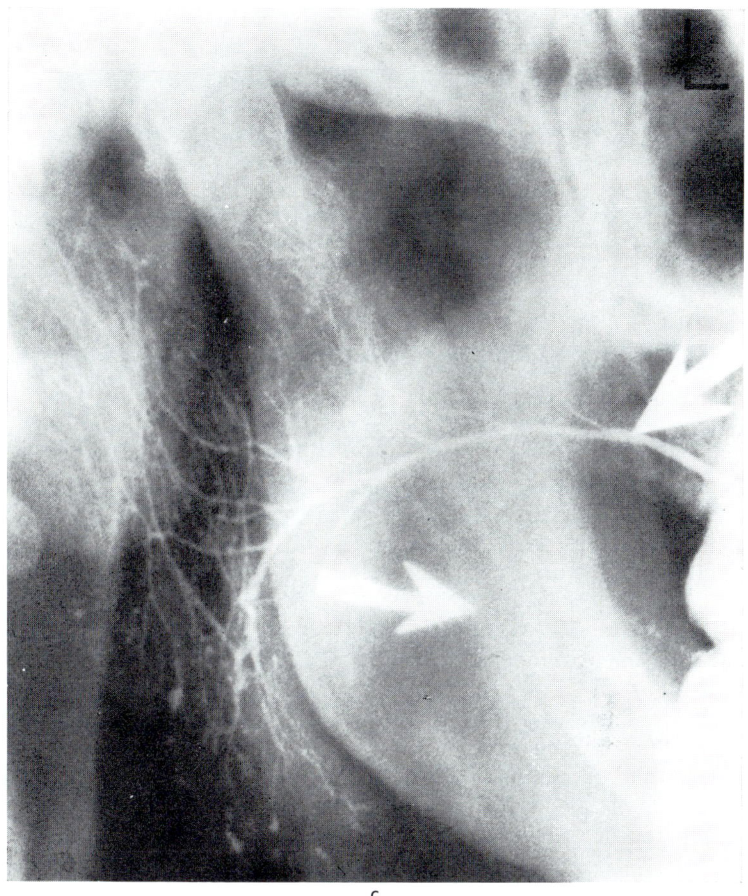

c

Fig. 183.—a, Primary acute parotitis (left) in a 21-year-old man. b, Sialogram of the left parotid gland of the same patient in the subacute stage. Flaky structure of the gland; duct and main branches are normal. c, Sialogram 2 years later. The aspect is normal again except for perhaps some peripheral ectasias (white arrows are of no significance).

infection via the duct during periods (for one reason or another) of reduced saliva production. The lesion, which is unilateral as a rule, is characterized by a very marked swelling of the parotid area causing a feeling of tension and a deep, dull pain, radiating to the whole

217

involved half of the face (*Fig.* 183 a). Often a collateral oedema occurs, sometimes there is trismus and the patient can only swallow with difficulty. The papilla salivalis is red and swollen and no saliva can be massaged from the duct. The patient has a raised temperature and feels ill. A sialogram in the acute stage must not be made (increase of tension and enhanced chance of squeezing infectious material into the gland). When the most acute symptoms have subsided the sialogram shows a fine 'fibrillary' structure, because the ductules are very narrowed due to oedema (*Fig.* 183 b). Moreover, they have very little resistance so that Lipiodol is easily discharged into the tissues. Often it takes a considerable time before the gland is empty again (disturbed function). When the inflammation has subsided, the structure of the gland returns to normal (*Fig.* 183 c). Another example of a normal sialogram is shown in *Fig.* 184.

Treatment consists of high doses of antibiotics and stimulation of secretion of the gland (pilocarpine, chewing-gum, acid drinks, and massage of the gland). Abscess formation is seldom encountered. Incision is hardly ever indicated (salivary fistula). If necessary, the swelling may be aspirated (culture!).

Acute Postoperative Parotitis.—This disease may occur as a complication of extensive operations. This postoperative form, however, is gradually seen less frequently (prevention of dehydration by better shock treatment).

Furthermore, acute parotitis may occur in association with serious thoracic and abdominal diseases (pneumonia, peritonitis) and is then looked upon as a bad sign. Treatment consists of antibiotics and stimulation of salivary secretion.

CHRONIC INFLAMMATION

Chronic (Recurrent) Parotitis.—This peculiar syndrome is characterized by periodic acute or subacute inflammation of one or both parotid glands. These exacerbations are predominantly of unilateral occurrence. Especially in children the disease is fairly often misdiagnosed as 'recurring' mumps.

In quiet stages there are no symptoms and nothing out of the ordinary can be felt in the gland. Sometimes the area anterior to the ear is slightly swollen and the gland may feel somewhat firmer than usual (*Fig.* 187 a). Intra-orally (especially at a later age) a dilated

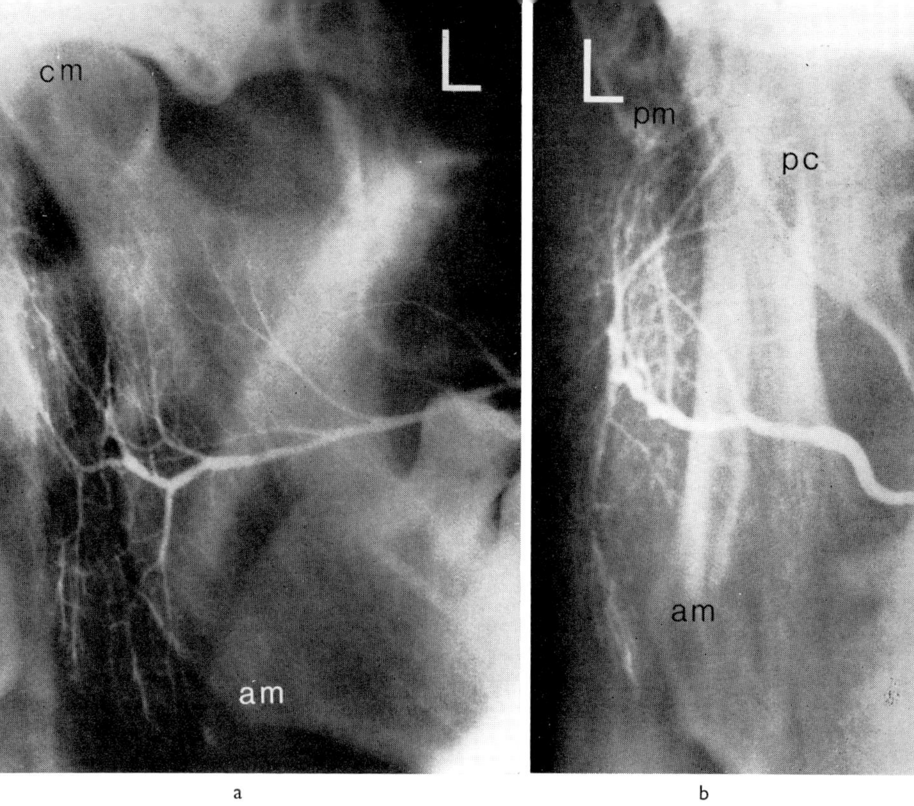

a   b

Fig. 184.—a, Sialogram of a normal parotid gland. Parma projection (cm = head of the mandible; am = angle of the mandible). b, Sialogram of a normal parotid gland. Anteroposterior projection (pm = mastoid process; pc = coronoid process of the mandible).

duct (and orifice) may raise suspicion of the lesion. The papilla salivalis is normal in colour; clear saliva can be massaged from the duct, in which, however, white flakes often occur (no marked pus; microscopically they consist of necrotic epithelial cells, leucocytes, and non-specific cocci). Sometimes massage seems to eliminate an obstruction, a small mucous plug emerges, followed by a flow of macroscopically almost normal saliva.

During acute exacerbations there is marked swelling of the parotid area (*Fig.* 185). Usually there is only slight pain, but it may be very severe in cases of a large swelling. The patient may then feel very ill and the temperature may be markedly raised. Sometimes complaints increase at meal times. As a rule the skin over the indurated parotid

219

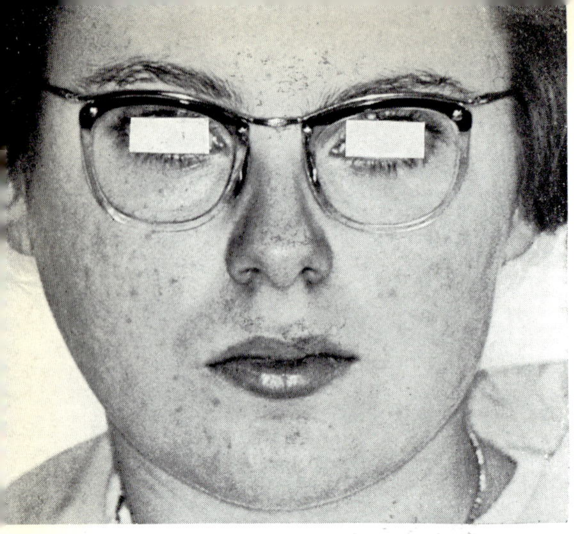

Fig. 185.—Subacute exacerbation of chronic parotitis (right) in a 14-year-old girl. Recurring since she was 8 years old.

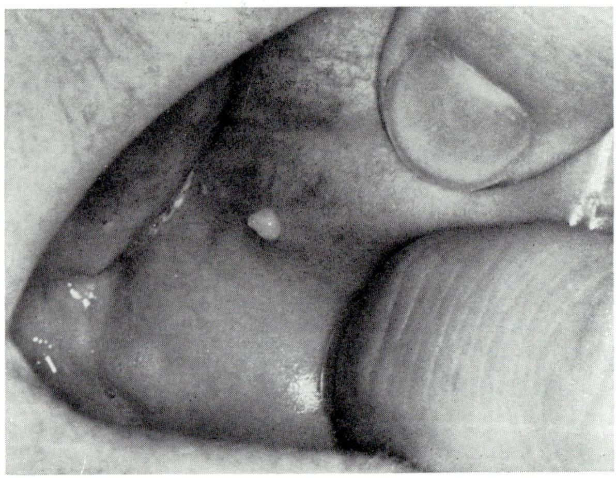

Fig. 186.—Acute exacerbation of chronic parotitis in a 55-year-old female patient. Inspissated, pus-like secretion can be massaged from the duct.

Fig. 187.—(*Above*) Six-year-old girl with bilateral chronic sialo-adenitis (*see below*). (*Below*) Slight swelling of the parotid gland area, both left and right. b, The sialogram of the left parotid gland of this patient shows small point-like ectasias (*Apfelblüten*, 'snowflakes'), diffusely distributed over the whole gland and even over the accessory parotid gland located in the cheek. The caudal part of the main duct is dilated. The picture of the right parotid gland is identical.

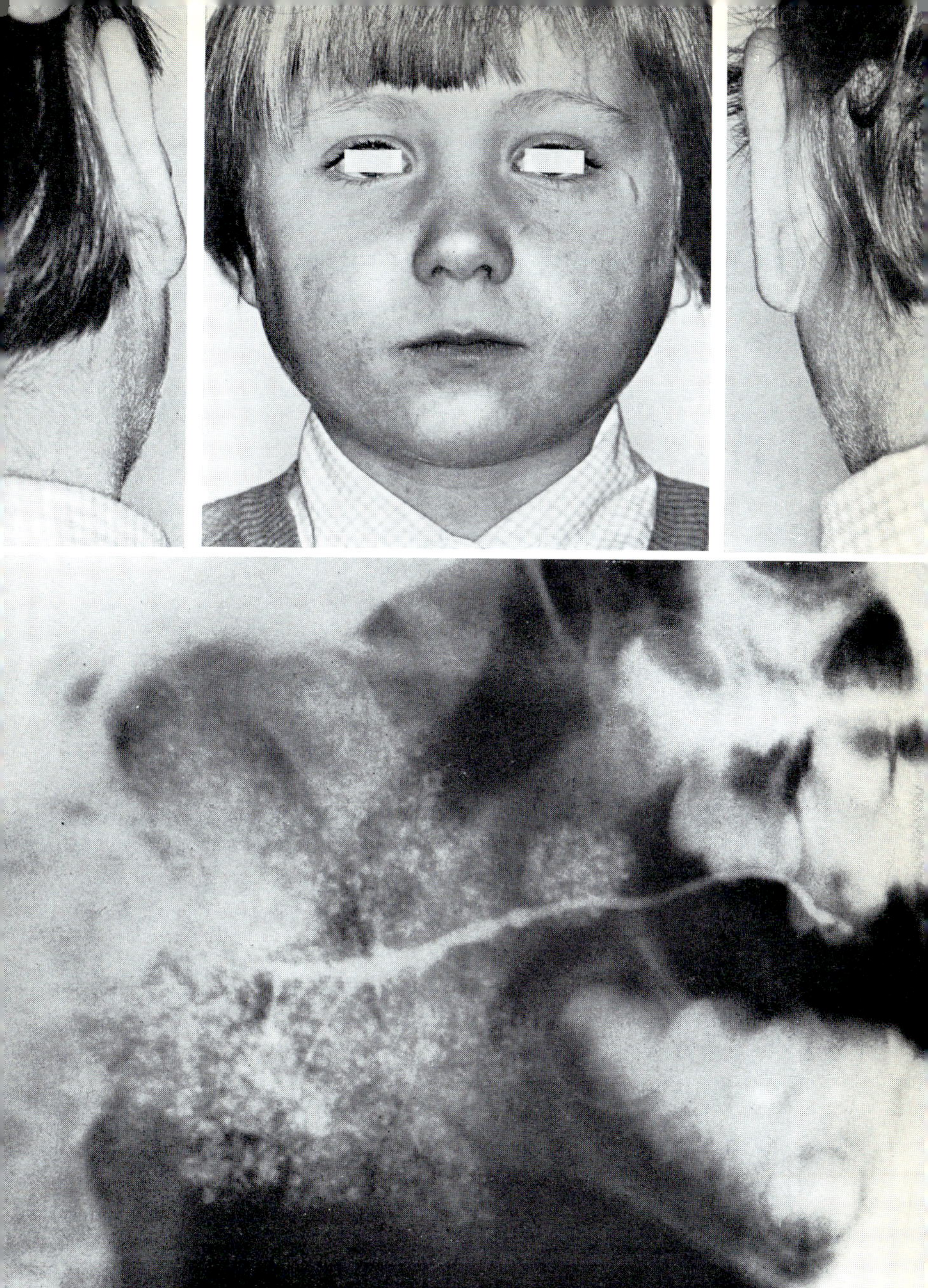

(*Fig.* 187)

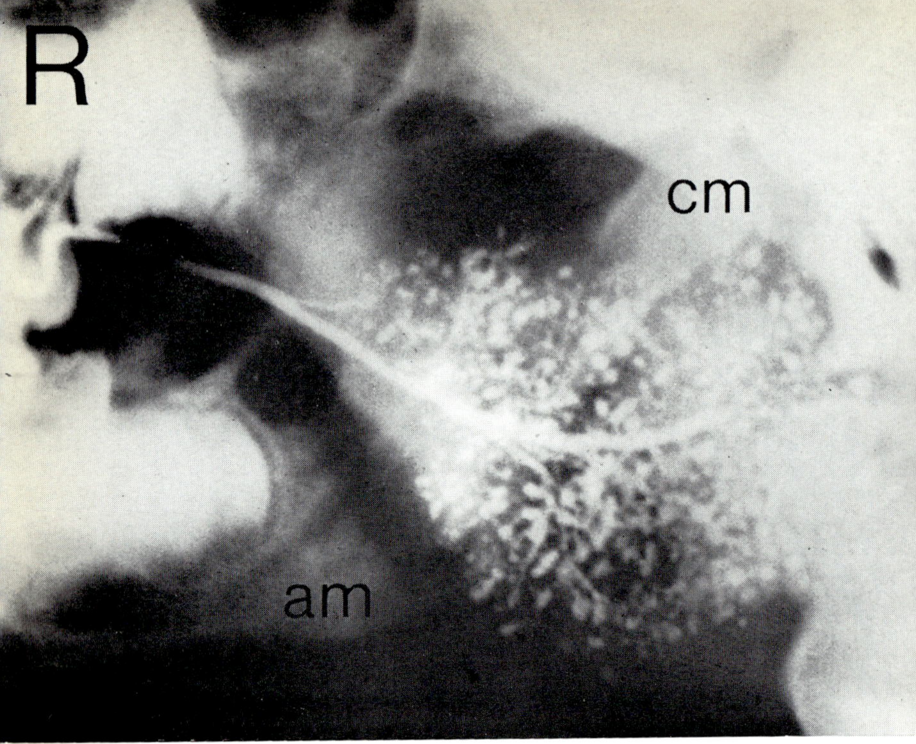

Fig. 188.—Chronic sialo-adenitis of the right parotid gland in a 4-year-old child ($\times$ 1·5). Marked ectasias. The picture of the left parotid gland was identical.

gland is mobile and generally not very hyperaemic. The papilla salivalis is normal; the orifice may be somewhat dilated. No saliva or only small quantities can be massaged from the duct at this stage. Later on the saliva may become milky-white or gelatinous (*Fig.* 186). Bacteriological examination is generally not very revealing (sterile culture; *Haemophilus influenzae, Streptococcus viridans,* etc.).

As all kinds of transitional stages from subacute to severe acute inflammations may occur, the clinical picture is variable.

The disease is encountered in babies, toddlers, and schoolchildren but may also occur in adults. Exacerbations may occur over many years and are sometimes very troublesome. We have the impression that there is a decrease in frequency in the course of time, without, however, disappearance of the distinct alterations in the gland.

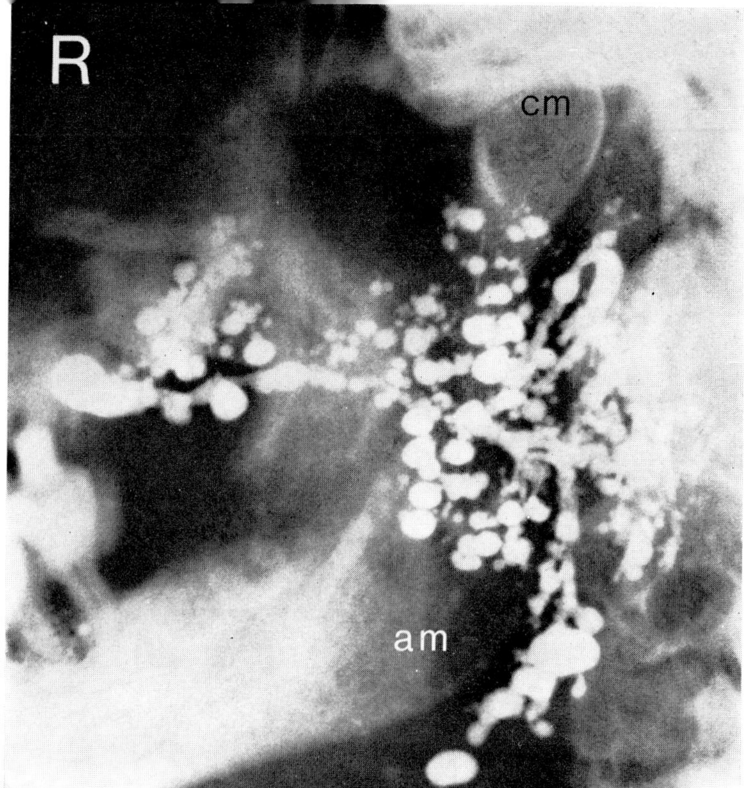

Fig. 189.—Chronic parotitis in a 59-year-old female patient. The sialogram
shows marked ectasias. Few complaints. Palliative treatment.

These changes can be seen plainly in the sialogram, which is prefer-
ably performed in a quiet stage or during a subacute stage. There
are terminal dilatations of the ducts, which give the very characteristic
picture of small, regularly disseminated accumulations of the contrast
medium (*Apfelblüten*, 'snowflakes'). The accessory lobes show
clearly an identical picture (*Figs.* 187 b and 188). At an older age
sometimes larger, irregular accumulations of the contrast medium
are to be seen, which may resemble small caverns (*Perlenschnuren*,
Traubenformen) (*Fig.* 189). In children the duct is usually normal
and in adults it is often dilated. Especially in the subacute stage there
is only a slight secretion of saliva and the contrast medium is only
slowly discharged. We have the impression that Lipiodol reduces
the inflammatory symptoms and therefore the symptoms.

When a sialogram is made of the parotid gland of the unaffected side, in the majority of cases the radiographic picture is identical. Presumably the lesion occurs bilaterally, but causes only unilateral symptons.

The histological picture of the gland shows a chronic inflammation with dilated ducts and massive infiltration with inflammatory cells.

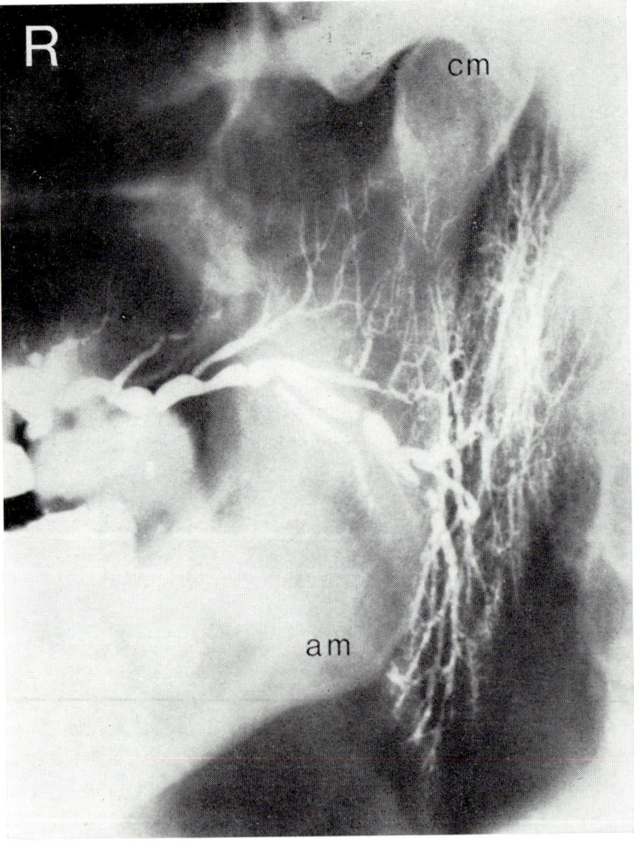

Fig. 190.—Chronic inflammation of the parotid gland, mainly located in the main duct and larger branches (sialodochitis), in a 35-year-old man. Moderate colon-like dilatation of the parotid duct (cm = head of the mandible; am = angle of the mandible).

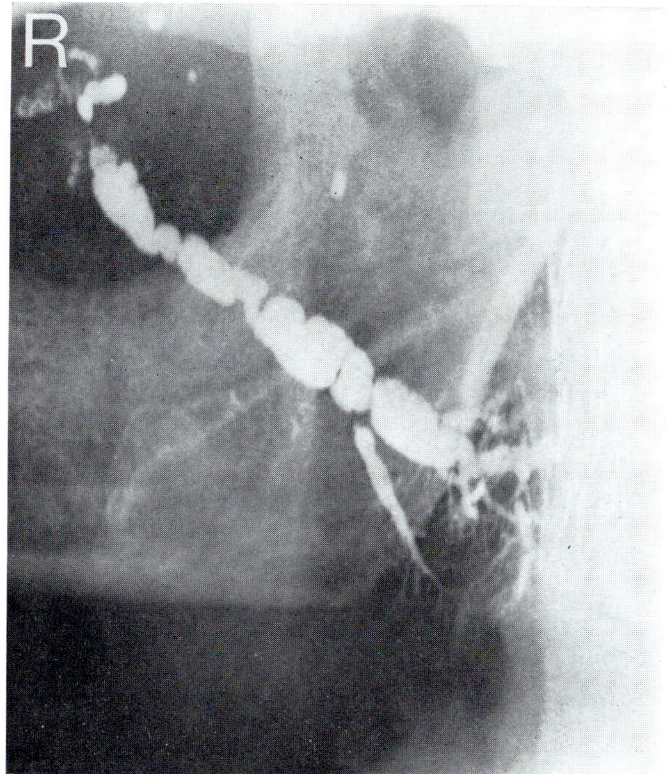

Fig. 191.—Chronic sialodochitis of the parotid gland with very conspicuous colon-like dilatations in a middle-aged woman.

The cause of the peculiar disease is as yet unknown. As the lesion is often encountered in babies a congenital disorder is postulated. Probably it is a question of a faulty structure of the gland with a great number of small sialectases (comparable with bronchiectases). Salivary secretion is not optimal. In a period with greatly reduced secretion a retrograde infection with oral bacteria may occur via the duct. Familial incidence, allergic conditions, and auto-immune disease have also been incriminated. The impression is that the lesion is more frequently seen in patients suffering from rheumatoid arthritis (*see* p. 229).

Possibly there are several causes for the same clinical and radio-graphic picture.

Therapy consists of treating the acute stages with antibiotics, of administration of preparations stimulating salivary secretion, and of careful massage of the gland in the direction of the duct. In the case of very frequently recurring inflammations continuous adminis-tration of an antibiotic may be necessary. Complete healing will probably never occur. It is of importance to reassure the patient. Operative removal of the gland is seldom indicated and may only be performed when the sialographic picture of the other gland is known.

Chronic Parotitis with Changes in the Ducts.—The clinical picture and the occurrence of acute symptoms make this form of parotitis resemble chronic (recurrent) parotitis. There are, however, differences: the sialogram is characterized by marked colon-like dilatations of the main duct and the larger branches (sialodochitis); the lesions of the terminal ductules in the form of 'snowflakes', already mentioned before, are completely absent or remain in the background (*Figs*. 190 and 191). The lesion is mainly encountered in patients of 30 years and older. The gland may show atrophy and reduced function.

Not much can be done therapeutically. Sometimes opening and resuturing of a duct, dilated at its orifice, may result in an increase of the salivary discharge and may therefore give relief of symptoms. It is, however, a technically difficult operation, where the result does not always come up to expectations.

Chronic Parotitis with Stone Formation.—Clinically the picture is characterized by salivary colics just before or at meal times. Secon-dary acute inflammatory reactions may occur. The radiograph usually revcals a small stone. Sometimes, however, the stone gives too little contrast to become visible and in these cases sialography is necessary to demonstrate its presence (*Fig.* 192). The duct may be dilated in the immediate surroundings of the stone. The lesion occurs almost exclusively in adults. Also in this lesion there is no char-acteristic picture of 'snowflakes'.

Actinomycosis. This infection of the parotid gland is rare. Involvement of the gland is usually caused by an actinomycosis

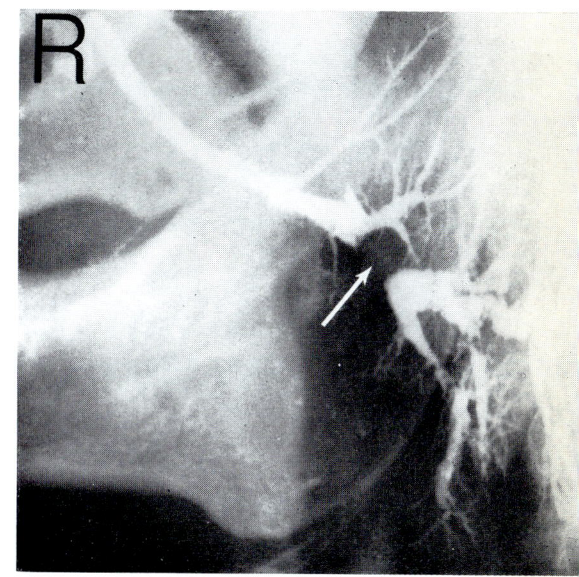

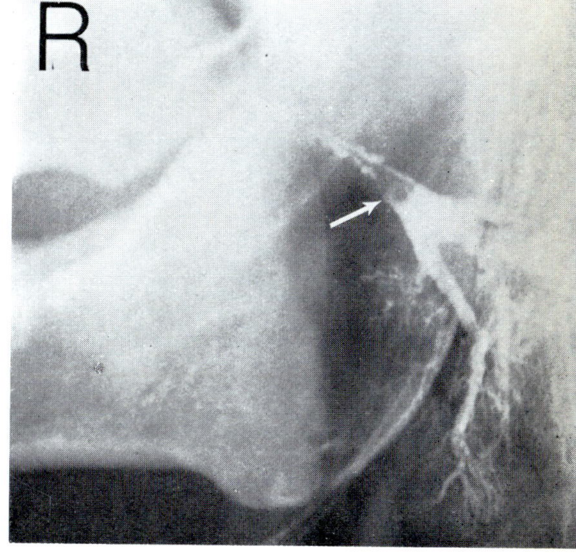

Fig. 192.—a, Small salivary stone in the parotid duct, visible as a filling defect in the contrast medium. The stone itself gave too little contrast to be visible in a normal film. The ductules between the obstruction and the gland are grossly dilated. b, After 1 day the duct is empty; the gland, however, is still filled, which is clearly demonstrating the obstructive effect of the stone. Removal of the stone is technically difficult, therefore parotidectomy was performed.

process in the adjacent tissues. The sialogram is characterized by irregular destruction. Both clinical picture and treatment are similar to those of cervicofacial actinomycosis (*see* p. 184).

Tuberculosis.—This is also a rarely occurring infection. The parotid gland is involved three times as often as the submandibular gland. Clinically the picture may resemble sialo-adenitis. Generally there is a painless, unilateral swelling and induration (*Fig*. 193 a). There is no discharge of pus via the duct and there are no symptoms related to secretional disorders. The sialogram may, if fibrosis is dominating, show a normal main duct with normal larger branches and peripheral sclerosis. More characteristic is the occurrence of large irregular accumulations of contrast medium (*Fig*. 193 b). In order to make a diagnosis it is necessary that the patient is examined for other foci of tuberculosis elsewhere in the body. Examination of the lungs is

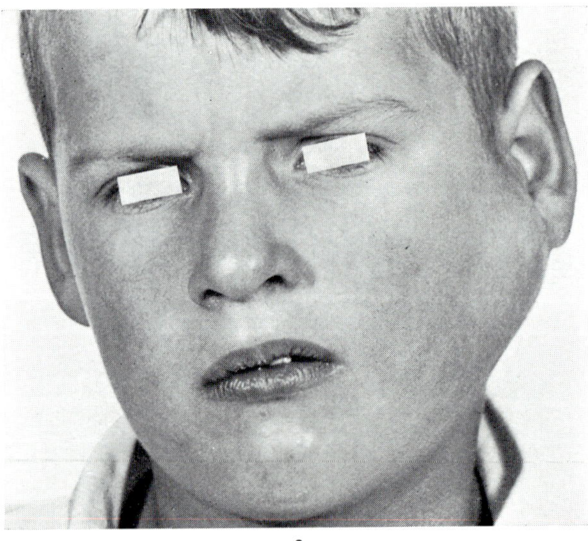

a

Fig. 193.—a, Six-year-old boy with marked swelling of the left parotid gland. Clinically the picture resembles an inflammation. b, The sialogram shows an 'abscess cavern' at the level of the mandibular angle, filled with contrast medium. From a differential diagnostic point of view an abscess, tuberculous cavern, and a malignant neoplasm have to be considered. Biopsy confirmed the diagnosis: tuberculosis (cm=head of mandible; × 2).

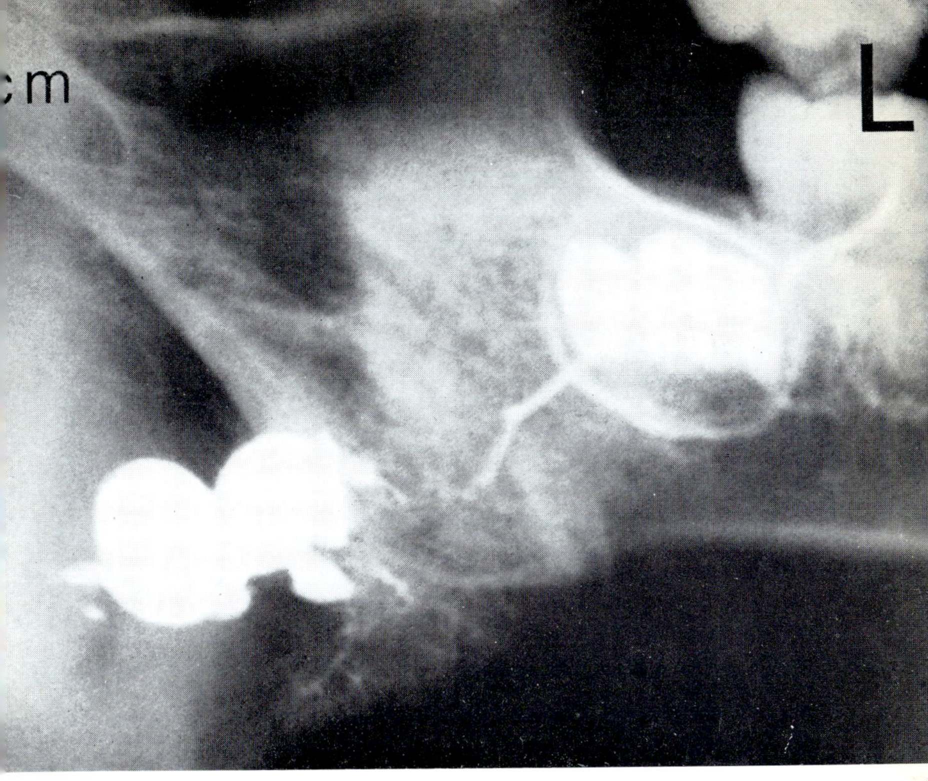

(Fig. 193 b)

usually negative. The patients do not feel ill. As a confirmation of the diagnosis a biopsy must be taken. Histologically granulomata are found, which may also be seen in sarcoidosis (Besnier-Boeck disease).

The cause is probably a haematogenous infection, especially of the lymphoid tissue located in the salivary gland. The glandular epithelium is only involved secondarily.

RARE LESIONS

Sjögren's Syndrome.—The sicca syndrome is characterized by a combination of dryness of the mouth, dryness of the eye (kerato-conjunctivitis), pharyngolaryngitis sicca, rhinitis sicca, and a lesion of the joints resembling rheumatoid arthritis. The parotid glands may be swollen and show acute inflammatory symptoms. The sialogram often resembles the picture of a chronic (recurrent) parotitis, as is described on p. 218. The lesion is of unknown origin, possibly an auto-immune disease.

Sialo-'adenoses'.—By this term is understood swellings of the parotid gland, not caused by inflammation or neoplasm. They may occur as an allergic condition, but also in cases of undernourishment, liver cirrhosis, diabetes, etc.

Uveoparotitis (Heerfordt's Disease).—The lesion is characterized by swelling of both parotid glands, combined with an inflammation of the choroid of the eye and sometimes with paralysis of the facial nerve. There is only slight pain, but a dry mouth is a common finding (xerostomia). The other salivary glands are usually not involved. The lesions develop in the course of days or weeks and may last for 2–6 months and then disappear spontaneously. In one-third of cases the lesion starts with erythema nodosum or erythroderma. The picture of the lungs is that of a generalized sarcoidosis, with compact swelling of the hilar glands. Fever is found in 25 per cent of cases, but the temperature is generally not above 38·5° C.

No method of treatment is known. Probably it is a rarely occurring form of sarcoidosis (Besnier-Boeck's disease).

Mikulicz's Syndrome.—This syndrome is of extremely rare incidence; it is characterized by a slowly increasing, symmetrical swelling of the parotid and lacrimal glands. There is no feeling of illness and no pain. In the course of months or years other salivary glands are also involved in the process. The swellings are of firm consistency and somewhat nodular; the skin and mucosa are of normal colour and freely movable. The glands may increase in size between three to six times. In two-thirds of cases the lesion is bilateral. The glands do not produce saliva or lacrimal fluid. The average age of the patients is 30–40 years. The lesion occurs equally in males and females.

Symptoms are associated with dryness of the eyes and of the mouth. Paresis of the facial nerve has been described. The blood-picture shows, in some cases, lymphocytosis or eosinophilia. Blood-chemistry: raised calcium content. The hilum of the lung is often broadened; the spleen and liver may be enlarged. The syndrome is often encountered in Besnier-Boeck's sarcoidosis (palatal biopsy may be of diagnostic value), in leukaemia, in lymphogranulomatosis, and in tuberculosis. It may, however, also occur as a separate entity. The prognosis of the latter form (sarcoidosis) is favourable. In the lymphatic myeloid form the prognosis is determined by the progress of the systemic disease.

CHAPTER 16

INFLAMMATIONS OF THE SUBMANDIBULAR GLAND

Acute Inflammations.—Primary acute inflammation of the sub-mandibular gland is extremely rare. In nearly all cases it is actually an acute exacerbation of chronic sialo-adenitis with stone formation. There is marked swelling of the gland, which can be palpated on the inner side of the mandible, the size of a pigeon's egg, firm-elastic, and generally with little pain (*Fig.* 176). Especially on bimanual palpation of the floor of the mouth the gland can be felt distinctly. Mucopurulent secretion can be massaged from the duct. The lesion is predominantly unilateral. In most cases the radiograph clearly shows a salivary calculus.

Treatment consists of combating the acute stage, and then the stone must be removed as soon as possible. There is a chance of recurrence.

Sometimes there may be difficulties from a differential diagnostic point of view in regard to mumps or in regard to a swollen and indurated submandibular lymph-node (*Fig.* 171). This non-specific lymphadenitis occurs predominantly in children, whereas acute inflammation of the submandibular gland is almost exclusively encountered in adults. The swollen lymph-node is usually located somewhat more superficially and somewhat more ventrally than the salivary gland. On bimanual palpation of the floor of the mouth the lymph-node and the salivary gland can sometimes be moved separately. The sialogram is normal and the radiograph does not show salivary stones.

Chronic Inflammations.—Chronic inflammations of the sub-mandibular gland occur almost always in combination with stone formation. Generally it is a question of a vicious circle. The stones are conducive to the occurrence of chronic inflammation and the latter to stone formation. Clinically the lesion becomes manifest as a slightly indurated gland with little pain.

Treatment consists of removal of the stone. Also after removal of the stone healing may be prolonged. It may appear from the sialogram that the duct and larger branches are definitely dilated (*Fig.* 178 b); this promotes stasis. Moreover, there is often reduced function owing to fibrosis of the gland. Both these factors, and the unfavourable location of the gland in regard to gravitation, render the duct liable to infection.

When marked changes are revealed by sialography (fibrosis, distinct dilatations of the ductules, intraglandular stones) and repeated occurrence of acute symptoms, it is advisable to remove the gland surgically.

CHAPTER 17

CYSTS OF THE SALIVARY GLANDS

CYSTS of the major salivary glands are relatively rare. Clinically and also in the sialogram the picture resembles a benign tumour.

A mucous cyst, originating from the submandibular gland, is known as a *ranula*. The cyst appears as a shining bluish swelling under the mucosa of the floor of the mouth and is filled with a very sticky mucoid fluid, which is clear or slightly yellowish (*Fig.* 195).

Therapy consists of marsupialization and suturing of the cut cyst margins into the floor of the mouth. Sometimes it is necessary to keep the opening, which is made as large as possible, patent by

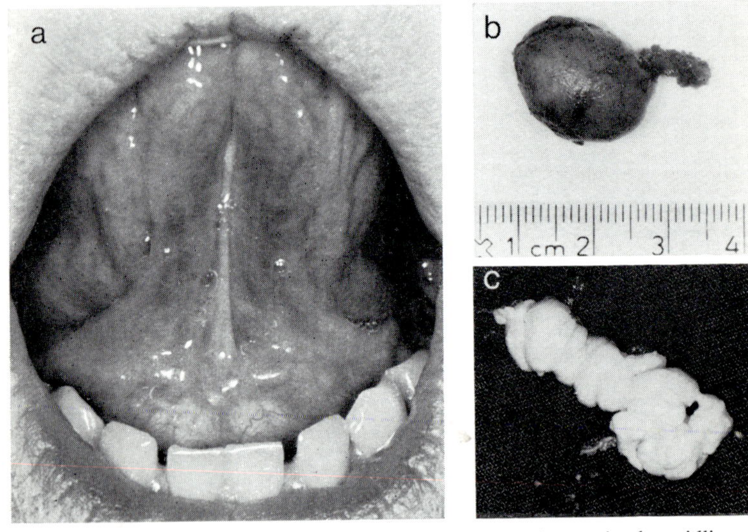

Fig. 194.—a, Painless swelling, the size of a pigeon's egg, in the midline of the floor of the mouth, shining yellowish through the mucosa, in a 5-year-old girl. Diagnosis: epidermoid cyst. (Differential diagnosis: cyst of the thyroglossal duct.) b, Extirpated cyst. c, Contents: yellowish-white pulpy mass.

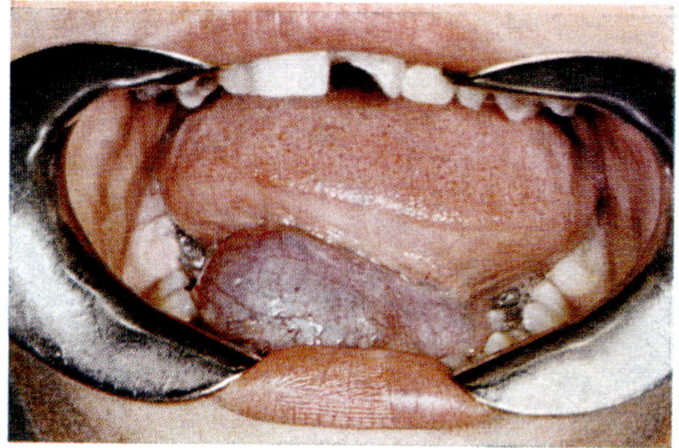

Fig. 195.—Ranula.

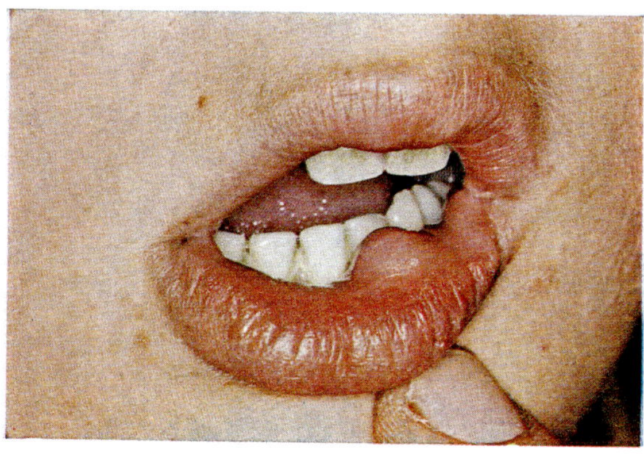

Fig. 196.—Mucous cyst of the lower lip.

means of a small obturator. Some authorities also advise the extirpation of the cyst together with the related sublingual gland.

In the case of a deep located cyst, which sometimes cannot easily be recognized as such, an epidermoid cyst must be considered in differential diagnosis. This cyst, however, is usually located in the midline (*Fig.* 194).

The mucous cyst of the lower lip, too, may be a retention cyst (mucocele) (*Fig.* 196). Often, however, discharge of mucus into the soft tissues occurs (possibly as a result of a trauma, for instance owing to lip biting), causing the formation of granulation tissue. The result is a cavity in the soft tissues, filled with mucus and surrounded by a wall of granulation tissue (mucus extravasation granuloma). It must be stated, however, that a mucocele or a mucus extravasation cyst is of rare occurrence after lip operations or larger lip wounds, which lends scant support to the often-mentioned traumatic aetiology.

Treatment of both lesions consists of extirpation, together with any related minor salivary gland. Recurrence is not uncommon.

CHAPTER 18

TUMOURS

Benign Tumours.—

'*Mixed Parotid Tumour*'.—The mixed tumour is the most important tumour of the salivary gland and is seen in the parotid gland in 90 per cent of cases. The lesion is almost exclusively encountered in adults. It is a slowly growing, painless, smooth, or nodular tumour of a firm-elastic consistency. A benign mixed tumour does not metastasize. The sialogram shows displacement of gland tissue (*balle dans la main*) (*Figs.* 197, 198, and 199). When taking a lateral radiograph

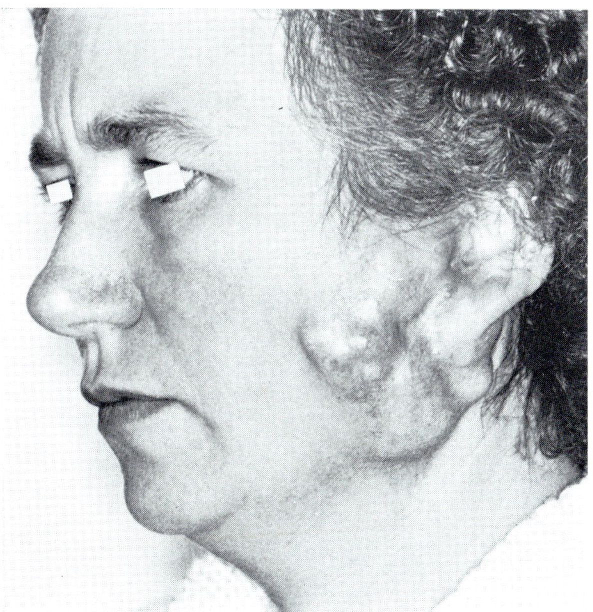

Fig. 197.—Nodular benign mixed tumour of the left parotid gland in a 39-year-old woman. Present (inclusive of recurrences) for 20 years.

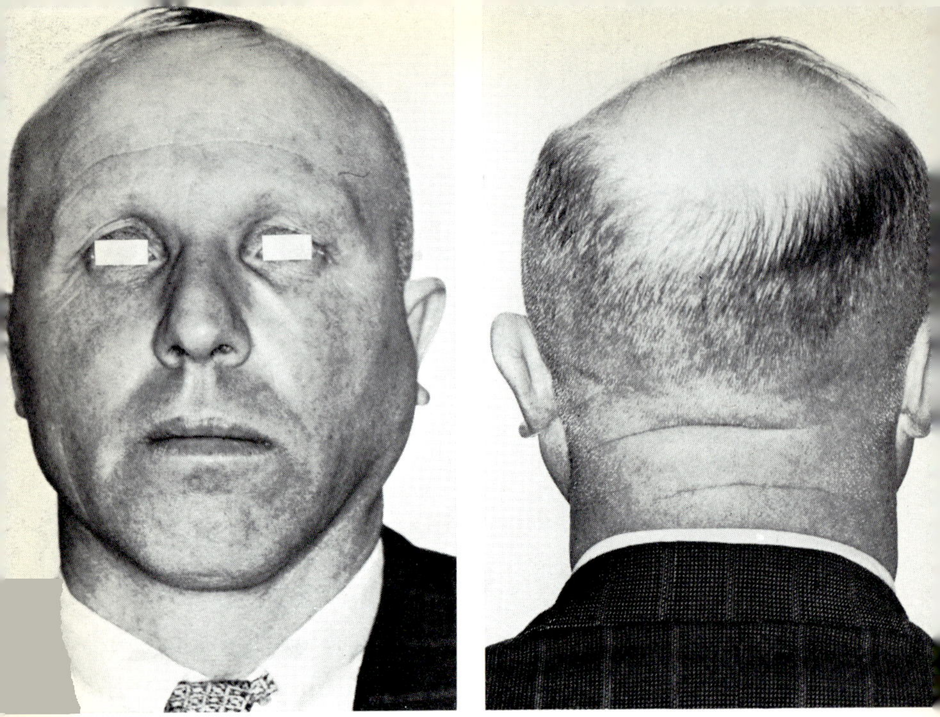

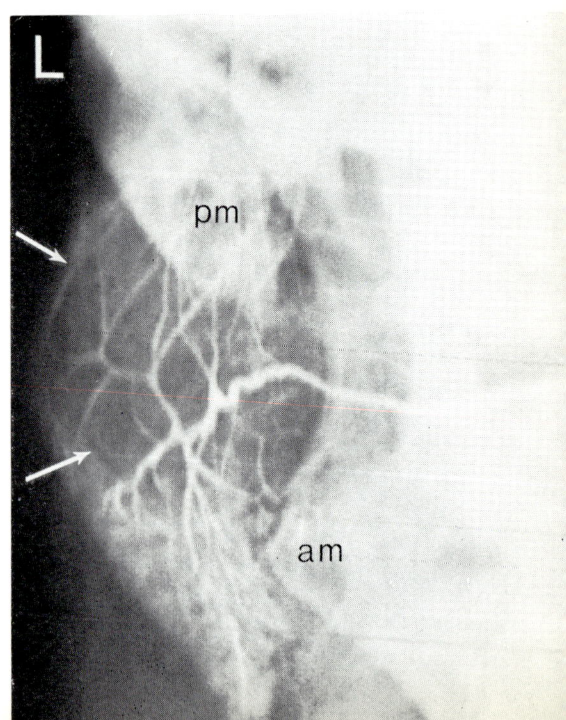

(*Fig*. 198 a)

(*Fig*. 198 b)

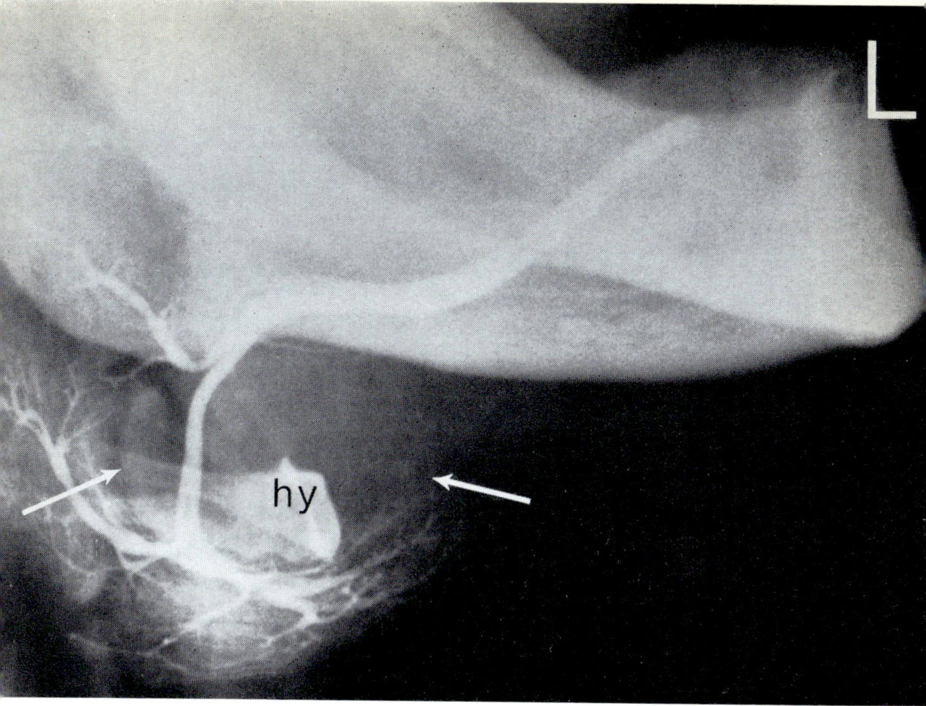

Fig. 199.—Benign neoplasm (mixed tumour) of the submandibular gland
with displacement of the gland (hy=hyoid bone).

care must be exercised that the cassette does not contact the tumour
too tightly, as a result of which, part of the ductular system may be
emptied, so that the picture will be false.

Treatment consists of excision of the tumour, which means for the
parotid gland total or partial parotidectomy. On occasions irradiation treatment is given of 5×400 r to prevent any inoculation
metastases. The facial nerve can be left undamaged when the
operation is performed by a surgeon who is very experienced in this
field. Puncture and biopsy are not advisable. Because the tumour

Fig. 198.—a, Firm, elastic, painless swelling anterior to the left ear.
Observed for the first time 3 years before. The ear lobe is pushed outwards,
which is characteristic of a swelling in or of the parotid gland. b, The
sialogram (anteroposterior projection) shows displacement of the glandular
tree. This tree embraces the big, globular tumour as a *balle dans la main*. It
is the picture of a benign (mixed) tumour (pm=mastoid process; am=
angle of the mandible).

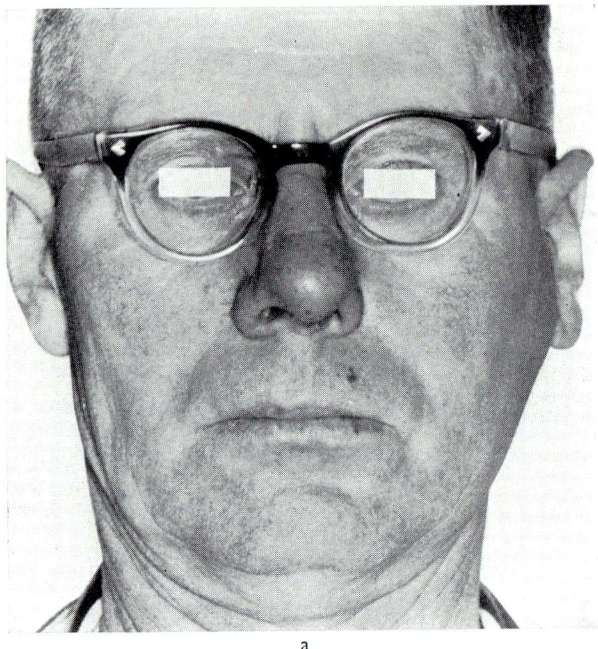

a

Fig. 200.—a, Circumscribed swelling anterior to the left ear in a 55-year-old man. Observed for the first time 6 months before; slowly growing, painful on palpation, occasional paraesthesiae of the cheek, anterior to the ear. b, The sialogram of the left parotid gland shows plainly a recess in the upper pole. The ductules terminate blind here, because the glandular tissue is displaced by tumour tissue. It is the picture of a malignant tumour (cylindroma). The arrows are glued to the skin for the localization of the tumour.

may show malignant degeneration, when present for a long time, and a large tumour causes, in general, more difficulties at operation (there is especially an enhanced chance that the facial nerve will be injured), the patient should be advised to have the mixed tumour removed as soon as possible.

Malignant Tumours.—
The *malignant mixed tumour* belongs to this group, but the carcinomas (among which is the cylindroma, which is the most feared

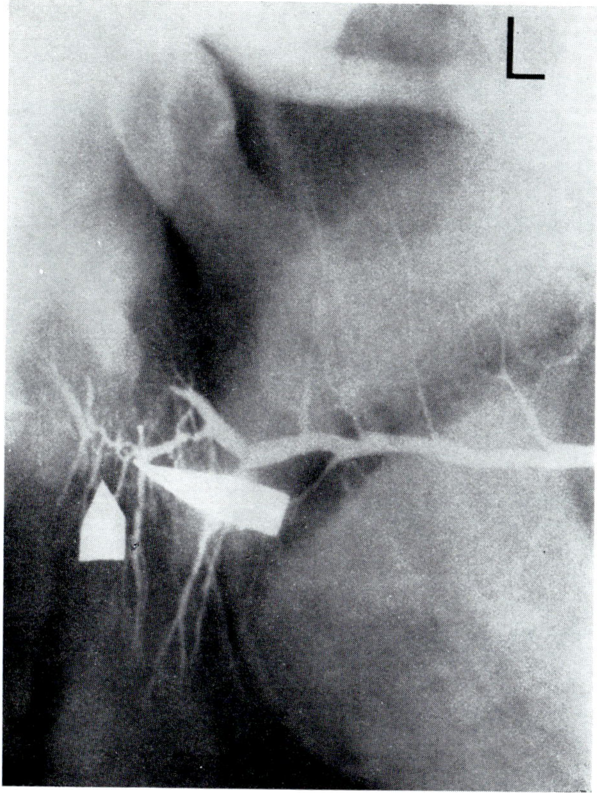

(*Fig.* 200 b)

carcinoma) form by far the biggest group. Clinically and radiographically they cannot be distinguished. The malignant tumours
may also be characterized by a firm-elastic swelling in the salivary
gland area. There is little difference between benign and malignant
tumours, especially in the early stages.

Malignant tumours may show:—

Rapid growth;

Spontaneous pain or tenderness;

Disturbances of the innervation (facial nerve);

Fixation to the skin with discoloration and ulceration;

Large size and persistence.

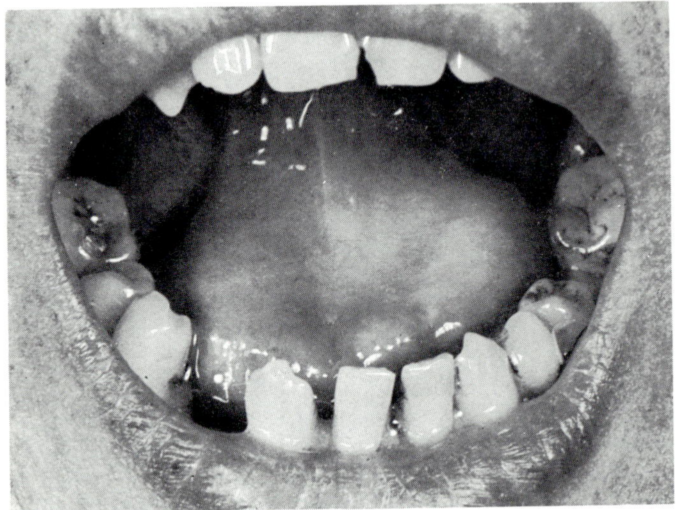

Fig. 201.—Cylindroma in the floor of the mouth in a 45-year-old man, presumably originating from the sublingual gland (*see also Fig.* 194).

A sialogram with irregular destruction of the ductule system (part of the gland is absent) (*Fig.* 200) or local irregular accumulations of Lipiodol; (*Fig.* 202) and in the course of time:—
Swollen and indurated lymph-nodes;
Limitation of movements of the lower jaw.
Treatment consists of excision of the gland *en bloc,* radical block dissection of the neck, and irradiation to prevent inoculation metastases (2000 r). In most cases the facial nerve cannot be spared. As rather a rare complication the auriculotemporal syndrome (Frey's syndrome) may occur, characterized by sweat secretion of

Fig. 202.—a, Growing tumour in the right parotid gland area in a 79-year-old man. Disturbance of the facial nerve is very suspicious of malignancy (planocellular carcinoma). b, Fistula from which pus-like secretion is discharged. c, Lateral sialogram with distinct destruction of the gland in the ventrocaudal quadrant. A main duct terminates abruptly (*see* left upper arrow); irregular accumulation of contrast medium indicates destruction of the gland. (Differential diagnosis: non-specific abscess and tuberculosis, *see Fig.* 193 b) (cm=head of mandible). d, The anteroposterior sialogram shows identical destruction, especially in the caudal part.

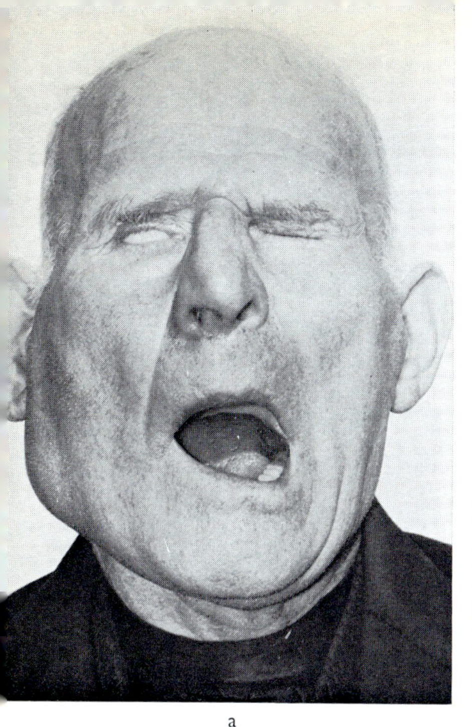
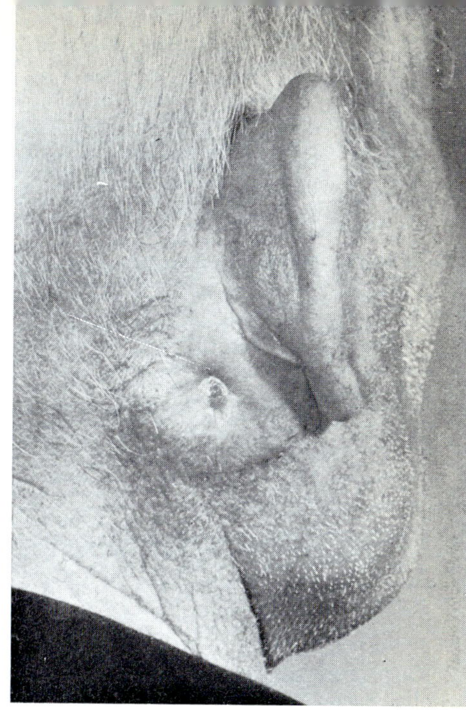

a

Fig. 202

b

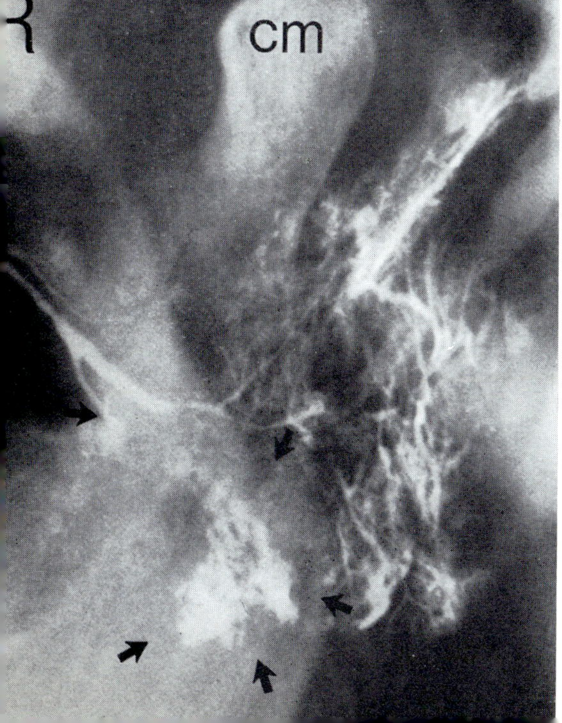

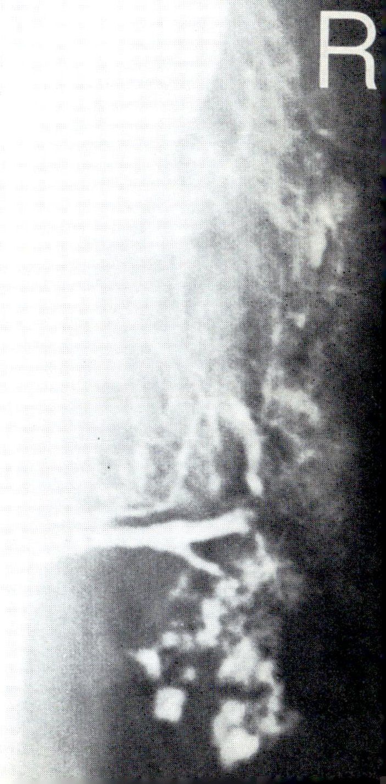

c

d

the skin in the lateral part of the face in the area innervated by the auriculotemporal nerve, when smelling or tasting food.

The cylindromata especially have a bad prognosis; they cannot easily be excised radically. Except in the major salivary glands they are also seen on the palate (*Figs.* 71 and 122 a) and in the floor of the mouth (*Fig.* 201).

In conclusion, it is useful to keep the following surgical maxim in mind: tumours of the parotid gland are malignant in 30 per cent of cases, tumours of the submandibular gland are malignant in 50 per cent of cases, and those of the sublingual gland in 100 per cent of cases!

APPENDIX

NOMENCLATURE

THE complete *permanent dentition* consists of thirty-two *teeth*, which are similar on each side and are symmetrically divided into the *lower and upper dental arches.*

The *deciduous dentition* has twenty teeth; in each quadrant there are only two deciduous molars (predecessors of the premolars). The permanent molars have no predecessors in the deciduous dentition.

In the *classification of the dentition* the lower and upper arches are bent open and stretched, resulting in two rows of teeth placed one above the other. By means of a cross the teeth are divided into *four quadrants.* The upper teeth are placed above the horizontal line and the lower teeth below. The teeth of both right halves of the jaws are placed on the left of the midline and those on the left are placed to the right of the midline (these places correspond with the position of the teeth as they are seen when looking into a patient's mouth).

Each quadrant has eight teeth, namely a central incisor, a lateral incisor, a cuspid or canine, a first and a second premolar, and finally a first, a second, and a third molar. Third molars are sometimes called 'wisdom teeth'.

In the classification of the dentition the permanent teeth are normally indicated by Arabic numerals and the deciduous dentition by capital letters.

Classification of the permanent dentition:

$$\text{R} \quad \frac{8\ 7\ 6\ 5\ 4\ 3\ 2\ 1 \ \big| \ 1\ 2\ 3\ 4\ 5\ 6\ 7\ 8}{8\ 7\ 6\ 5\ 4\ 3\ 2\ 1 \ \big| \ 1\ 2\ 3\ 4\ 5\ 6\ 7\ 8} \quad \text{L}$$

One single tooth may also be indicated by means of a numeral in combination with part of this cross, for instance $\underline{6|}$ = right upper first permanent molar and $\overline{|3}$ = lower left permanent canine.

The place of a tooth in the classification of the dentition may also be indicated by a $+$ (upper jaw) or a $-$ (lower jaw). When this sign is written to the right of the numeral a tooth in the right half of the jaw is meant and when the sign is written to the left the tooth is located in the left half of the jaw (Haderup system), for instance $+1$ ($=$ left upper permanent central incisor) or $8-$ ($=$ lower right third molar).

Classification of the deciduous or temporary dentition:

$$R \frac{E\ D\ C\ B\ A\ |\ A\ B\ C\ D\ E}{E\ D\ C\ B\ A\ |\ A\ B\ C\ D\ E} L$$

The recent Fédération Dentaire International General Assembly in Bucharest resolved to adopt a two-digit system of tooth designation submitted by the Special Committee on Uniform Dental Recording. In the two-digit system the first digit indicates the quadrant and the second digit the type of tooth within the quadrant. Quadrants are allotted the digits 1–4 for the permanent teeth and 5–8 for the deciduous teeth in a clockwise sequence, starting at the upper right side. Teeth within the same quadrant are allotted the digits 1–8 (deciduous teeth, 1–5) from the midline backwards. The digits should be pronounced separately. Thus, the permanent canines are teeth 1–3, 2–3, 3–3, and 4–3.

Permanent Teeth

(upper right)	(upper left)
18 17 16 15 14 13 12 11	21 22 23 24 25 26 27 28
48 47 46 45 44 43 42 41	31 32 33 34 35 36 37 38
(lower right)	(lower left)

Deciduous Teeth

(upper right)	(upper left)
55 54 53 52 51	61 62 63 64 65
85 84 83 82 81	71 72 73 74 75
(lower right)	(lower left)

Each tooth has an *incisal edge* or an *occlusal surface*, a *buccal, lingual,* or *palatal surface,* furthermore a *mesial surface* (i.e., that facing the median line following the curve of the dental arch) or a *distal surface* (facing away from the median line following the curve of the dental arch).

A tooth consists of a *crown* and one or more *roots* (radices). The upper molars have three roots (two buccal and one palatal root) and the lower molars two roots (a mesial and a distal root).

Frequently used Terminology:—

Conservative dentistry: Operative dentistry: that part of dentistry which deals with restoration of hard dental tissues (fillings, root-canal treatment (endodontics), oral hygiene, etc.).

Prosthodontics: Prosthetic dentistry: the branch of dentistry dealing with suitable substitutes for the coronal portions of teeth, for one or more lost or missing natural teeth (crowns, bridges, partial and full dentures).

Orthodontics: That branch of dentistry dealing with the prevention and correction of irregularities of the teeth and malocclusion, and with associated facial problems.

Dowel crown: A restoration replacing the entire coronal portion of a tooth deriving its retention from a post extending into a treated (filled) root canal.

Jacket crown: A resin or porcelain restoration that is applied over the specially prepared clinical crown of a tooth and terminates at or under the gingiva.

Bridge: A non-removable prosthesis restoring the continuity of the dental arch by one or more artificial teeth suspended between and attached to abutment teeth which furnish support and stability to the restoration.

Endodontic treatment: Root-canal treatment: devitalization of a (usually inflamed) tooth pulp and/or preparation and filling of the root canal when the pulp has become necrotic.

Occlusion: Any contact between lower and upper dental arch.

Interdigitation: The fitting together of the cusps of opposing teeth in occlusion.

Articulation: The contact relationship of the occlusal surfaces of the teeth while in action.

Tele-roentgenogram: Radiographic picture of the skull (mostly *en profile*) while the head is fixed in a cephalometer and the radiographic tube at such a distance that parallelism of the rays is nearly secured (distance: patient–tube 3·75 m.; minimal disfiguration is produced).

BIBLIOGRAPHY

ADAMS, C. W., and HUDGINS, J. H. (1959), 'Pulmonary Infarction after Dental Extraction. Report of Two Cases with Recovery', *J. Am. med. Ass.*, **170**, 412.

ANGELOPOULOS, A. P., and TILSON, H. B. (1966), 'Malignant Transformation of the Epithelial Lining of the Odontogenic Cysts', *Oral Surg.*, **22**, 415.

ARCHER, W. H. (1958), *A Manual of Dental Anesthesia*, 2nd ed. Philadelphia and London: Saunders.

BACKER DIRKS, O., and DE KLOE, W. (1967), 'Yoghurt en Tandcaries', *Ned. Tijdschr. Geneesk.*, **111**, 361.

BELL, W. A. (1959), 'Sclerosing Osteomyelitis of the Mandible and Maxilla', *Oral Surg.*, **12**, 391.

BERTRAM, U. (1967), 'Xerostomia', *Acta odont. scand.*, **25**, Suppl. 49.

BHASKAR, S. N. (1965), *Synopsis of Oral Pathology*, 2nd ed. St. Louis: Mosby.

BLOOM, J., CHACKER, P. M., and THOMA, K. H. (1962), 'Cherubism and other Intra-osseous Giant-cell Lesions', *Oral Surg.*, **15**, Suppl. 2, 74.

BOERING, G. (1966), 'Arthrosis Deformans van het Kaakgewricht', Academisch Proefschrift. Leiden: Stafleu-Tholen.

— — and BEKS, J. W. F. (1963), 'Cerebrospinal Rhinorrhoea in Cases of High Facial Fractures', *Archvm chir. neerl.*, **15**, 111.

— — and HAMMING, H. D. (1965), 'Osteomyelitis Sicca Mandibulae', *Maandschr. Kindergeneesk.*, **33**, 70.

— — and HUFFSTADT, A. J. C. (1962), 'De Buccal-inlay-operatie', *Ned. Tijdschr. Geneesk.*, **106**, 1331.

— — — — (1967), 'The Use of Derma-fat Grafts in the Face', *Br. J. plast. Surg.*, **20**, 172.

BRONS, R., and JONGEBREUR, J. W. (1966), 'Cystis Nasoalveolaris', *Ned. Tijdschr. Geneesk.*, **110**, 1311.

BURKET, L. W. (1967), *Oral Medicine, Diagnosis and Treatment*, 5th ed. Montreal: Lippincott.

CAWSON, R. A. (1965), 'Symposium on Denture Sore Mouth, I. An Aetiological Review', *Dent. Practnr dent. Rec.*, **16**, 135.

— — (1966), 'Chronic Oral Candidiasis and Leucoplakia', *Oral Surg.*, **22**, 582.

COMROE, B. J., COLLINS, L. H., and CRANE, M. P. (1954), *Internal Medicine in Dental Practice*. Philadelphia: Lea & Febiger.

DAWSON WATTS, K. (1968), 'Sarcoid of the Gingivae: A Case Report', *Br. J. oral Surg.*, **6**, 108.

DINGMAN, R. O., and NATVIG, P. (1964), *Surgery of Facial Fractures*. Philadelphia and London: Saunders.

EDITORIAL (1966), 'Tetracyclines and the Teeth', *Lancet*, **1**, 917.

ERICSON, S. (1967), 'Sialographic Study of the Parotid Glands in Rheumatoid Arthritis', *Odont. Revy*, **18**, 163.

FELTKAMP, T. E. W., and VAN ROSSUM, A. L. (1968), 'Antibodies to Salivary Duct Cells, and other Antibodies, in Patients with Sjögren's Syndrome and other Idiopathic Autoimmune Diseases', *Clin. exp. Immunol.*, **3**, 1.

FICK, J. M. (1966), 'Yoghurt en Tandcaries', Academisch Proefschrift, Utrecht. Utrecht: Tholen.

GÄSTRIN, U., and JOSEPHSON, S. (1966), 'Tetracyclines and the Teeth', *Lancet*, **2**, 492.

GLICKMAN, I. (1964), *Clinical Periodontology*, 3rd ed. Philadelphia and London: Saunders.

GOLD, L. (1955), 'The Classification and Pathogenesis of Fibrous Dysplasia of the Jaws', *Oral Surg.*, **8**, 628, 735, 856.

GORLIN, R. J. (1965), 'The Multiple Basal-cell Nevi Syndrome', *Cancer*, **18**, 89.

— — and CHAUDRY, A. P. (1961), 'Odontogenic Tumors. Classification, Histopathology and Clinical Behavior in Man and Domesticated Animals', *Ibid.*, **14**, 73.

— — and PINDBORG, J. J. (1964), *Syndromes of the Head and Neck*. New York and London: McGraw-Hill.

HERMANS, E. H., GROSFELD, J. C. M., SPAAS, J. A. J., and BIJLSMA, J. B. (1965), 'De Vijfde Facomatose', *Ned. Tijdschr. Geneesk.*, **109**, 696.

HILSON, D. (1957), 'Malformation of Ears as Sign of Malformation of Genito-urinary Tract', *Br. med. J.*, **2**, 785.

HOVINGA, J. (1968), 'Replantatie en Transplantatie van Tanden', Academisch Proefschrift, Amsterdam.

HOWE, G. L. (1961), *The Extraction of Teeth*. Bristol: Wright.

HUFFSTADT, A. J. C. (1966), 'Enige Facetten van de Behandeling van Patiënten met Cheilognathopalatoschisis', *Ned. Tijdschr. Geneesk.*, **110**, 993.

KILLEY, H. C. (1971), *Fractures of the Middle Third of the Facial Skeleton*, 2nd ed. Bristol: Wright.

— — (1971), *Fractures of the Mandible*, 2nd ed. Bristol: Wright.

— — and KAY, L. W. (1965), *The Impacted Wisdom Tooth*. Edinburgh and London: Livingstone.

— — — — (1966), *Benign Cystic Lesions of the Jaws*. Edinburgh and London: Livingstone.

KUSEN, G. (1960), 'Fracturen van de Processus Condylaris Mandibulae', Academisch Proefschrift, Utrecht.

KUTSCHER, A. H., ZEGARELLI, E. W., and HYMAN, G. A. (1964), *Pharmacotherapeutics of Oral Disease*. New York and London: McGraw-Hill.

LUCAS, R. B. (1964), *Pathology of Tumours of the Oral Tissues*. London: Churchill.

MCCARTHY, P. L., and SHKLAR, G. (1964), *Disease of the Oral Mucosa*. New York and London: McGraw-Hill.

MACSWEEN, R. N. M., GORDIE, R. B., ANDERSON, J. R., and others (1967), 'Occurrence to Salivary Duct Epithelium in Sjögren's Disease, Rheumatoid Arthritis and other Arthritides', *Ann. rheum. Dis.*, **26**, 402.

MERKX, C. A. (1959), 'Fractures of the Facial Skeleton. Case Report', *Archvm chir. neerl.*, **11**, 343.

MEYER, W. (1961), *Zahnärztliche Operationslehre*. Munich and Berlin: Urban & Schwarzenberg.

MOORE, C. (1965), 'Smoking and Cancer of the Mouth, Pharynx and Larynx', *J. Am. med. Ass.*, **191**, 283.

MÜHLEMANN, H. R., and SCHMID, H. (1958), 'Anticaries Dentifrices under Laboratory Conditions', *J. Dent. Belge*, **49**, 353.

NEILL, D. J. (1965), 'Symposium on Denture Sore Mouth. An Aetiological Review', *Dent. Practnr dent. Rec.*, **16**, 135.

NETTER, F. H. (1959), *The Ciba Collection of Medical Illustrations*, Vol. 3, Part I: *Upper Digestive Tract*. New York: Ciba.

NYSINGH, J. G. (1960), 'Zygomatico-maxillaire Fracturen', Academisch Proefschrift, Utrecht.

PANDERS, A. K. (1970), 'Fibro-osseuze en Fibro-osseuze-cementeuze Dysplasie van de Kaken', Academisch Proefschrift, Groningen.

POTTER, E. L. (1946), 'Bilateral Renal Agenesis', *J. Pediat.*, **29**, 68.

RASMUSSEN, P. (1965), *Facial Pain*. Copenhagen: Munksgaard.

RAUCH, S. (1959), *Die Speicheldrüsen des Menschen*. Stuttgart: Thieme.

REDON, H. (1955), *Chirurgie des Glandes Salivaires*. Paris: Masson et Cie.

REHSTEINER, H. P. (1960), 'Untersuchungen über den Einfluss der Schwangerschaft auf den Gebisszustand', *Schweiz. med. Wschr.*, **90**, 1307.

ROORDA, L. A. M. (1960), 'Aspiratie als Oorzaak van Longverwikkelingen na Tandheelkundige Ingrepen', Academisch Proefschrift, Groningen.

ROWE, N. L., and KILLEY, H. C. (1955), *Fractures of the Facial Skeleton*. Edinburgh and London: Livingstone.

RUSSEL, H. B. (1963), 'De Beketenis van Genetische Factoren voor de Ontwikkeling van het Tand-kaakstelsel. Een Tweelingenonderzoek', Academisch Proefschrift, Utrecht.

SCHULER, J. (1966), '"Krakende kaken"', Psychiatrische Beschouwingen over het Syndroom van het Pijnlijke, slecht Functionerende Kaakgewricht', Academisch Proefschrift, Groningen.

SCHULTE, J. E. (1958), 'Erfelijk Syndroom van Peutz-Jeghers', *Ned. Tijdschr. Geneesk.*, **102**, 2392.

SCHWACHMAN, H., and SCHUSTER, A. (1956), 'Tetracyclines; Applied Pharmacology', *Pediatr. Clins N. Am.*, **3**, 295.

SHAFER, W. G. HINE, M. K., and LEVY, B. M. (1963), *A Textbook of Oral Pathology*. Philadelphia and London: Saunders.

SILLEVIS SMITT, P. A. E. (1960), 'Gingivitis Gangraenosa (Plaut-Vincent)', Academisch Proefschrift, Amsterdam.

TEMPEST, M. N. (1966), 'Cancrum Oris', *Br. J. Surg.*, **53**, 949.

THERON, A. (1959), 'Apthae with Special Reference to the Chronic Recurrent Variety of Mikulicz', Academisch Proefschrift, Groningen.

THOMA, K. H. (1958), *Oral Surgery*, 3rd ed. London: Kimpton.

— — and GOLDMAN, H. M. (1960), *Oral Pathology*, 5th ed. London: Kimpton.

— — and ROBINSON, H. B. G. (1960), *Oral and Dental Diagnosis*, 5th ed. Philadelphia and London: Saunders.

TIECKE, R. W. (1965), *Oral Pathology*. New York: McGraw-Hill.

TOAFF, R., and DAVID, R. (1966), 'Tetracyclines and the Teeth', *Lancet*, **2**, 282.

VAN DER KWAST, W. A. M. (1957), 'Over de Hyperplasie van de Gingiva als Neven-effect van het Anti-epilepticum Fenytoïne', Academisch Proefschrift, Groningen.

VAN DER LINDEN, F. P. G. M. (1965), 'Schadelijke Invloeden van Tetracycline op de Vorming van Melkgebit en Blijvend Gebit', *Ned. Tijdschr. Geneesk.*, **109**, 1909.

VAN DER VELD, R. G. M. (1967), 'Gingivitis Ulcerosa', *Ned. Tijdschr. Tandheelk.*, **74**, 738.

BIBLIOGRAPHY

Van Dop, F. (1964), 'Seboglandulae Buccales et Labiales', *Ned. Tijdschr. Tandheelk*, **71**, 686.

— — (1967), 'De Epulis', Academisch Proefschrift, Groningen. Leiden: Stafleu-Tholen.

Vriezen, Th. C. (1967), 'Lichen Planus Mucosae Oris', *Ned. Tijdschr. Geneesk.*, **111**, 1469.

— — (1967), 'Dentogene Fistels in het Gelaat', *Ibid.*, **111**, 65.

— — (1970), 'Odontogene Ontstekingen', Academisch Proefschrift, Groningen.

Waldron, C. A., and Shafer, W. G. (1966), 'The Central Giant-cell Reparative Granuloma of the Jaws', *Am. J. clin. Path.*, **45**, 437.

World Health Organization (1961), *Periodontal Disease, Tech. Rep. Ser.*, No. 207. Geneva.

Worth, H. M. (1963), *Principles and Practice of Oral Radiologic Interpretation.* Chicago: Year Book Medical Publishers.

INDEX